T0358167

THE STEPCHILDREN OF SCIENCE
PSYCHICAL RESEARCH AND PARAPSYCHOLOGY IN
GERMANY, c.1870–1939

THE WELLCOME SERIES
IN THE HISTORY OF MEDICINE

Forthcoming Titles:

The Wellcome Series in the History of Medicine series editors are
V. Nutton, R. Cooter, M. Neve and E.C. Spary.
Please send all queries regarding the series to Michael Laycock,
The Wellcome Trust Centre for the History of Medicine at UCL,
183 Euston Road, London NW1 2BE, UK.

THE STEPCHILDREN OF SCIENCE
PSYCHICAL RESEARCH AND PARAPSYCHOLOGY IN GERMANY, c.1870–1939

Heather Wolffram

Amsterdam – New York, NY 2009

First published in 2009
by Editions Rodopi B.V., Amsterdam – New York, NY 2009.

Editions Rodopi B.V. © 2009

Design and Typesetting by Michael Laycock,
The Wellcome Trust Centre for the History of Medicine at UCL.
Printed and bound in The Netherlands by Editions Rodopi B.V.,
Amsterdam – New York, NY 2009.

Index by Indexing Specialists (UK) Ltd.

British Library Cataloguing in Publication Data
A catalogue record for this book is available from the British Library

ISBN 978-90-420-2728-2
E-Book ISBN 978-90-420-2729-9

'The Stepchildren of Science:
Psychical Research and Parapsychology in Germany, c.1870–1939' –
Amsterdam – New York, NY:
Rodopi. – ill.
(Clio Medica 88 / ISSN 0045-7183;
The Wellcome Series in the History of Medicine)

Front cover:

Polish psychic Stanislawa P. produces ectoplasm in Munich,
in the presence of A. Schrenck-Notzing. Digitally coloured.
Courtesy of the Mary Evans Picture Library.

© Editions Rodopi B.V., Amsterdam – New York, NY 2009
Printed in The Netherlands

All titles in the Clio Medica series (from 1999 onwards) are available to
download from the IngentaConnect website: http://www.ingentaconnect.co.uk

Contents

List of Images

List of Figures

List of Abbreviations

ADW	Archiv des Diakonischen Werk der Evangelischen Kirche in Deutschland (Berlin)
CA-AC-S	Apologetische Centrale des Central-Ausschusses für die Innere Mission
EZB	Evangelisches Zentralarchiv Berlin
GStA	Geheimes Staatsarchiv Preußischer Kulturbesitz
IGPP	Institut für Grenzgebiete der Psychologie und Psychohygiene
SdArMü	Stadtarchiv München
StArMü	Staatsarchiv München
UAL	Universitätsarchiv Leipzig
UAT	Universitätsarchiv Tübingen
UBL	Universitätsbibliothek Leipzig
ZA	Zeitungsausschnitte

Glossary

Apport – The paranormal transference of an object from one place to another or the appearance of an article from an unknown source usually in the presence of a medium.

Clairvoyance – The faculty of perceiving events in the future or beyond normal sensory contact.

Ectoplasm – A viscous substance that exudes from the body of a medium during a spiritualistic or somnambulistic trance and forms the material for the manifestation of spirits and other forms.

Hypnosis – The induction of a state of consciousness, usually via optical fixation, in which a person loses the power of voluntary action and is highly responsive to suggestion or direction.

Materialisation – The manifestation, by means of ectoplasm, of apparitions or other forms, many of which possess human physical characteristics, e.g., hands, heads and limbs.

Medium – A person able to communicate between the dead and the living, or, in non-spiritualist interpretations, a person with the ability to manipulate natural laws.

Mesmerism (also known as **animal magnetism**) – A system of therapeutics based on the idea that ill health is a result of an imbalance of magnetic fluid within the body, which a mesmerist can redistribute by means of magnetic strokes. In some patients the application of mesmerism leads to a state of (artificial) somnambulism.

Physical phenomena – Physical manifestations of mediumship, such as apports, ectoplasm, levitation, materialisation, and telekinesis.

Psychical phenomena – Mental manifestations of mediumship, such as clairvoyance, psychometry and telepathy.

Psychometry – The ability to discover facts about an event or person from inanimate objects associated with them.

Somnambulism – A state of sleep, or half-waking trance, spontaneously or artificially induced – i.e., through mesmerism or hypnosis – in which complex intellectual tasks can be carried out and in which paranormal abilities such as clairvoyance and telepathy are sometimes exhibited.

Telekinesis – The ability to move objects at a distance by mental power or other non-physical means.

Telepathy – The communication of thoughts or ideas by means other than the known senses.

Acknowledgements

In completing this book I have benefited from the support of a large number of institutions and people. I would like to take the opportunity to thank them here.

For the generous financial support they provided, my thanks are due to the German Academic Exchange Service (DAAD), the Graduate School at the University of Queensland, the Centre for the History of European Discourses at the University of Queensland, the Australian Universities Europe Network, and the Parapsychology Foundation in New York.

In Germany, I would like to acknowledge the assistance of archival staff at the Archiv des Diakonischen Werkes der EKD, the Bayerisches Hauptstaatsarchiv, the Evangelisches Zentralarchiv in Berlin, the Geheimes Staatsarchiv Preussischer Kulturbesitz in Berlin, the Monacensia Literaturarchiv in Munich, the Stadtarchiv in Munich, the Universitätsarchiv Leipzig, the Universitäts-Sondersammlungen Leipzig, and the Universitätsarchiv Tübingen. To Eberhard Bauer at the Institut für Grenzgebiete der Psychologie und Psychohygiene (IGPP) in Freiburg, I owe a particular debt of gratitude. His interest in, and enthusiasm for, my project as well as his knowledge of this field, helped focus my work early on. Thank you also to Uwe Schellinger and Andreas Fischer also of the IGPP for their assistance with the Hellwig and Schrenck-Notzing Nächlaße.

At the University of Queensland I wish to thank Andrew Bonnell and Sarah Ferber, who were wonderful supervisors and who remain mentors and good friends. Peter Cryle, Simon Devereaux, Marion Diamond and Andrea MacKenzie were also enthusiastic supporters of my work for which I thank them. A number of friends at the University of Queensland experienced the highs and lows of this project with me. Thank you especially to Nicola Petzl, Susannah Helman, and Robert Hogg as well as Andrea Humphreys, Trudy Jacobsen, Catherine McTavish and Yorick Smaal.

At the National University of Singapore, I wish to thank Gregory Clancey, who made me welcome in the Science, Technology and Society (STS) Research Cluster within the Faculty of Arts and Social Sciences. In STS and the Departments of History and English, thank you also to my colleagues Ai Lin Chua, Thomas Dubois, Brian Farrell, Ross Forman, Sorelle

Henricus, Edith Kaneshiro, Albert Lau, Nurenee Lee and John Whalen-Bridge.

For their comments and suggestions on the dissertation out of which this book evolved, I am grateful to Francesca Bordogna of Northwestern University in Evanston and Sylvia Paletschek of Albert Ludwig University in Freiburg. At The Wellcome Trust Centre for the History of Medicine at University College London, my thanks go to those involved with the *Clio Medica* series, in particular Mike Laycock, as well as Roger Cooter, Michael Neve, Vivian Nutton and Emma Spary.

I would also like to thank both Carfax Publishing and Wiley for allowing me to reprint previously published material: Carfax Publishing for 'Supernormal Biology: Vitalism, Parapsychology and the German Crisis of Modernity, *c.*1890–1933', *European Legacy*, 8, 2 (2003), 149–63, which forms part of Chapter 4; and Wiley for 'Parapsychology on the Couch: The Psychology of Occult Belief in Germany, *c.*1870–1939', *Journal of the History of the Behavioral Sciences*, 42, 3 (2006), 237–60, which became Chapter 6.

Finally, my greatest debt is to my family, Marie, Michael, Paul and Victoria, and my partner, Ian, who have provided unflagging love and support.

For Marie and Michael

Introduction

An unusual experiment

On a winter evening in 1922, a small group of people, among them several doctors, a psychiatrist, two zoologists and a writer, participated in an unusual experiment at the palatial Karolinenplatz residence of the Munich-based physician Freiherr (Baron) Albert von Schrenck-Notzing (1862–1929), a renowned specialist in both nervous diseases and sexual pathology. The aim of this experiment, conducted amidst an eclectic mix of household items, medical instruments and photographic equipment, was to observe, record, and analyse the strange psychological and physical phenomena associated with the experimental subject: an Austrian medium named Willy Schneider (1903–71). Seated in a semi-circle facing the young man, the participants held hands, talked and sang, straining their eyes in the dim red light that enveloped the laboratory in the hope of seeing an ectoplasmic limb or a telekinetic movement. 'Ectoplasm', a word borrowed from the biological sciences, was used by researchers in this field to describe the pale, malleable substance that often issued from mediums' orifices during a trance, while 'telekinesis' referred to the movement of objects at a distance by mental or ectoplasmic means.[1] Both phenomena – examples of so-called physical rather than psychical mediumship, of which telepathic and clairvoyant ability were characteristic – were considered particular talents of the adolescent Willy Schneider.

For several hours, the increasingly restless participants encouraged and cosseted the somnambulistic medium's female trance personality, pleading with the recalcitrant 'Mina' to show them some phenomena. In response, Willy writhed and moaned as if in the process of childbirth, until, at last, a handkerchief rose from the floor to make swift assured movements around the room, a typewriter began to clatter noisily in a corner, and a white shimmering apparition appeared shaped like a human forearm. While a number of the more novice attendees, who on this occasion included the writer Thomas Mann (1875–1955), found themselves both bewildered and amused by the levitation of household objects and the overtly sexual behaviour of the young male medium, others, including their host Schrenck-

Notzing, sought not only to vouchsafe the reality of these phenomena, but to establish their cause.[2]

The photographs and witness reports produced during and immediately after this experiment were intended to provide tangible evidence of what had taken place in the Baron's laboratory. Such proof was crucial in order to counter claims that those present were either hypnotised or delusional. The cameras, lining the wall behind the participants, were thus set up to capture the elusive phenomena produced by the medium.[3] These photographs, which Schrenck-Notzing contended were an objective, unmediated record of events, appeared to offer incontestable evidence of the ectoplasmic material that issued from and was reabsorbed into the medium's body as well as the telekinetic movement of the objects that littered the floor.[4] The experimental reports written by those in attendance either immediately after or within days of leaving the laboratory served a similar function – who could doubt the written testimony of this group of scientists, doctors and cultural luminaries, all of whom swore to the reality of the phenomena they had witnessed in the presence of Willy Schneider? Unlike their more capricious English, French and American contemporaries, surely these German scholars might be expected to approach such sensational phenomena with Teutonic reserve and rationality.[5]

While the photographs and experimental reports derived from this experiment seemed to establish that a handkerchief had indeed floated mysteriously around the room and that an unseen hand had clumsily manipulated the typewriter, such evidence did not constitute an explanation for these anomalous phenomena, which remained open to a range of hypotheses, including supernatural, fraudulent and natural forces. For many of those who witnessed the new personalities and materialised forms manifested by somnambulists and mediums during the late nineteenth and early twentieth centuries, such paranormal phenomena were explained through recourse to the theory of spirits or spirit possession. There were other observers, however, who maintained that all such phenomena could be explained naturalistically, as a result either of fraud and delusion or unknown mental powers.

Unlike many of his contemporaries, Schrenck-Notzing did not seek the aetiology of Willy Schneider's telekinetic movements and teleplastic protrusions in either the spirit world or the murky realm of fraud and delusion. He argued instead that such phenomena could be explained naturally and scientifically. While the Baron allowed the participants to indulge Willy's trance personality, the coquettish Mina, he did not believe she was a real spirit, regarding her simply as a psychological remnant of the medium's spiritualist training.[6] Given the ostensibly organic nature of Willy's phenomena and the explicitly sexual sounds and gyrations that accompanied

12

their production, Schrenck-Notzing and others in this field were convinced that the true cause of these strange occurrences would be located in the laws of biology, psychology and physics.[7] In pursuit of such scientific explanations, Willy's pulse and blood pressure were taken several times before and during the experiment to measure and record any organic changes wrought by his strange somnambulistic powers.

The possibility that fraud and delusion played a role in the mediumistic productions witnessed in the Karolinenplatz laboratory was, like the spirit hypothesis, rejected by Schrenck-Notzing and his colleagues. A significant amount of time was spent before the experiment searching the medium's body for hidden props and ensuring that the boy would remain both visible and restrained throughout the proceedings. Luminous material and pins were affixed to the medium's costume and his hands and feet were held during the experiment by two participants known as controls, making it difficult for the young man to manually fake his phenomena.[8] While the dim lighting in the laboratory made errors in sensory perception a possibility, Schrenck-Notzing tried to habituate his medium to increasing amounts of illumination and to the blinding magnesium flash-bulbs of the cameras.[9] To counter claims that the suggestive atmosphere of his laboratory caused delusions or hallucinations among those who attended his experiments, the Baron also encouraged Willy to provide tangible evidence of his manifestations. As the typewriter began to clatter during this experiment, Schrenck-Notzing exclaimed, 'Write, Mina... Do something useful. We will listen to you, and then we shall have the writing, to prove that we are not hypnotised, as some of your enemies say.'[10] Perhaps the most effective means of vouchsafing the medium's phenomena against claims of fraud and delusion, however, was the Baron's use of scientific and cultural authority. There were few critics, after all, who wanted to imply collusion or mental instability on the part of the scientific and cultural luminaries who had sworn to the reality of Willy's mysterious powers.

Although Schrenck-Notzing was never eager to theorise about such phenomena, concentrating instead on careful observation and the collection of data, he clearly subscribed to a natural or animist explanatory paradigm.[11] As an alternative to those theories involving spirits and deceit, the Baron and many of his colleagues, both in Germany and abroad, drew on ostensibly non-mechanistic currents in the contemporary physical and biological sciences. During the early twentieth century, understandings of matter, time and space began to alter in the field of physics and experiments in areas such as embryology became suggestive of the purposive or vitalistic nature of life, enabling those who studied paranormal phenomena to adapt and utilise these new ideas. These researchers argued that in some gifted individuals, mental energy could be projected outside the body where it was transformed into an ephemeral form of matter capable of mimicking human appendages like arms and hands.[12] These teleplastic limbs could act in the physical world by moving objects or leaving impressions in wax or flour before de-materialising and being re-absorbed back into the medial organism from whence they had come. For Schrenck-Notzing, whose experiments with Willy Schneider took place at the height of such theoretical speculations, the best explanation for what had occurred in the Karolinenplatz laboratory appeared to be that the medium had somehow projected and materialised his psychological processes outside of, but in connection with, his body.

While Schrenck-Notzing may have satisfied himself and some of his contemporaries as to the purpose and explanation of events in his laboratory, what is the historian to make of this unusual experiment? Can it be seen, for example, as a manifestation of deeper historical processes through which marginalised individuals sought to come to terms with or help shape modernity? Alternatively, can it be regarded as an example of so-called pseudo-science; a threat to both the integrity and authority of contemporary scientific knowledge? Or, can it be understood as a manifestation of the psychological processes and inner conflicts of those who became involved in such experiments?[13] While all of these approaches offer the historian compelling ways of understanding what Schrenck-Notzing and his colleagues were trying to achieve, this book takes a slightly different approach. It attempts to understand the Baron's experiment not only as a signifier of broader social, cultural, political and psychological currents, but as part of an effort to construct and protect the boundaries of a new scientific discipline.

A border science?

Those members of Germany's educated 'Bildungsbürgertum' [middle classes] who, like Schrenck-Notzing, submitted the elusive phenomena of somnambulism and mediumship to scientific analysis during the late nineteenth and early twentieth centuries, imagined themselves as pioneers of a new science; a science as radical in its implications for psychological, biological and physical knowledge as the work of Eduard von Hartmann (1842–1906) or Sigmund Freud (1856–1939) were for the understanding of the mind or Albert Einstein's (1879–1955) theory was for Newtonian physics. These researchers argued that like the study of the unconscious or the doctrine of relativity, the study of mediumship and allied states such as magnetic somnambulism would make fluid the borders between science and metaphysics.[14] Such borders had grown increasingly rigid during the nineteenth century as science had fallen under the spell of a materialist philosophy that denied the significance of those phenomena it could not quantify. This emphasis on the material basis of life and mind had the effect of excluding large swathes of human experience from the realm of scientific research; an exclusion that was particularly noticeable in fields like psychology where experimentation became increasingly restricted to measuring physiological responses to external stimuli. According to those Germans who experimented with mediums, their research into somnambulism, telepathy, materialisation and telekinesis, was capable of demolishing the arbitrary boundaries erected by scientific materialism to a holistic understanding of mind, body and matter.[15] In the eyes of these researchers this made them practitioners of a border science; not because they were pariahs operating outside the realm of legitimate science, but because they were pioneers altering and expanding the reductive materialist boundaries that others had inscribed on the scientific landscape.

The pursuit of this nascent discipline, known initially as psychical research, but from the mid-1920s onwards increasingly as parapsychology, did not remain uncontested.[16] The claim that these new disciplines were capable of re-mapping scientific terrain or altering relations on the scientific family tree, led to sustained critique. While many scientists dismissed such research as a combination of credulity and fraud, refusing to engage in serious debate about it, others, particularly in new fields such as psychology, felt the need to vigorously combat its claims. The psychologist Wilhelm Wundt (1832–1920), for example, considered one of the founders of experimental psychology, argued for the peripheral or illegitimate nature of these putative sciences, labelling them as the 'stepchildren of science'.[17] Although doubtless intended to signify the outsider status of these nascent disciplines, Wundt's remark captured something important about the scientific study of the paranormal – its insistent claim to the chattels of its more legitimate siblings. Indeed, for scientists like Wundt, the difficulty with psychical research and, later, parapsychology lay not just in the fact that the scientific and social terrain these disciplines sought to colonise led their proponents to transgress the borders between so-called legitimate and illegitimate science, but that in so doing they encroached upon the territory and epistemic authority claimed by other fields, most particularly, psychology. The response of psychologists to this threat ranged from critiques of psychical research and parapsychology, which focused on scientific expertise and authority, to those that made psychical researchers and parapsychologists the focus of psychological analysis.

This book, *The Stepchildren of Science*, explores this disputed terrain, assessing the epistemological, cultural and social issues that arose from the claims of psychical research and parapsychology to scientific legitimacy in the German context. Using the experimental protocols, theoretical writings, photographs and correspondence of those dedicated to the scientific study of the paranormal, it examines the attraction of this field for the men and women who frequented the medium-haunted parlours and laboratories of Imperial and inter-war Germany. It also addresses the motives of opponents, like Wundt, who regarded the study of mediumship as a pursuit simultaneously outside of, but encroaching dangerously on, the realm of science. While the sciences were strengthened by increasing precision, specialisation and professionalisation during the late nineteenth and early twentieth centuries, they still felt the need to respond vehemently to any perceived form of scientific dilettantism; seeking to distance themselves from the taint of illegitimacy.[18]

These epistemological and territorial struggles were not confined, however, to scientists and psychical researchers. As this book will demonstrate, the attempt to establish the legitimacy of psychical research and parapsychology as scientific disciplines also involved a deliberate distancing of the study of the paranormal from its less scientific relations. Just as scientists in fields like psychology, biology and physics worked hard to demarcate their disciplines from the study of the paranormal and to sanitise areas in which contamination was perceived, so too did psychical researchers and parapsychologists attempt to distinguish their science from that of the spiritualists and occultists.[19] In so doing, psychical researchers and parapsychologists restricted both the membership of their scientific community and the range of acceptable research foci and methodologies, lessening their conflict with neighbouring disciplines perhaps, but vastly increasing the number and frequency of their internecine disputes.

The Stepchildren of Science is not, however, simply an intellectual history of psychical research and parapsychology in Germany, it also aims to provide a cultural analysis. While focusing on the professional and epistemological conflicts arising from the claims of psychical research and parapsychology to scientific status, it considers the manner in which scientists and parapsychologists used public forums such as the salon, the stage and the courtroom to mould the German public's understanding of the paranormal. The public comprehension of, and response to, the scientific study of mediumship was, as this book will show, determined not only by these public debates, but also by the attitudes of Germany's religious, legal and political institutions. The responses of these groups to psychical research and parapsychology, as we will see, coincided and departed in interesting ways from their responses to the contemporaneous modern occult movement. Ultimately, then, in its attempt to provide an account of the scientific study of the paranormal in the German context, this book tries to reconcile the 'Grenzgebiete der Wissenschaft' [border areas of science], with both the intellectual and cultural history of the *Kaiserreich*, the Weimar Republic and the Nazi period.

Central to the historical analysis offered here is the contention that psychical research and parapsychology in late nineteenth- and early twentieth-century Germany, are best understood as border sciences. This emphasis on the border status of these disciplines distinguishes this book from recent studies of mesmerism, occultism and psychical research, in which historians of science, including Matthew Brower, Sofie Lachapelle and Alison Winter, have consciously avoided the use of terms such as 'fringe' or 'pseudo-science'.[20] Stressing that the very definition and demarcation of scientific orthodoxy and authority, centre and periphery, was at stake in debates over these disputed disciplines during the nineteenth and early twentieth centuries, these scholars have demonstrated the limited utility of such anachronistic and misleading labels.[21] What historians of science have found useful in conducting such studies, however, are analyses of discipline formation and professionalisation. The ambiguity surrounding scientific and medical orthodoxy during the mid-nineteenth century led not only to the epistemological and methodological negotiations from which modern scientific disciplines formed, but a process of professionalisation intended to secure the status and authority of these fields against the claims of amateurs and other usurpers.[22] Lay and alternative medicine, for example, as the work of scholars such as Paul Weindling and Nils Freytag has shown, were understood by nineteenth-century medical practitioners to act as both a stimulus to medical advance and an impediment to the medical profession's monopolisation of healthcare, leading to a series of long and often futile campaigns against charlatanry.[23] Similarly, mesmerism, occultism and psychical research – the disciplinary formation of which historians of science have shown can be studied just like those of their more legitimate siblings – acted as antagonists in the processes of discipline formation and professionalisation, encroaching on, democratising and popularising territory claimed by sciences like biology, psychology and physics.[24] In highlighting the fluidity of concepts like orthodox and fringe, amateur and professional in this period, these scholars have more convincingly explained the violent reaction of scientists and doctors to nascent disciplines like mesmerism, occultism and psychical research, than those who have regarded them as self-evidently beyond the margins of science.[25]

While many of these studies locate the significance of mesmerism, occultism and psychical research in debates over the limits of scientific orthodoxy and authority, concentrating on their disciplinary claims and formation, a number of these works also seek to understand the attraction of these disputed disciplines by engaging with their content. Older studies, particularly of psychical research and parapsychology, tended to ignore the knowledge claims made within these fields, seeing the interest of both scientists and ordinary citizens in paranormal phenomena as symptomatic of a personal 'crisis of faith' or a more widespread 'flight from reason'.[26] More recent work on the histories of psychical research and parapsychology, however, has demonstrated the cross-fertilisation between the ideas and problems that scientists encountered in their research and their interest in the phenomena produced by mediums. For example, several historians of science working on psychical research in the English context, in particular Richard Noakes and Courtenay Grean Raia, have explored the way in which the experimental work of scientists such as William Fletcher Barrett (1844–1925), Cromwell Varley (1828–83) and Oliver Lodge (1851–1940) helped shape their interpretations of paranormal phenomena.[27] Rather than viewing the interest of these scientists in psychical research as divorced from their more mainstream scientific work, these historians have demonstrated the congruence between their experimentation in both fields; a congruence that enabled such scientists to construct internally consistent cosmologies out of materials as diverse as ectoplasm and energy physics, telepathy and mechanism.[28]

In their emphasis on epistemological disputes, discipline formation, and knowledge creation it is clear that those historians of science currently working on mesmerism, occultism and psychical research have been influenced by sociological studies of the putative pseudo-sciences. Beginning in the late 1970s, sociologists of science, including Harry Collins, Trevor Pinch and Roy Wallis, took an interest in both historical and contemporary examples of pseudo-science as part of their efforts to understand what demarcated science from non-science.[29] In their studies of paranormal metal-bending, mesmerism, phrenology and parapsychology, these scholars discovered that classic demarcation criteria, such as falsification and repeatability, were not reliable ways of distinguishing science from non- or pseudo-science; indeed it became clear through these studies that demarcation was a dynamic process that altered depending on historical and cultural exigencies. This discovery has increasingly led sociologists like Thomas Gieryn to claim that non-science (commonsense, pseudo-science, politics and religion) is differentiated from science by a range of complex social and cultural manoeuvres, dubbed 'boundary-work'.[30]

According to Gieryn, the borders of science at any given historical moment are dependent upon who is struggling for credibility, what is at risk, in front of which audience this contest occurs, and in which institutional arena.[31] Sociologists have asked, therefore, how scientific boundaries are established, sustained, enlarged, policed and breached in the pursuit or denial of epistemic authority.[32] In pursuing such questions, Gieryn and others have identified several genres of boundary-work – including expulsion, expansion and protection of autonomy – seeking to study these genres by concentrating on both historical and contemporary credibility contests.[33] As David Hess, in his study of contemporary new ageism, parapsychology and scepticism, has shown all three forms of boundary-work are significant in the attempts of psychical research and parapsychology to define their borders, not only in relation to science but also with respect to their occult siblings.[34]

One of the most striking features of this recent work on scientific boundaries is its explicit engagement with metaphors. Gieryn, for example, points to the way that science is rhetorically conceived of as a cultural space with specific features and borders.[35] The language used to expel opponents or to broaden science's mandate, he argues, is very often cartographic, for example, 'borders', 'boundaries', 'territory', 'oceans' and 'mountains' feature in the rhetoric of scientific boundary-work. In a similar fashion, Hess has demonstrated how cartographic metaphors are used both within and outside new ageism, parapsychology and scepticism as a means of demarcation, sanitisation and justification and how pathology metaphors are utilised in this same arena to describe both putative sciences and their practitioners.[36] While this might suggest that science's metaphoric borders and boundaries are only used in an exclusionary manner, Hess shows that they can also be employed to connote a ground-breaking project. Both contemporary and historical practitioners of the so-called pseudo-sciences, it appears, have used frontier images, resonant with a faith in progress and evolution, in order to characterise their disciplines as pioneering rather than peripheral.[37]

It is in this context, then, that this book's claims about the border status of psychical research and parapsychology in Germany begin to make sense. Indeed, psychical research and parapsychology were understood by their proponents and opponents alike as border sciences. For those who engaged in mediumistic research this liminal quality was part of its appeal; experimenting with those phenomena that fell outside the scope of psychology, biology and physics, they believed they were expanding the frontiers of science. Critics of this project, on the other hand, understood the border status of psychical research and parapsychology to be a result of their proponents' inability to agree upon phenomena, epistemology and method; a problem that disqualified research into the paranormal from being or becoming a science. The insistence of psychical researchers and parapsychologists on transgressing the borders of other sciences, however, ensured that they could not simply be ignored by psychologists and scientists, who sought to combat this trespass not only by arguing that their opponents' science was diseased, but that their minds were. For these reasons, this book argues, the border status of paranormal research is central to understanding psychical research and parapsychology in the German context.

Historical approaches to occultism,
psychical research and parapsychology

In its exploration of psychical research and parapsychology not only within the scientific realm, but also within German social and political culture, *The Stepchildren of Science,* covers ground well trod by social historians in the last thirty-five years. Early historical analyses, as has been mentioned, tended to view an interest in occultism, spiritualism and psychical research, as a manifestation of a Victorian 'crisis of faith' precipitated by a process of secularisation.[38] In many cases such studies intimated social, religious and political conservatism on the part of adherents, characterising their engagement with the paranormal as atavistic and anti-modern.[39] More recent work on occultism and the study of mediumship, including that of Joy Dixon and Alex Owen, however, has rejected such analyses pointing both to the uneven and incomplete nature of secularisation and to the important explanatory factors such as gender and class that are ignored by the 'crisis of faith' and 'flight from reason' hypotheses.[40] Indeed, these sophisticated socio-political analyses demonstrate not only the multiple attractions of these disputed disciplines, but their practice across the social and political spectrum.[41]

While the last three and a half decades have seen growing interest in occultism and its offspring, in the British, American and French contexts, historians have been slower to appreciate the broad significance of the modern occult revival in Germany.[42] In large part this has been the result of an historiographical tradition that regards occultism in Germany as an ideological forebear of National Socialism. Studies of German occultism from the early 1950s until the mid-1980s, such as those conducted by Joachim Besser, Wilfried Daim, George Mosse and James Webb, tended to focus on Ariosophy, an ideology that derived from the thought of the Austrians Jörg Lanz von Liebensfels (1874–1954) and Guido von List (1884–1919), and which combined occultism, racism, anti-Semitism and nationalism.[43] This research established a number of links between Ariosophy and Nazism, including, most prominently, the fact that the meeting at which the German Worker's Party was founded in 1919 was hosted by a Munich-based ariosophical group. In 1985, however, Nicholas Goodrick-Clarke reassessed this relationship, arguing that while a connection did exist between the Thule Society, the Germanenorden and the early Nazi Party, Hitler's interest in Ariosophy was confined to the racial and pan-German aspects of this doctrine.[44] In concluding that Ariosophy was a symptom rather than an influence in its anticipation of Nazism, Goodrick-Clarke opened the way for a broader understanding of modern occultism in the German context.

Given the perceived connection between occultism and Nazism it is perhaps unsurprising that German psychical research and parapsychology – which bore little connection to *völkisch* or racist ideologies – have received scant attention from historians. One of the few works to have considered the emergence of psychical research in Germany is Adolf Kurzweg's 1976 doctoral dissertation. This work provides a valuable analysis of the intellectual currents and epistemological problems that led to the foundation of the Psychologische Gesellschaft [Psychological Society] in Munich and the Berliner Gesellschaft für Experimental-Psychologie [Berlin Society for Experimental Psychology]; both of which acted as venues for the emergence of psychical research in the German context. [45] Recent histories of German occultism and spiritualism, having moved beyond a search for the occult roots of Nazism, have also made important contributions to our understanding of psychical research and parapsychology as they developed in Germany. Ulrich Linse has conducted several studies in this area, pointing to the wider significance of occultism in Germany and arguing for its close relationship to both modernity and rationality. His book on faith-healing in Berlin, for example, rejects the 'flight from reason' hypothesis, arguing that modern occultism was an attempt at a rational and scientific exploration of the mystical. [46] Linse's work on spiritualist publishing is also important in highlighting the crucial role of publishers in fostering communities not only among German spiritualists but also among German psychical researchers. [47] In his book on the emergence of spiritualism in Germany, which employs Linse's work on spiritualist publishing, Diethard Sawicki considers a number of antecedents of spiritualist belief, including magnetic somnambulism and magnetic spiritism. [48] Sawicki's work demonstrates that these antecedents not only provided explanatory paradigms through which to understand table-turning and spiritualism in the second half of the nineteenth century, but also helped mould German psychical research and its research agendas. Magnetic somnambulism and magnetic spiritism are also important features of Nils Freytag's study of superstition in nineteenth-century Prussia and its Rhine provinces. [49] This book considers, in part, the reaction of the medical community and the authorities to animal magnetism, hypnosis and spiritualism. What is of particular interest here is the struggle of late nineteenth-century hypnotists, a number of whom were involved in psychical research, to gain acceptance for hypnotic therapy by distancing it from animal magnetism, lay therapy, and spiritualism and by using it to explain historical examples of the paranormal, including witchcraft, stigmata and magic.

Corinna Treitel's study of occultism during the late nineteenth and early twentieth centuries sets out to show that German occultism was not necessarily linked with the politics of the far right or with an outright rejection of modernity.[50] It demonstrates not only that occultism was attractive to Germans from across the social and political spectrum, but that the occult offered them practical and empirical ways of engaging with, critiquing, and reforming modernity. Treitel considers psychical research and parapsychology in terms of their relationship to, and boundary disputes with, psychology, giving particular attention to the way that these new disciplines opened up and utilised the creative unconscious. While occultism and creativity are important themes in Treitel's book, they are explored in greater depth in Priska Pytlik's study of occultism, modernity and literature.[51] This work describes the occult and psychical research milieu in Germany during the late nineteenth century, gauging its influence on the aesthetics of writers such as Alfred Döblin (1878–1957), Thomas Mann, and Rainer Maria Rilke (1875–1926). It also outlines the central debates within nascent German psychical research, giving particular attention to the animism versus spiritism controversy, which ultimately proved divisive for the Munich-based Psychologische Gesellschaft. The birth and eventual dissolution of this society are also important features of Tomas Kaiser's dissertation on Carl du Prel (1839–99), one of the leading intellectual figures in both German occultism and spiritualism during the late nineteenth century.[52] Kaiser's work provides an enormously useful overview of the occult philosopher's life, writings and associations. While his study certainly makes a significant contribution to the understanding of the early history of psychical research in Germany, what is most intriguing is the author's claim that du Prel can be seen as a prototypical scientific populariser. Like recent work on French psychical research, then, Kaiser's study links psychical research and occultism to scientific popularisation; a movement with which the professionalising sciences in the late nineteenth century had an uneasy and sometimes combative relationship.[53]

These studies have demonstrated the broader significance of occultism in the German context, not only revealing the ambiguities in Nazism's relationship to the occult and its practitioners, but opening up whole new areas of enquiry, including the interplay of occultism and the arts, and the congruence between scientific popularisation and occult propaganda. They have also added to our knowledge of German psychical research and parapsychology, examining their early institutionalisation in societies and periodicals, outlining the central debates within this community, and highlighting the tensions between these nascent disciplines and the sciences. None of these works, however, focus exclusively on psychical research and parapsychology. There remains room, therefore, for a more thoroughgoing study of psychical research and parapsychology in the German context; a study that will outline their emergence and development as well as their struggle to gain scientific legitimacy.

Introduction

The Stepchildren of Science

The Stepchildren of Science is an attempt, using the tools of intellectual and cultural history, to analyse and understand the scientific study of the paranormal in Germany during the Imperial and inter-war periods. Rather than focus exclusively on psychical research and parapsychology as excrescences of deeper social, cultural and political currents or as tools for dealing with and creating 'the modern', as do many recent studies of occultism, it aims to understand the difficulties surrounding the epistemic claims of these fields as problems of discipline formation.[54] This volume maintains that in order to fully understand the extreme reactions that the pursuit of these nascent disciplines inspired, we must see them as border sciences, that is, disciplines that by their very nature encroached on the territory and epistemic authority of other fields, necessitating vigorous bouts of boundary-work (demarcation, sanitisation and exclusion). Like the sciences on which they encroached, however, the scientific legitimacy and disciplinary cohesion of psychical research and parapsychology were dependent on a form of double boundary-work; an expansionist move that entailed the use of the methods and instruments of neighbouring disciplines for the study of phenomena that lay beyond their borders and an exclusionary move, which required that they distance themselves from their occult siblings. In so doing, this book argues, psychical research and parapsychology found themselves disciplinary stepchildren, stuck between occultism and science.[55]

In providing a slightly different perspective on the occult sciences and a fuller exploration of psychical research and parapsychology in the German context, this book hopes both to fill a historiographical gap and contribute to the exciting contemporary discourse on occultism, science and modernity. *The Stepchildren of Science* therefore focuses on the period *c.*1870 to 1939; chronological parameters that are dictated not only by the work of other historians, but by historical events. The publication of the journal *Psychische Studien* [*Psychical Studies*] in 1874 and the debate that followed Johann Karl Friedrich Zöllner's (1834–82) experiments with the American medium Henry Slade (1835–1905) at the end of the 1870s mark the birth of scientific interest in the study of the paranormal in Germany. The outbreak of the Second World War also represents a watershed for parapsychology in the German context. The last indications that parapsychologists remained active in their campaign to gain official recognition date from the years 1938 and 1939. Following the commencement of hostilities it is clear that parapsychologists, like their counterparts in the occult movement, became targets of government persecution.

The methodology adopted in this book privileges both place and conflict. While the chapters follow a roughly chronological pattern a number of them – particularly Chapters 3 and 5 – utilise a certain site, such as the laboratory or the courtroom, in order to offer an insight into the scientific study of the paranormal in the contexts in which it took place. It is hoped that this approach will offer the reader a sense of what it was like to attend an experiment with a medium or the passion with which parapsychologists and their critics fought each other in the legal arena. It also has the advantage of demonstrating the significance of psychical research and parapsychology within a broader social and cultural milieu. An emphasis on conflict throughout much of this book – particularly Chapters 2, 5 and 6 – is intended to illustrate the highly controversial nature of parapsychology's claim to be a legitimate science. The disagreements and credibility contests that were an habitual feature of psychical research and parapsychology in this period illustrate what was at stake in the scientific study of somnambulism and mediumship. These conflicts, often of a litigious nature, took place not only between parapsychologists and their critics from fields including medicine, psychology and science, but also between parapsychologists and occultists, whose religious and commercial aspirations threatened to damage parapsychology's chances of official recognition.

The Stepchildren of Science relies on a wide range of primary sources from both within and outside the psychical research and parapsychological communities in Germany in the hope of providing a deeper understanding of the significance of these border sciences during the late nineteenth and early twentieth centuries. Books, articles, experimental protocols, photographs, newspaper stories and memoirs, as well as personal correspondence and records are used. A number of the archival collections utilised here have not been used for a study of this nature before. In some cases this is because these important sources are not yet indexed. Of particular note in this regard are the papers of Albert von Schrenck-Notzing and the jurist Albert Hellwig (1880–1950) held at the Institut für Grenzgebiete der Psychologie und Psychohygiene [Institute for the Border Areas of Psychology and Psychohygiene] in Freiburg. Other sources made use of here include the papers of the philosopher and psychologist Traugott Konstantin Oesterreich (1880–1949) at the University of Tübingen, and the correspondence of the biologist and philosopher Hans Driesch (1867–1941) at the University of Leipzig. The attitude of the authorities and other interest groups towards parapsychology and occultism have been derived from governmental papers in state archives and newspaper clippings and correspondence in city and church archives.

The book begins by examining the contexts from which psychical research emerged in the late nineteenth century, pointing to its mesmeric antecedents, its response to, and confrontation with, a materialist psychology, and its complex and sometimes uncomfortable relationship with both modern occultism and medical hypnotism. These early chapters also introduce many of the institutions, publications, people and debates that played an important role in both the emergence of psychical research and in the development of parapsychology. The focus then shifts both temporally and thematically to consider the work and influence of the most prominent and controversial figure in German parapsychology during the early twentieth century, Albert von Schrenck-Notzing. Making use of the Baron's laboratory, *The Stepchildren of Science* explores the experiential and theoretical elements of experimental parapsychology, as well as the power relations that existed within this space and the broader parapsychological community. Following this analysis, it turns to consider the parapsychological scene after Schrenck-Notzing's death in 1929, looking in particular at the influence of the vitalist philosopher Hans Driesch. The examination of Driesch's vitalism and its implications lead into a discussion of the official responses to psychical research and parapsychology in Germany from the late nineteenth century through to the National Socialist era. The final chapters deal with the bitter and often sensational struggles for epistemic authority over the paranormal that occurred in the early twentieth century. The first of these credibility contests takes place in the courtroom, where parapsychologists and their opponents acted as expert witnesses in occult trials during the inter-war period. The second occurs within the realm of psychology where psychologists and parapsychologist did battle over the ontological status of paranormal phenomena and the mental stability of those who studied them. In this way both sides sought to transform their opponents from epistemic competitors into objects of psychological analysis.

Notes

1. The term 'ectoplasm' appears to have been coined by the French physiologist and psychical researcher Charles Richet (1850–1935) during experiments with the Italian materialisation medium Eusapia Palladino (1854–1918) in 1894. He speculated that the material that issued from the medium's body was actually her own vital protoplasm projected outside of her body. See, C.G. Raia, 'From Ether Theory to Ether Theology: Oliver Lodge and the Physics of Immortality', *Journal of the History of the Behavioral Sciences*, 43, 1 (2007), 19. The term 'telekinesis' (in German 'Fernwirkung'), meaning literally 'motion at a distance', was coined by Alexander Aksakow (1832–1903) in 1890. See L.A. Shepard (ed.), *Encyclopedia of Occultism and Parapsychology*, 3rd edn (Detroit: Gale Research, 1991), 1167.

2. The descriptions provided here derive from Thomas Mann's essay, 'Okkulte Erlebnisse', which provides a comprehensive account of one of Schrenck-

Notzing's experiments as well as a discussion of contemporary theories of mediumship and its phenomena. This essay, which Mann also presented as a paper on a number of occasions, formed the basis for the series of séances that occur towards the end of Mann's 1924 novel *The Magic Mountain.* 'Okkulte Erlebnisse' first appeared in *Neue Rundschau* for March 1924. See T. Mann, 'An Experience in the Occult', in *Three Essays,* H.T. Lowe-Porter (trans.), (London: Adelphi, 1932), 219–61.

3. On the role of photography in parapsychological experiments, see R.H. Kraus, *Beyond Light and Shadow: The Role of Photography in Certain Paranormal Phenomena: An Historical Survey* (Munich: Nazraeli Press, 1995).

4. For examples of such photographs, see A. von Schrenck-Notzing, *Phenomena of Materialisation: A Contribution to the Investigation of Mediumistic Teleplastics,* E.E. Fournier d'Albe (trans.), (London: Kegan Paul, Trench, Trubner & Co., 1920)

5. Mann, *op. cit.* (note 2), 226.

6. *Ibid.,* 237

7. *Ibid.,* 239–240

8. *Ibid.,* 232–233

9. Schrenck-Notzing, *op. cit.* (note 4), 21.

10. Mann, *op. cit.* (note 2), 251.

11. P. Pytlik, *Okkultismus und moderne: Ein kulturhistorisches Phänomen und seine Bedeutung für die Literatur um 1900* (Munich: Schöningh Verlag, 2005), 47–8.

12. S. Lachapelle, 'A World Outside Science: French Attitudes Towards Mediumistic Phenomena, 1853–1931' (unpublished PhD dissertation: University of Notre Dame, 2002), 326–37.

13. R. Hayward, *Resisting History: Religious Transcendence and the Invention of the Unconscious* (Manchester: Manchester University Press, 2007), 3–4.

14. Thomas Mann noted 'in this doctrine of relativity the border-line between mathematical physics and metaphysics has become fluid.' Mann, *op. cit.* (note 2), 223–4.

15. 'Programm der psychologischen Gesellschaft in München', *Sphinx,* 2, (1887), 32–6.

16. While I use the term 'psychical research' [psychische Forschung] here, there were a number of words used to describe the scientific study of mediumship in Germany prior to the First World War. One of the more popular was 'scientific occultism' [wissenschaftliche Okkultismus], see E. Bauer, 'Periods of Historical Development of Parapsychology in Germany – An Overview', *Proceedings of the Parapsychological Association 34th Convention* (Parapsychological Association, 1991), 10. The word parapsychology was coined in 1889 by the psychologist Max Dessoir, but did not come into use until the mid-1920s when Schrenck-Notzing renamed a major periodical in

the field *Zeitschrift für Parapsychologie* [*Journal for Parapsychology*]. See M. Dessoir, 'Die Parapsychologie', *Sphinx,* 7 (1889), 341–4.

17. W. Wundt, *Hypnotismus und Suggestion,* 2nd edn (Leipzig: Wilhelm Engelmann, 1911), 5.

18. T. Kaiser, 'Zwischen Philosophie und Spiritismus: Bildwissenschaftliche Quellen zur Leben und Werk des Carl du Prel' (unpublished MPhil dissertation: Universität Lüneburg, 2005), 20.

19. On sanitisation, see R. Wallis, 'Science and Pseudo-Science', *Social Science Information,* 24, 3 (1985), 598.

20. See M.B. Brower, 'The Fantasms of Science: Psychical Research in the French Third Republic, 1880–1935' (unpublished PhD dissertation: Rutgers University, 2005); Lachapelle, *op. cit.* (note 12); A. Winter, *Mesmerized: Powers of Mind in Victorian Britain* (Chicago: University of Chicago Press, 1998).

21. Winter, *op. cit.* (note 20), 4–6.

22. For nascent human sciences like sociology and psychology this involved distancing themselves from their precursors in literature and philosophy and embracing, as far as was feasible, the methods of the natural sciences; a process that stranded these disciplines between the humanities and the sciences. See W. Lepenies, *Between Literature and Science: The Rise of Sociology,* R.J. Hollingdale (trans.), (Cambridge: Cambridge University Press, 1988), 7. Similarly, recent studies of psychical research have represented it as a discipline, inhabiting the space between the competing claims of literature, philosophy, psychology and science for the jurisdiction of the mind. Brower, *op. cit.* (note 20).

23. N. Freytag, *Aberglauben im 19. Jahrhundert: Preußen und seine Rheinprovinz zwischen Tradition und Moderne (1815–1918)* (Berlin: Duncker & Humblot, 2003); P. Weindling, *Health, Race and German Politics between National Unification and Nazism, 1870–1945* (Cambridge: Cambridge University Press, 1989).

24. For a study which considers the disciplinary formation of psychical research, see S.H. Mauskopf and M.R. McVaugh, *The Elusive Science: Origins of Experimental Psychical Research* (Baltimore: Johns Hopkins University Press, 1980); On the democratisation and popularisation of science through mesmerism and séances, see Winter, *op. cit.* (note 20), 26; Lachapelle, *op. cit.* (note 12), 222.

25. Winter, *ibid.*; Lachapelle, *ibid.*; Brower, *op. cit.* (note 20).

26. Guided by the assumption that a straightforward process of secularisation had taken place in the course of the nineteenth century, historians viewed the emergence of spiritualism, occultism, theosophy and psychical research as the result of a widespread 'crisis of faith'. According to this hypothesis, individuals uncomfortable with the implications of scientific naturalism took

'flight from reason', finding in occultism a crutch for their religious beliefs. 'The flight from reason' is the phrase that the historian James Webb used to describe the modern occult revival. Like the crisis of faith analysis this theory assumed a crisis of consciousness during the nineteenth century brought on by rationalism and materialism and resulting in a rejection of reason, see J. Webb, *The Occult Establishment* (La Salle: Open Court, 1976), 7–10.

27. R. Noakes, '"The 'Bridge which is between Physical and Psychical Research": William Fletcher Barrett, Sensitive Flames, and Spiritualism', *History of Science,* xlii (2004): 419–64; R. Noakes, 'Ethers, Religion and Politics in Late-Victorian Physics: Beyond the Wynne Thesis', *History of Science,* xliii (2005): 1–41; R. Noakes, 'Cromwell Varley Frs, Electrical Discharge and Victorian Spiritualism', *Notes and Records of the Royal Society,* 61 (2007): 5–21; Raia, *op. cit.* (note 1), 19–43.

28. Raia, *op. cit.* (note 1), 22.

29. See, for example, H.M. Collins and T.J. Pinch, *Frames of Meaning: The Social Construction of Extraordinary Science* (London: Routledge, 1982); T.J Pinch, 'Normal Explanations of the Paranormal: The Demarcation Problem and Fraud in Parapsychology', *Social Studies of Science,* 9, 3 (1979): 329–48; R. Wallis, (ed.) *On the Margins of Science: The Social Construction of Rejected Knowledge,* Sociological Review Monograph No. 27 (Keele: University of Keele Press, 1979); Wallis, *op. cit.* (note 19), 585–601.

30. T. F. Gieryn, *Cultural Boundaries of Science: Credibility on the Line* (Chicago: The University of Chicago Press, 1999), x

31. *Ibid.,* x–xi

32. *Ibid.,* xi.

33. *Ibid.,* 15–17

34. D. Hess, *Science in the New Age: The Paranormal, Its Defenders and Debunkers, and American Culture* (Madison: University of Wisconsin Press, 1993), 145.

35. Gieryn, *op. cit.* (note 30), x.

36. Hess, *op. cit.* (note 34), 62.

37. *Ibid.,* 30.

38. There are a number of excellent older studies that utilise the 'crisis of faith' analysis, for example, see F.M. Turner, *Between Science and Religion: The Reaction to Scientific Naturalism in Late Victorian England* (New Haven: Yale University Press, 1974); R.L. Moore, *In Search of White Crows: Spiritualism, Parapsychology and American Culture* (Oxford: Oxford University Press, 1977); J. Oppenheim, *The Other World: Spiritualism and Psychical Research in England, 1850–1914* (Cambridge: Cambridge University Press, 1985). For a comprehensive discussion of the secularisation thesis and the 'crisis of faith' analysis in relation to modern occultism, see A. Owen, *The Place of*

Enchantment: British Occultism and the Culture of the Modern (Chicago: University of Chicago Press, 2004), 10–13.

39. On British psychical research as the conservative response of a Cambridge educated élite to the professional, social and moral ambitions of middle-class scientific naturalists, see B. Wynne, 'Physics and Psychics: Science, Symbolic Action, and Social Control in Late Victorian England', in B. Barnes and S. Shapin (eds), *Natural Order: Historical Studies of Scientific Culture* (Beverly Hills: Sage Publications, 1979), 167–86. For responses to Wynne's hypothesis, see J.P. Williams, 'The Making of Victorian Psychical Research: An Intellectual Elite's Approach to the Spiritual World' (unpublished PhD dissertation: University of Cambridge, 1984); and Noakes, 'Ethers, Religion and Politics', *op. cit.* (note 27), 1–41.

40. For examples of studies that privilege gender in their attempts to understand the modern occult revival, see J. Dixon, *Divine Feminine: Theosophy and Feminism in England* (Baltimore: Johns Hopkins University Press, 2001); A. Owen, *The Darkened Room. Women, Power and Spiritualism in Late Victorian England* (London: Virago Press, 1989).

41. On the social and political flexibility of modern occultism in the German context, see C. Treitel, *A Science for the Soul: Occultism and the Genesis of the German Modern* (Baltimore: The Johns Hopkins University Press, 2004).

42. For examples of works on French spiritism and occultism, see T. Kselman, *Death and Afterlife in Modern France* (Princeton: Princeton University Press, 1993); J. Monroe, 'Evidence of Things Not Seen: Spiritism, Occultism and the Search for a Modern faith in France, 1853–1925' (unpublished PhD dissertation: Yale University, 2002); L.L Sharp, 'Rational Religion, Irrational Science: Men, Women, and Belief in French Spiritism, 1853–1914' (unpublished PhD dissertation: University of California at Irvine, 1996); B. Verter, 'Dark Star Rising: The Emergence of Modern Occultism, 1800–1950' (unpublished PhD dissertation: Princeton University, 1997).

43. J. Besser, 'Die Vorgeschichte des Nationalsozialismus in neuem Licht', *Die Pforte: Monatsschrift für Kultur* 2, 21/22 (1950), 763–84; W. Daim, *Der Mann, der Hitler die Ideen gab: Jörg Lanz von Liebenfels*, 3rd edn (Vienna: Ueberreuter, 1994); G.L. Mosse, 'The Mystical Origins of National Socialism', *Journal of the History of Ideas*, 22 (1961), 81–96. See also: G.L. Mosse, *The Crisis of German Ideology: Intellectual Origins of the Third Reich* (London: Weidenfeld and Nicolson, 1964); J. Webb, *The Occult Underground* (La Salle: Open Court Publishing, 1974); Webb, *op. cit.* (note 26), 275–344.

44. N. Goodrick-Clarke, *The Occult Roots of Nazism: Secret Ayran Cults and their Influence on Nazi Ideology: The Ariosophists of Austria and Germany, 1890–1935* (New York: New York University Press, 1985), 192–204.

45. A. Kurzweg, 'Die Geschichte der Berliner "Gesellschaft für Experimental-Psychologie" mit besonderer Berücksichtigung ihrer Ausgangssituation und des Wirkens von Max Dessoir' (unpublished PhD dissertation: Free University of Berlin, 1976). There has also been some work on the emergence of psychical research in Germany conducted by historians of medicine at the University of Bonn, but this work, commissioned by the Instiut für Grenzgebiete der Psychologie und Psychohygiene in Freiburg, remains unpublished. See, for example, B. Wolf-Braun, *Mesmerismus, Hypnotismus und die Parapsychologische Forschung: 'Rapport' und 'Mentalsuggestion' als Gegenstand der Wissenschaft im ausgehenden 19. und frühen 20. Jahrhundert* (Final report for the Institut für Grenzgebiete der Psychologie und Psychohygiene, University of Bonn, 1999).

46. U. Linse, *Geisterseher und Wunderwirker: Heilsuche im Industriezeitalter* (Frankfurt am Main: Fischer, 1996).

47. U. Linse, 'Der Spiritismus in Deutschland um 1900', in M. Bassler and H. Châtellier (eds), *Mystik, Mystizismus und Moderne in Deutschland um 1900* (Strasburg: Presses Universitaires de Strasbourg, 1998); U. Linse, 'Das Buch der Wunder und Geheimwissenschaften: Der spiritistische Verlag Oswald Mutze in Leipzig im Rahmen der spiritistischen Bewegung Sachsens', in M. Lehmstedt and A. Herzog (eds), *Das Bewegte Buch: Buchwesen und soziale, nationale und kulturelle Bewegungen um 1900* (Wiesbaden: Harrassowitz, 1999).

48. D. Sawicki, *Leben mit den Toten: Geisterglauben und die Enstehung des Spiritismus in Deutschland, 1770–1900* (Munich: Schöningh, 2002).

49. Freytag, *op. cit.* (note 23).

50. Treitel, *op. cit.* (note 41), 40–55.

51. Pytlik, *op. cit.* (note 11).

52. Kaiser, *op. cit.* (note 18)

53. Lachapelle, *op. cit.* (note 12).

54. In its focus on the boundary disputes between psychology and the study of the paranormal – which increasingly involved the 'psychologisation' and 'pathologisation' of psychical research and parapsychology in the Imperial and inter-war periods – this book also hopes to make a small contribution to Rhodri Hayward's argument about the role of psychology and psychical research in the construction of 'historicist' conceptions of self. Unable to come to terms with the paranormal ontologically, this book will show German psychologists attempted to transform paranormal phenomena and those who studied them into legitimate objects of research, thereby undermining their threat not only to psychology, but also to stable notions of history and self. See, Hayward, *op. cit.* (note 13).

55. This is similar to the claim that Lepenies has made about sociology, which he regards as stranded between literature and science by its attempts, on the

one hand, to mimic science and, on the other, to distance itself from literature. See Lepenies, *op. cit.* (note 22), 7.

1

The Emergence of Psychical Research in Imperial Germany

Introduction

At a meeting of the Psychologische Gesellschaft [Psychological Society] in Munich during September 1887, the physician Albert von Schrenck-Notzing presented the findings of a series of forty experiments in which a range of obscure phenomena associated with hypnosis had been investigated.[1] Placing the talented young somnambulist Lina Matzinger into a state of hypnotic lethargy, members of the society, who included the philosopher Carl du Prel, the former colonial propagandist Wilhelm Hübbe-Schleiden (1846–1916), and the artists Albert von Keller (1844–1920), Gabriel von Max (1840–1915) and Wilhelm Trübner (1851–1917), sought to conduct three distinct kinds of experiment. The first, which took their impetus from the English Society for Psychical Research, involved the transference of thoughts.[2] Seated behind or in another room from the hypnotised Lina, the experimenters attempted to mentally transmit instructions to her. In one such experiment, Lina was ordered to take a specific book from a table covered in reading material and place it in the pocket of a jacket hanging in another room; a task she completed with astonishing success.[3] In related tests, the experimenters tried to transmit physiological responses, such as pain, and sensations, such as taste, to the somnolent girl, piercing their skin with pins and placing a range of sweet and sour substances on their tongues.[4] Lina responded to these strange experiments with a range of appropriate cries and grimaces. The men investigating these phenomena concluded from this series of tests that the transference of thoughts and sensations from one person to another without the mediation of the known senses was possible and that this ability was heightened in certain states of hypnosis.[5] The second group of experiments sought to transfer one of the five senses to another part of the body. In a state of deep hypnosis, a blindfolded Lina demonstrated the ability to read a book pressed against her skull, leading the experimenters to speculate that her sight had been transferred to the intersection of her sagittal and crown sutures (see Image 1.1 overleaf).[6] Similarly, witnesses noted Lina's ability to read material pressed against her mid-section, indicating perhaps the transfer

Image 1.1

Lina Matzinger reads a book without the mediation of the senses, Munich, 1887. Reproduced with permission from the Institut für Grenzgebiete der Psychologie und Psychohygiene e. V., Freiburg im Breisgau (IGPP collection).

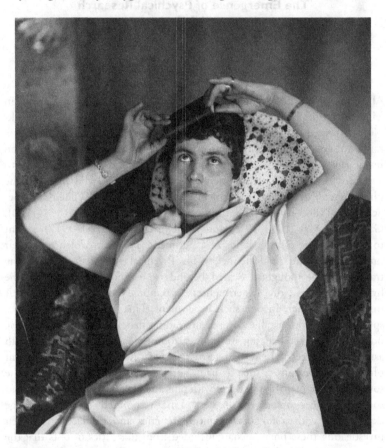

of her sight to the pit of her stomach. The third set of experiments attempted to elicit emotional and physical responses to visual and aural stimuli. Placed in front of a picture or exposed to music, the somnambulistic Lina exhibited a profound mimetic passion and plasticity which experimenters such as Albert von Keller tried to capture on photographic plates.[7] The suggestions provided by those in attendance saw the hypnotised girl assume the role of a priestess, mimic prayer and religious ecstasy, as well as a variety of angry, threatening poses. Examining the photographs that resulted from these experiments, the members of the Psychologische Gesellschaft claimed that the creative ability Lina displayed in somnambulism went far beyond that possible in the waking state, making the phenomena she exhibited of both practical and psychological significance.[8]

Contextualising these experiments for his audience, Schrenck-Notzing explained that they derived their *raison d'être* from key sections of the nascent society's programme in which hypnotic experimentation had been touted as the basis of a new form of psychology and as an aid to artistic expression.[9] Taking their impetus from the hypnotic experiments conducted at the medical schools in Nancy and Paris, the artists, philosophers and physicians who founded the Psychologische Gesellschaft in 1886, declared themselves dedicated above all else to establishing what they called 'experimental psychology'. This new discipline, which used the abnormal states and somnambulistic feats of Lina and her ilk to demonstrate the influence of mind upon body, was intended to free contemporary psychology from its slavish adherence to materialism and to bring to an end its subordination to physiology, allowing a more complete understanding of the human mind. As Lina's dramatic turn as priestess and ecstatic illustrated, however, the 'experimental psychology' practised by the Psychologische Gesellschaft was also envisaged as a stimulus to cultural endeavour.[10] For the preponderance of artists who became members of the society, for example, this new science offered both practical assistance in the form of somnambulistic models and psychological insight into the link between the unconscious mind and creative ability. For others, however, the significance of Lina's hypnotic performances went beyond the scientific and the cultural. Although not apparent in the report of the empirically minded Schrenck-Notzing – who saw in the experimental exploration of Lina's somnambulistic abilities a means of extending scientific knowledge – the society's programme, authored by Carl du Prel, the Psychologische Gesellschaft's leading figure, also stressed the profound social and philosophical implications of its project.[11] In the opinion of du Prel, Lina's telepathic talents provided the basis not just for an 'experimental psychology' but for a transcendental one. This new science built upon a foundation of somnambulism would, du Prel and his followers insisted, vouchsafe the existence of the soul, expose the moral bankruptcy and scientific paucity of the dominant materialist *Weltanschauung*, and ensure social stability.[12]

While du Prel's use of hypnotic experimentation to forge a transcendental worldview garnered support among select members of the Psychologische Gesellschaft, those intellectuals and physicians who founded the Berliner Gesellschaft für Experimental-Psychologie [Berlin Society for Experimental Psychology] in 1888, among them the ethnologist Adolf Bastin (1826–1933), the chemist Heinrich Biltz (1865–1943), the philosopher Max Dessoir (1867–1947), the art historian Friedrich Goeler

von Ravensburg (1854–96) and the colonial director Albrecht Wilhelm
Sellin (1841–1933), approached the strange phenomena of somnambulism
in much the same manner as Schrenck-Notzing. The Berlin society's
programme, like that of their Munich-based colleagues, revealed a distaste
for the dominance of materialism within the psychological sciences and a
desire to establish an 'experimental psychology' that would differ from those
older forms of psychology based on introspection and the physiological
psychology of Wilhelm Wundt.[13] Modelling their group on the Society for
Psychical Research, the members of the Berliner Gesellschaft für
Experimental-Psychologie sought to understand those phenomena,
including somnambulism, clairvoyance and telepathy that existed on the
border between the normal and the pathological, an aim highlighted by
Dessoir's coining of the term 'parapsychology' in 1889.[14] While this word did
not come into common use until the 1920s, it clearly described the
disciplinary space and function that the science promoted by the Berlin
society was intended to fill. Dessoir wrote:

> If we designate something whose scope goes beyond or alongside normal
> experience with *para-* by analogy with words like *para*genesis, *para*goge,
> *para*graph, *para*cope, *para*cusis, *para*logism, *para*nois, *para*ergon, etc., then we
> can perhaps refer to those phenomena which do not figure in the normal
> functioning of the psyche as parapsychic, and to the science which concerns
> itself with these phenomena as 'parapsychology'.[15]

Like their colleagues in Munich, the members of the Berliner
Gesellschaft für Experimental-Psychologie pursued their new discipline with
the aim of expanding psychology's empirical knowledge, using hypnosis to
push beyond the borders of consciousness into a realm which science had
tended to ignore because of its apparent relationship with superstition, fraud
and delusion.[16] In so doing, both societies became important venues for the
emergence of psychical research in Germany during the *Kaiserreich*.

While the central aims espoused in the programmes of the Munich and
Berlin societies suggest that German psychical research can be understood as
a response to the mechanistic turn that occurred within psychology in the
late nineteenth century, closer perusal of these documents and the
experiments these societies conducted indicate the equal importance of other
social and epistemological factors. As we have seen, for example, sections of
the Psychologische Gesellschaft's programme moved beyond the promotion
of a new form of psychology, in which the examination of unconscious or
abnormal phenomena was facilitated by hypnosis, to suggest that such
phenomena might form the basis of a transcendental worldview. The series
of investigations described by Schrenck-Notzing, likewise betrayed a

concern not only with the scope of human mental abilities, but also with their practical application in areas such as medicine and art. Similarly, the programme of the Berlin society revealed the interest of its members in both rigorously controlled psychological experiments with somnambulistic subjects, and the investigation of spontaneous cases in spiritualist séances and occult circles.[17] These examples suggest that psychical research emerged in Germany not just as a reaction to the psychology practised by Wundt and his associates, but to broader social and epistemological concerns about scientific materialism, as well as a profound interest in and, in some cases, affinity with the ideas and phenomena associated with modern occultism.

With these factors in mind, this chapter seeks to examine the multiple and overlapping contexts in which psychical research emerged at the end of the nineteenth century. It provides an introduction to the people, publications and societies that featured prominently in the development of this nascent discipline in Germany and links them to the broader social, cultural and philosophical milieu. The chapter begins by discussing the difficult and often combative relationship between German psychical research and psychology. As the programmes of the Munich and Berlin societies demonstrate, proponents of psychical research, or so-called 'experimental psychology', sought to define their discipline by contrasting it with the physiological psychology on the ascendancy in Germany's universities. In so doing, they found themselves embroiled in a series of boundary disputes with psychologists over the constitution of scientific expertise and authority. Turning to an exploration of modern occultism and its antecedents – the versatility of which allowed them to act as a panacea for a materialistic worldview, as a means of accessing the creative unconscious and as tools for social reform and self-help – this chapter considers the way in which the personnel, publications and interests of the occult movement overlapped with and helped foster psychical research. What follows is an exposition of the 'transcendental psychology' of the philosopher Carl du Prel. While du Prel hoped to use the study of somnambulism to overthrow materialism and promote a new worldview, men such as Schrenck-Notzing pursued psychical research as a means of expanding the borders of science. The disjuncture between du Prel's spiritist approach and the animist 'experimental psychology' of his colleague led, as we will see, to an irrevocable split within this society, dictating the shape and dimensions of German psychical research in the decades that followed.

The confrontation with psychology

According to the programme of the Psychologische Gesellschaft, which appeared in the occult journal *Sphinx* in January 1887, psychology, with its potential for profound insight into human nature, was the most important of the sciences, central to the understanding of both humanity and nature.[18] This programme, which outlined the society's purpose and aims, went on to argue, however, that in its late nineteenth-century incarnation, where every mental event was explained physically, psychology had become a mere appendix of physiology and the mind as an independent entity had disappeared. This materialist form of psychology, the society complained, was demonstrably false.[19] The critique of contemporary psychology that emerged from the Berliner Gesellschaft für Experimental-Psychologie was less explicit. While the programme applauded the rejection of self-observation within modern psychology and the use of the more exacting methods of physiology to gain empirical knowledge, it lamented the restriction of this science to the measurement of involuntary twitches and timed responses in the waking state.[20] This approach, the Berlin society's programme pointed out, shut off from investigation all those mental phenomena native to the unconscious sphere. The complaints outlined in these documents, prefacing, as they did, the introduction and underlining the necessity of the new discipline that these societies promoted, were unambiguously directed at that species of mental science known as experimental or physiological psychology. Epitomised by the work of Wilhelm Wundt, this materialist approach to the mind had emerged mid-century as a result of efforts to have psychology recognised within Germany's universities as a discipline not only distinct from philosophy but meticulous in its empiricism.

The attempt during the second half of the nineteenth century to transform psychology from a sub-discipline of philosophy into an empirical science saw an emphasis on mental events for which there were physiological correlates. Higher functions, including thought, were set aside in favour of phenomena, such as sensation, reaction time and attention span, which could be classified and measured using methods derived from physiology.[21] This new discipline rejected self-observation and introspection, aiming instead for the independence of the observer from the object; a goal achieved in part by the transference of psychology to a laboratory environment.[22] Equipped with instruments for tracing and gauging stimulus and response, the psychological laboratory allowed access to individual consciousness in a manner previously unimagined. This form of psychology, which bore a closer relationship to physiology than it did to philosophy, had had its beginning with Gustav Fechner's psychophysics and had developed through the work of the so-called 'high-priest' of psychology, Wundt, into what contemporary critics, such as those who formed the membership of the Munich and Berlin societies, called 'a psychology without soul'.[23]

While the roots of experimental psychology can be located in the 1860s in the work of men such as Gustav Fechner (1801–87), Hermann

Helmholtz (1821–94), Rudolf Hermann Lotze (1817–81) and Ernst Weber (1830–1902), this new discipline only began to enjoy an institutional presence from the late 1870s, at which time Wundt established his laboratory in Leipzig.[24] Wundt used Fechner's law (1860), which expressed the relationship between mental and physical events as an equation – the strength of sensation is proportional to the logarithmic value of the intensity of sensation – as the basis for his experimental exploration of the mind.[25] This approach meant that the study of the unconscious, along with abnormal and developmental psychology, fell outside the scope of this new science, the focus of which were those mental phenomena associated with healthy conscious individuals. Beside these normal psychological phenomena with their physiological correlates, however, stood another group of mental events that appeared to demonstrate the independence of the mind from the body.[26] These phenomena, usually associated with unconscious or altered states, stood in a completely different relationship to physiological events, than did those of conscious ones. Communication between the subject and his or her body and environment in states of somnambulism, for instance, were radically different to those of the waking state. According to their programmes, it was these gaps in physiological psychology that inspired the Psychologische Gesellschaft and the Berliner Gesellschaft für Experimental-Psychologie to embark upon their pursuit of what they labelled 'experimental psychology'.

The Munich and Berlin societies sought to make an empirical study of those phenomena, including somnambulism, telepathy and clairvoyance, that were most commonly associated with abnormal states such as hypnosis and occult practices such as mediumship. If the patina of superstition and fraud could be removed from such phenomena, these groups maintained, what remained would be a range of unconscious psychological events and abilities that could not be explained simply in physiological terms and which would vastly enrich the understanding of the mind.[27] The experiments conducted by the Psychologische Gesellschaft and the Berliner Gesellschaft für Experimental-Psychologie thus set out both to study such phenomena under experimental conditions and to demonstrate the limitations of a physiological approach. Thought-transference, for example, when not dismissed out of hand by scientists, had been explained as a physiological phenomenon. As the theories of the physiologists Wilhelm Preyer (1841–97), F.C.C. Hansen and Alfred Lehmann (1858–1921) explained, this strange ability was a result of unconscious gestures, muscular movements and number preferences.[28] The 1887 tests carried out with Lina by members of the Munich society set out to disprove this theory. Placing the hypnotised girl in another room, out of visual or aural contact with anyone else, the experimenters tried to exclude the possibility that Lina was merely responding to the unconscious twitches and muscular movements of those around her.[29] Du Prel, whose home acted as a laboratory for many of these experiments, claimed that these precautions ensured that there was no possibility that Lina's apparent telepathy was a result of 'muscle-reading'; confirming for him the reality of thought-transference and the limitations of the physiologists' theory.[30] Through such experiments the Munich and Berlin societies imagined themselves expanding psychological knowledge beyond the limits set for it by the physiological approach to the mind.

Psychical research, however, did more than fill the gaps and highlight the erasures of physiological psychology. It encroached on territory that the more established discipline claimed as its own. The appropriation of the term 'experimental psychology', for example, was a distinct irritant to psychologists like Wundt, who feared that his empirical science might be confused with the mawkish mysticism and irrationality of the psychical researchers. Psychologists such as Wundt and Hugo Münsterberg (1863–1916), as we will see in subsequent chapters, used their published work to try to sever this connection and to combat what they saw as the outlandish and unscientific claims associated with this illegitimate form of 'experimental psychology'. There were, however, a number of occasions when the confrontation between psychology and psychical research escaped the confines of scholarly discourse and became a matter of public debate. These altercations were important because they demarcated the territory over which psychology and psychical research would do battle during the late nineteenth and early twentieth centuries and introduced the arguments that would be rehearsed *ad nauseam* as a means of expanding and protecting disciplinary boundaries.

Predating the foundation of the Munich and Berlin societies, the first of these credibility contests began during the winter of 1877–8, when Johann Karl Friedrich Zöllner, one of the founding figures in the field of astrophysics and a respected professor at the University of Leipzig, attended a series of séances with the American medium Henry Slade. The fruit of these sittings, according to Zöllner, who witnessed in Slade's presence both slate writing and the mysterious appearance of knots in loops of leather, was a new science called 'Transzendentalphysik' [transcendental physics]; a term he borrowed from the philosopher Immanuel Fichte (1797–1879).[31] Convinced that the strange phenomena manifested by mediums like Slade could offer empirical proof of the existence of a fourth dimension – a concept postulated within non-Euclidean mathematics – Zöllner embarked on a further series of tests hoping to elicit definitive proof of this theory.[32] These experiments, which for the most part took place in Zöllner's home, were abundant in phenomena. Apart from slate writing and knot tying, witnesses noted the appearance of limb-like impressions in both wax and flour and examples of apparent clairvoyance on the part of the medium.[33] Such phenomena were experienced not only by Zöllner, but also at different times by his friends Gustav Fechner (1801–87), Wilhelm Scheibner (1826–1908) and Wilhelm Weber (1804–91), and other members of the university including Wilhelm Wundt, Carl Ludwig (1816–95) and Carl Thiersch (1822–95). From his observations of, and discussions with, Slade, Zöllner concluded that these phenomena were not the result of physical manipulation by the medium, rather they were the work of some invisible agency in the fourth dimension with which Slade had an affinity.[34] This was the position he made public in the third volume of his *Wissenschaftliche Abhandlungen* [*Scientific Treatise*]. [35]

The publication of Zöllner's theories provoked outrage on the part of the scientific community, who filled entire journals and newspapers with their vitriolic responses to his work. While a number of Zöllner's friends, including Fechner and Weber, continued to support him, men such as Emil du Bois-Reymond (1818–96), Ernst Häckel (1834–1919), Hermann Helmholtz and Rudolf Virchow (1821–1902) were extremely disapproving and dismissive of this apparent misapplication of scientific energy.[36] Zöllner's use of his position as a university professor to popularise what amounted to spiritualism was particularly repugnant to Wundt. Zöllner's treatise and an article by the philosopher Hermann Ulrici (1806–84), which maintained that the scientific authority of Zöllner, Fechner and Weber vouchsafed Slade's phenomena, were a provocation to the psychologist, whose nascent discipline hinged on a number of factors that were threatened by Zöllner's transcendental physics.[37] In a paper entitled *Der Spiritismus eine sogenannte wissenschaftliche Frage* [*Spiritualism, a So-Called Scientific Question*], Wundt attempted to highlight Zöllner's misapplication and misrepresentation of the scientific method. He argued, for example, that scientific expertise and authority were non-transferable; one's expertise in astrophysics, for instance, did not make one's observations in other fields, such as observational psychology, reliable. Wundt also stressed the predictable function of natural law and causation, arguing that it was far more likely that the witnesses to Slade's phenomena were mistaken, than that natural law had been contravened.[38] These complaints, although they largely failed to dissuade public interest in spiritualism, were significant because they identified the areas of tension, in particular the nature of scientific authority and expertise, around which many subsequent boundary disputes between psychical research and psychology would revolve.

The second disciplinary confrontation examined here took place during the 1880s and 1890s; its key protagonists were the philosopher Eduard von Hartmann, author of *Philosophie des Unbewußten* [*Philosophy of the Unconscious*] (1868), and Aleksandr Aksakov (1832–1903), editor of the

41

occult journal *Psychische Studien*. Hartmann, whose work on the unconscious enjoyed considerable popularity among Germany's intellectual elite, provoked this debate by publishing an analysis of spiritualism in which he attributed the phenomena exhibited by spiritualist mediums to unknown mental powers, and the materialisations witnessed by séance participants to hallucination.[39] In this book, entitled *Der Spiritismus* (1885), Hartmann set out an argument in which the medium was likened to a powerful mesmerist, capable of transferring ideas to those around her and creating a shared hallucination.[40] Séance participants were made susceptible to such hallucinations, Hartmann maintained, by a willingness to believe in spiritualism and the half somnambulistic state into which they were lulled by the suggestive environment. The position adopted by Hartmann – that when the phenomena associated with spiritualism were not a result of delusion or fraud they could be explained psychologically in terms of hidden mental powers and suggestion – became known as animism.

In response to this work, Aksakov, who was one of Germany's most active propagandists for spiritualism, defended the spiritist hypothesis. This hypothesis stated that the phenomena produced by mediums, most particularly materialisation, should be attributed to spirits. While Aksakov welcomed Hartmann's study, arguing that its psychological analysis made an important contribution to the understanding of spiritualism, he maintained that not all cases of mediumship or materialisation could be explained with reference to unconscious powers and hallucination.[41] The evidence that Aksakov used to disprove Hartmann's hallucination hypothesis was spirit photography. Photographs taken during séances, in which both the medium and the materialised form were visible, Aksakov argued, proved conclusively that materialisation was an objective phenomena rather than a form of mass hallucination.[42] Aksakov's writings on this topic initially appeared in the *Psychische Studien*, but were eventually published in book form in 1890 as *Animismus und Spiritismus* [*Animism and Spiritualism*]. The spiritist hypothesis and Aksakov also found defenders among the occultists who contributed to the journal *Sphinx*, where Hartmann was portrayed variously as obtuse or dishonest for his refusal to recognise his logical errors.[43] Hartmann responded to these critiques in 1891 in a book entitled *Die Geisterhypothese des Spiritismus und seine Phantome* [*The Ghost Hypothesis of Spiritulism and its Phantoms*] in which he updated his analysis by employing the concepts of suggestion and autosuggestion, as well as hallucination.

As Priska Pytlik has argued, the significance of this debate went beyond the immediate exchange between Hartmann, Aksakov and their supporters, highlighting the theoretical fissures that separated those who studied the phenomena of mediumship for the insights it offered into the human psyche, and those who took an interest in such phenomena for metaphysical or spiritual reasons.[44] A prime example of this broader significance, as Pytlik makes clear, was the split of the Psychologische Gesellschaft in 1889, where the differences between the animist Schrenck-Notzing and the spiritist du Prel proved irreconcilable.[45] The Hartmann–Aksakov debate, however, is also important for another reason. Hartmann's analysis, although it falls short of postulating a subliminal consciousness, can be understood as an effort to integrate the paranormal into the personal and historical record through psychology.[46] It is representative of those attempts, which began during the late nineteenth century in the German context, first to 'psychologise' the phenomena associated with spiritualism and psychical research, and then later to 'pathologise' their proponents. 'Psychologisation' and 'pathologisation' were a means not only of dealing with the disruptive influence of paranormal phenomena, but as we will see in subsequent chapters, of dealing with the disciplinary threat to psychology posed by both psychical research and parapsychology. The Hartmann–Aksakov debate thus helps highlight the positions and the rhetoric that spiritists, psychical researchers, parapsychologists and psychologists were to adopt in the boundary disputes of the late nineteenth and early twentieth centuries.

Modern occultism

Psychical research in the German context emerged during the 1870s, concomitant not only with the physiological turn in psychology, but also with the ascendancy of modern occultism. As the programme of the Psychologische Gesellschaft noted, the strange mental phenomena on which the members of the society sought to found their new experimental science were frequently associated with contemporary occult practices such as spiritualism.[47] While such practices might be dismissed *a priori* by adherents of a materialist psychology, members of the Munich and Berlin societies proposed to undertake an unbiased exploration of this area. In the programme of the Berliner Gesellschaft für Experimental-Psychologie, for example, Max Dessoir and Goeler von Ravensburg outlined their intention to conduct a thoroughgoing and unprejudiced scientific examination of spiritualist phenomena when suitable opportunities arose.[48] In so doing, they believed they might establish some connection – as had been done for mediumistic writing and hypnotic double consciousness – between spiritualist phenomena, hypnosis and telepathy.[49] The links between psychical research and occultism were, of course, deeper and more complex than this call for a neutral examination of occult phenomena suggested. Psychical research and modern occultism in the German context, for example, shared a common heritage in the mesmeric experiments conducted by Romantic philosophers and physicians in the first half of the nineteenth century. The boundaries between what constituted psychical research on the one hand, and what might be considered occultism on the other, were also difficult to distinguish and define. Not only did these boundaries move over time, but they were construed differently by competing groups, all of whom claimed the epistemic authority of science. Those who engaged in occult practice or who considered themselves psychical researchers might also blur such distinctions by combining an interest in hermetic knowledge or faith healing with fastidious hypnotic research, or by moving from occultism to psychical research and vice versa, as did figures like du Prel. Given the symbiotic, if volatile, relationship between psychical research and the occult sciences, it is clear that an exploration of the occult milieu is required in order to fully comprehend the emergence of psychical research in Germany during the late nineteenth century.

Modern occultism, evident in Germany as elsewhere from the late 1840s until the late 1930s, consisted of the revival of old forms of esoteric knowledge, such as astrology and Rosicrucianism, the birth of new occult sciences, such as theosophy, and the rise of popular religious practices such as spiritualism.[50] While modern occultism was undoubtedly an amalgam of old and new practices, it possessed characteristics that were distinctly modern. It was modern, for instance, in both its embrace of science, through which its practitioners hoped to annihilate both philosophical and scientific materialism, and in its 'openness', which at times sat uneasily with those definitions of occultism that stressed hidden knowledge and lengthy initiation. Combining the hermetic and mystical traditions of east and west with the rhetoric of science, modern occultism attempted to forge a rational form of spirituality without accepting the assumptions upon which a rationalist worldview was dependent.[51] The historian Alex Owen, in seeking to understand this curious fusion of occultism and science, has examined the relationship between 'enchantment', in the Weberian sense, and modern culture, arguing that the late nineteenth century saw a new notion of 'enchantment' in which rationality was a guiding principle.[52] This 'rational enchantment' was evident in a range of modern occult practices, including spiritualism and psychical research, where experiment and empiricism played an important role in epistemic claims.

The modern occult movement was also more 'open' and more accessible than its predecessors. While some of the occult sciences retained their exclusivity, demanding of their adherents a long and complex initiation into secret knowledge, a number of the more prominent contemporary occult practices stressed that anyone, regardless of gender, class or education, could gain such knowledge for themselves. The spread of modern occultism took place through public lectures, lay experimentation and popular periodicals, mimicking in many ways the popularisation of the sciences that took place during the second half of the nineteenth century. Indeed, leading figures within the occult movement in Germany, most prominently du Prel, have been seen as prototypes of the scientific populariser.[53] Such figures existed on the fringes of, and in tension with, the academic world, publishing prolifically not only as a means of scientifically educating a middle-class public but as a way of supporting themselves outside of the universities and the professions.[54]

Modern occultism was 'open' in another way also. As Corinna Treitel has shown in the German context, modern occultism was a very public and frequently commoditised enterprise, which offered exhibitions, periodicals and epistemological debate to a mass audience. The attraction of the occult for this audience, however, lay not in its ubiquity, but in its practicality and its versatility.[55] Occult practices could be used to determine an appropriate career path, to find lost items, to catch criminals, to provide a scientific foundation for religious or political belief, and to make contact with the dead. Indeed, because it was capable of catering to such a wide range of interests and needs, modern occultism found a home in the living quarters of factory workers with socialist sympathies, as well as in the parlours of Germany's social and intellectual élite who debated the ontological implications of spirit materialisation.

The lure of modern occultism for Germans from across the social and political spectrum and the key to its versatility were, above all, located in a phenomenon known as mediumship; this was the generative core not only of a range of occult practices, including psychical research, but also of certain areas of dynamic psychiatry where it provided fodder for theories about multiple personalities and the subconscious.[56] Mediums, individuals who, dependent on one's point of view, either possessed the ability to communicate with the spirits or to access unconscious and unexplored mental states, provided the raw material from which much of the modern occult movement was constructed. In a state of either self-induced or hypnotic somnambulism, mediums produced a number of strange phenomena, including putative clairvoyance, telepathy, spirit communication and materialisation. Studied and manipulated to form the basis of a wide range of occult sciences, including spiritualism, theosophy, and ariosophy, these phenomena helped bolster religious belief, liberated marginalised individuals from social constraints, and revealed an immense reservoir of untapped creative energies. The phenomena produced by Lina Matzinger – actually referred to using the older mesmeric appellation of 'somnambulist' in the writings of the Psychologische Gesellschaft – was used, for example, by some members of the Munich society to support a monistic or spiritist worldview, by others to explore the mysteries surrounding consciousness, and by the artists, who featured so prominently on the society's membership list, to aid in the composition and execution of a more spiritual form of art. As the Munich society's use of the term somnambulist suggested, however, mediumship was not a new phenomenon.

Mesmeric antecedents

While histories of modern occultism and mediumship commonly locate their emergence in the second half of the nineteenth century, linking them closely with spiritualism, these phenomena had their antecedents in the mesmeric experiments of the German Romantics. Many of the strange mental abilities, including the transference of the senses and thought-transference, demonstrated in the experiments of the Munich and Berlin societies, as well as in contemporary spiritualist séances, had been features of animal magnetism. In testing Lina's ability to read a book balanced on her head or on her stomach, for example, the Psychologische Gesellschaft attempted to reconstruct the experiments conducted by magnetists such as Justinus Kerner (1786–1862) who had placed folded messages on the stomach of his famous somnambulist Friederike Hauffe (1801–29), the so-called seeress from Prevorst.[57] Similarly, those experiments in which Schrenck-Notzing and his associates sought to transmit the bitter taste of coffee or the pungent aroma of a cigar to the somnolent Lina were attempts to provide experimental proof of the strong rapport that many mesmerists had noted between their somnambulistic subjects and themselves.[58] The research agenda proposed by the Berliner Gesellschaft für Experimental-Psychologie, while focused primarily on hypnosis and suggestion, also made the reality of bio-magnetism an object of inquiry.[59] Mesmerism, importantly, provided not only many of the phenomena, methodologies and terms utilised by the occultists and psychical researchers of the second half of the nineteenth century, but also the paradigms – natural, spiritual and demonic – through which occult manifestations and practices were interpreted.

Mesmerism, also known as 'animal magnetism', was a form of physical therapy proposed by the German physician Franz Anton Mesmer (1734–1815). During 1774, Mesmer conducted a series of experiments in which he placed magnets on the body of a female patient experiencing hysterical symptoms, including cramps and convulsions.[60] While the application of magnets seemed to provoke a painful crisis in the patient, her condition appeared markedly improved on the cessation of treatment. For Mesmer, the success of these experiments provided tangible evidence of the magnetic fluid he had long speculated existed not only within the universe, but also within the human body, leading him to abandon the therapeutic application of magnets in favour of using the magnetic power of his own person.[61] Within a few years, Mesmer's controversial new therapy – now applied through magnetic strokes above the body or through proximity to

46

magnetised water or objects, but still accompanied by a cathartic crisis – had travelled to France where it became popular despite the extreme hostility of the Parisian medical community.[62] While a series of Royal Commissions into mesmerism in 1784 concluded that there was no evidence for the existence of an animal-magnetic fluid and that any cures were a result of imagination, the same year saw the discovery of a significant corollary of mesmerism, which the French magnetiser Armand Marie Jacques de Chastenet, the Marquis de Puységur (1751–1825), named 'magnetic somnambulism'.

'Magnetic somnambulism' or 'magnetic sleep' was a state in which the magnetised person manifested a sleep-waking consciousness, a rapport with the magnetiser, suggestibility, amnesia upon waking, and a marked alteration of character.[63] These were all hallmarks of the magnetic sleep into which Puységur accidently placed the peasant Victor Race as he tried to cure his fever. While magnetic somnambulism helped alleviate Race's physical discomfort, its true significance appeared to be the alternate consciousness it revealed below the threshold of his waking state. This second consciousness seemed to possess a discrete memory, separate from that of the waking personality, and a very different character from that normally exhibited by Race.[64] The other significant feature of this somnambulistic personality was its heightened mental abilities, which included apparent thought-transference and clairvoyance. Through further experimentation, Puységur and other mesmerists discovered that magnetic somnambulism could be induced in other subjects, many of whom exhibited the same strange mental phenomena as Victor Race. These magnetisers were also quick to realise that magnetic sleep offered not just an efficacious form of treatment, but one that did not require the violent crises central to Mesmer's understanding of animal magnetism. For these reasons, magnetic somnambulism quickly became an integral part of magnetic treatment and theory spreading throughout France and into Germany.[65]

The reception of mesmerism in Germany during the first half of the nineteenth century was distinguished by a fixation on the heightened mental abilities, such as clairvoyance, exhibited in magnetic sleep; a fixation that can be explained by looking at the proponents of mesmerism in the German context, the majority of whom were adherents of *Naturphilosophie*.[66] For these men, who sought to develop an holistic worldview in which the differences between mind and matter, religion and science, and mystical experience and historical knowledge could be reconciled, mesmerism and its strange somnambulistic phenomena offered a means of bridging the gap between these poles, that is, between the 'day-side' and 'night-side' of nature.[67] This melding of mesmerism and *Naturphilosophie* in the German context saw it become not only a form of physical therapy, but, depending on the predisposition of the magnetiser, either a means of psychological introspection or a path to metaphysical and sacred knowledge.[68] The physiologist and painter Carl Gustav Carus (1789–1869) and the theologian David Friederich Strauss (1808–74), for example, regarded the clairvoyant visions of somnambulists as the result of unconscious processes, while the psychiatrist Dietrich Georg Kieser (1779–1862) saw the mental journeys of somnambulists to heaven or other planets as a species of dream fantasy.[69] In contrast, the poet and physician Justinus Kerner believed that the clairvoyance he witnessed among his somnambulistic patients could be explained as a form of spirit communication or possession.[70]

While the spirit hypothesis by no means enjoyed a monopoly among the German Romantics as an explanation for somnambulistic phenomena, Kerner's writings about clairvoyant somnambules, in particular, the seeress of Prevorst, proved extremely influential. Through his treatment of, and experiments with, the seeress Friederike Hauffe, as well as the somnambulists Christina Kapplinger and Caroline S., Kerner developed a theory of magnetic spiritism in which the illnesses these women suffered and the extraordinary abilities they exhibited were attributed to spirits.[71] Although all of these cases contributed to the development of magnetic spiritism it was Hauffe's that became best known through both Kerner's 1829 book *Die Seherin von Prevorst* [*The Seeress from Prevorst*] and the writings of the other Romantics who visited her in Kerner's home.[72] Hauffe who had undergone a profound spiritual experience while attending the funeral of a local dignitary, on the same day she was married, and who suffered from both depression and muscular spasms, existed in an almost perpetual state of somnambulism when Kerner was asked to treat her in 1826. While he began her treatment by abstaining from magnetic therapy, Kerner found that Hauffe's condition worsened until she was once again mesmerised. In the magnetic state, Kerner not only saw a marked improvement in his patient's physical and mental wellbeing, but also discovered her remarkable clairvoyant and prophetic powers. Like other somnambulists, Hauffe displayed a range of clairvoyant abilities, including the power to diagnose disease, to read without the use of her eyes, and foretell the future, but somnambulism also appeared to provide her with access to the spirit realm where she gained knowledge of a complex metaphysical system consisting of seven sun circles and one life circle.[73] For Kerner, his patient's experiences proved that there existed an unseen world in which both evil and good spirits did battle, causing illness or offering healing and knowledge. The magnetic state provided access to this realm, where the somnambulist and the physician might combine physical therapy and exorcism to become protagonists in the spiritual mêlée.

If Puységur's treatment of Victor Race had suggested the existence of an alternate consciousness, Kerner's treatment of Friederike Hauffe helped sustain the old idea that strange or aberrant mental phenomena were a result of supernatural agency.[74] The promotion of this theory through the story of the seeress of Prevorst had lasting repercussions. Hauffe's revelations, for example, provided a model for other somnambulists who produced similar cosmologies. Indeed, the seeress' system of magnetic sun and life circles helped shape the metaphysical discourse not only of her near contemporaries but also of late nineteenth- and early twentieth-century spiritualists, including the medium upon whom C.G. Jung based his doctoral dissertation.[75] Spiritualists and psychical researchers in the latter part of the century also maintained a fascination with the seeress, whose history continued to provide material for those with an interest in both psychological and metaphysical analyses of somnambulists. German occult journals often featured articles about Hauffe, an example of which was du Prel's contribution to *Sphinx*, accompanied by illustrations by the artist Gabriel von Max, a member of the Psychologische Gesellschaft, who also painted the somnolent Lina Matzinger.[76] While magnetic somnabulism did not dominate early nineteenth-century analyses of mesmerism it did provide a tradition within the German context through which modern spiritualism and other forms of occultism could be understood and developed during the second half of the century.

Mesmerism did, of course, provide other traditions and paradigms for understanding spiritualism and modern occultism upon their arrival in the German-speaking states. Table-turning, for example, which enjoyed a brief craze amongst Germans during 1853, was interpreted not only, and not even primarily, as the work of ill-disciplined spirits, but as a result of the magnetic fluid that coursed through and out of participants' bodies or unconscious muscular movements.[77] Spiritualism, similarly, was initially understood in terms that could have been used to describe the manifestations of somnambulists, like the seeress of Prevorst. Adherents linked mediums' phenomena to good spirits, often deceased relatives, while churchmen warned that such phenomena were demonic in origin and those who preferred a naturalistic explanation claimed that spiritualist mediums simply channelled their unconscious selves.[78] It is also clear that mesmerism as practiced and understood by the Romantics helped shape the research agendas and explanatory paradigms of German psychical researchers. Both the Psychologische Gesellschaft and the Berliner Gesellschaft für Experimental-Psychologie began by examining phenomena that had featured among magnetic somnambulists. Two of the leading figures of the Berlin society, Max Dessoir and Albert Moll (1862–1939), for example, tested the existence of a magnetic rapport between magnetiser and somnambulist in some of their early experimental work.[79] Similarly, the range of explanations that had existed among German mesmerists for the strange phenomena of somnambulistic sleep was apparent in these societies. In the Psychologische Gesellschaft, for instance, there were those who attributed all such phenomena to unconscious processes, while others believed they might offer access to a metaphysical realm.

Clearly, the occult sciences that developed in the second half of the nineteenth century, including spiritualism, theosophy and psychical research, shared a common heritage. The magnetic traditions that provided research agendas and explanatory paradigms for these practices, however, linked them not only to mesmerism, but also to each other. Thus, the sections that follow explore the attraction of spiritualism, theosophy and psychical research for the Germans who practised them, the dissemination of their ideas through occult organisations and publications, and the relationship between modern occultism and the contemporary reform milieu. They also highlight the epistemological and sociological links between these nascent occult sciences, making clear the difficulty for psychical researchers who wished to distance their discipline from occultism.

Spiritualism

One of the earliest and most enduring manifestations of the modern occult revival was spiritualism, a movement that revolved around the use of mediums in their capacity as conduits to the other world. With a large following in both America and Europe, estimated at several million worldwide by 1880 and at more than ten thousand in Germany alone between 1895 and 1914, spiritualism not only helped liberate religious subjectivity from dogma, privileging personal experience over blind faith, but provided experimental evidence of a realm beyond the material.[80] The main cultural venue for this movement, which inhabited the domestic sphere rather than the church, was the spiritualist 'circle', composed chiefly of family members and close friends who joined hands around a table in order to contact their loved ones in the beyond ['Jenseits'].[81] In this context, a dead child might assure its mother that it was happy and well cared for, while a departed husband might offer his widow emotional support and financial advice, both remaining active members of the family. Spiritualism's ability to sustain the strong emotional ties between family and friends after death thus played a large part in its appeal. The attraction of spiritualism, however, went beyond its capacity to assuage grief. Many people, for example, were converted by its use of science as a support for religious belief. The spiritualist séance helped fulfil a need no longer satisfied by theology's command simply to 'Believe!' offering the individual tangible evidence of life after death in the form of spirit materialisation or direct voice communication; a prime example of the kind of 'rational enchantment' of which the historian Alex Owen has spoken.[82] Spiritualism also proved attractive to those normally prevented from taking an active role in religious and cultural life. While mediumistic talent was by no means exclusive to women, female mediumship was significant for its elevation of women to positions of spiritual power and cultural authority. As mediums, middle-class women as well as domestic servants could pronounce on matters of ontological and political importance in a manner quite impossible outside of this role.[83] Spiritualist mediums also proved interesting to those unconcerned with religion by revealing the existence of a creative unconscious. Artists and writers, for example, made use of the highly expressive bodies of mediums, as well as phenomena such as somnambulism and automatic writing as sources of inspiration.[84]

The birth of modern spiritualism occurred in Hydesville, New York, in 1848 in the home of John Fox, a blacksmith and Methodist, whose daughters Margaret and Kate found they could communicate with the spirit of a murdered pedlar via a series of knocks and raps.[85] Given the extraordinary nature of this discourse, news of the girls' discovery spread quickly throughout the community, neighbours and friends suggesting more efficient means of communication, including a system, which became known as spirit telegraphy.[86] This involved the recitation of the alphabet during which the spirit would rap on the wall or table to indicate a letter and spell out a word.[87] Interest in this dialogue with the other world multiplied swiftly, aided in part by the Fox sisters who moved to Rochester and began to publicly exhibit their spirit conversations. Within a few years similar communications were occurring all over the United States and spiritualist mediums, who both mimicked and expanded upon the Fox sisters' repertoire, had begun to offer their services to an eager public.[88] Taking on ever more complex forms, including automatic writing, slate writing and direct voice communication, spiritualism was transported during the early 1850s, first to England and then to continental Europe where it was practised both on the stage and in domestic circles.[89]

Although, the reverberations of the spirit raps were felt in Germany in the early 1850s, as evidenced by a short-lived table-turning craze, spiritualism failed to inspire an enduring interest among Germans until the 1870s.[90] In part, this was due to a lack of novelty. For a German audience there was nothing particularly new about the phenomena associated with nascent spiritualism, most of which had been associated with the magnetic somnambulists of the early nineteenth century, and which could be understood using the mesmerists' explanatory paradigms. This disinterest may also have been a result of spiritualism's failure to meet Germans' discursive needs. Those opposed to materialism during the 1850s and 1860s tended to be concerned not with its metaphysical implications, but with its anticlerical and democratic consequences, issues that spiritualism in its earliest German incarnations did not directly address.[91] It was not until the last quarter of the nineteenth century, as the consequences of both a materialist worldview and industrial modernism became more apparent, that spiritualism began to take hold in Germany, providing support for flagging religious beliefs and a vehicle for social, political and philosophical reform.

In the 1870s and 1880s, spiritualism was largely restricted to Saxony and German-speaking areas of northern Bohemia, where the membership of this movement was derived chiefly from the petite bourgeoisie and proletariat.[92] Historians have contended that Saxony became a centre for spiritualism at this time because of the combination in this region of religious dissent, strong Protestantism, and rapid industrialisation and urbanisation.[93] The dissenting and Protestant traditions, for example, provided the context for the emergence of a form of revelatory spiritualism in which baptism played a role and a prayer-based spiritualism practised by dedicated Protestants, both of which helped revitalise and authenticate religion for their adherents.[94] In contrast, the social and political dislocation caused by industrialisation and urbanisation in Saxony fostered a politically minded variety of spiritualism, including a species of club spiritualism that was influenced by anti-clerical and reformist ideas.[95] With the help of the medium and editor Bernhard Cyriax and the publisher Oswald Mutze, who proved to be some of the most prolific propagandists of spiritualism in Germany during the 1880s, the ideas and practices generated in Saxony's spiritualist organisations spread throughout the country and across the social spectrum.[96]

By the early 1890s, new spiritualist clubs had formed in Berlin, Leipzig, Hamburg and Breslau, the social composition and purpose of which differed from those that had developed in Saxony. These groups, whose membership was mainly middle class, attempted to differentiate themselves from spiritualist groups with dissenting or socialist pretensions, rejecting overt political and reformist agendas, to concentrate on scientific materialism, the off-spring of which they believed were metaphysical despair and social disintegration.[97] For these middle-class adherents, spiritualism provided a means of critiquing the materialist worldview and proving empirically the existence of a spiritual realm. This form of spiritualism found its propagandists in men such as Aksakov, whose journal *Psychische Studien* became an organ for the ideas and debates of both educated spiritualists and psychical researchers, and du Prel, whose many publications in both the occult and mainstream press promoted spiritualism as an epistemological and social antidote to the excesses of materialism and industrial modernism.[98]

Theosophy

Theosophy, as it emerged in Germany during the late nineteenth century, shared many of the same preoccupations and some of the same personnel as spiritualism.[99] Like the spiritualist movement, for example, theosophy provided the spiritual solace that for many Germans was increasingly difficult to find in the nation's churches. Theosophy replaced organised religion for some, offering in its stead an eclectic mix of mystical traditions free of rigid dogma, while for others it supplemented their Christianity, opening their eyes to other religious traditions.[100] Just as spiritualism was politicised and reformist in some of its incarnations, so too was theosophy. It was not unusual, for instance, to find theosophists who were also committed feminists or vegetarians. Theosophists also shared the spiritualists' concerns about materialism, locating Germany's social ills in the materialists' stubborn refusal to acknowledge the transcendental in human beings.[101] Du Prel, for example, whose attraction to spiritualism derived from his deep concern with a materialist *Weltanschauung*, was interested in theosophy for the same reason, briefly acting as the vice president of the Theosophische Societät Germania [German Theosophical Society].[102] Where theosophy differed from spiritualism, however, was in ascribing its insights to occult rather than spiritual sources. While the mediumship of theosophy's co-founder Helena Petrovna Blavatsky (1831–91), had much in common with that of magnetic somnambulists and spiritualist mediums, it did not provide her with access to the spirit world, allowing her instead to receive messages from a group of mysterious Tibetan Mahatmas or Masters known as the Great White Brotherhood.[103]

With the lawyer Henry Steel Olcott (1832–1907), Blavatsky, a Russian émigré, founded the theosophical movement in New York in 1875. Based on the teachings of the Mahatmas, whose messages provided insight into a comprehensive system of occult knowledge, theosophy's central tenet was a commitment to the construction of a universal brotherhood of humanity without distinction of race, creed, sex, caste or colour.[104] Its other major objects were to encourage the study of comparative religion, philosophy and science, and to investigate the unexplained laws of nature and the mental powers latent in human beings.[105] While theosophy purported to be a form of universal wisdom, the knowledge of which had supposedly been scattered among the religions of the world, it contained an undeniable emphasis on eastern mystical traditions, primarily Buddhism. It was for this reason perhaps that the movements' leaders relocated to Adyar in southern India in 1879. Theosophy's appropriation of eastern religion has also been the reason that historians have linked the movement not only to the histories of reformist politics and alternate religion – a connection apparent in the

Theosophische Societät's three main tenets and in the activities of its members – but also to the history of imperialism.[106]

Theosophy's links to imperialism as well as reformist politics and alternate religion were particularly apparent in the German context, where one of the movement's leading figures, Wilhelm Hübbe-Schleiden, a former colonial propagandist, pursued a liberal agenda through his occult writings and an alternate religion through his promotion of theosophy and a transcendental worldview.[107] Hübbe-Schleiden joined the international Theosophical Society in 1884, at the same time assuming the presidency of the newly founded Theosophische Societät Germania, whose members aimed at the reform of German culture via occult means.[108] For Hübbe-Schleiden and his colleagues, who included Carl du Prel, Gustav Meyrink (1868–1932), Carl Kiesewetter (1854–95), Ernst Häckel and Gabriel von Max, such reform entailed a critique of scientific materialism and the construction of a 'vollständige Weltanschauung' [complete worldview] through the study of the latent powers of the human mind.[109] While this society was dissolved, following the discovery in December 1885 that Blavatsky had committed fraud, its aims continued to be pursued through Hübbe-Schleiden's occult journal *Sphinx*. This periodical, which first appeared in 1886, published not only theosophical material, such as comparative and historical studies of world religions and mysticism, but occult writings more broadly, including the experimental reports and proceedings of the newly formed Psychologische Gesellschaft.[110]

Psychical research

The circle of scholars, artists and intellectuals who gathered around the *Sphinx* in 1886, many of whom were refugees from the failed Theosophische Societät Germania, sought a means of pursuing an experimental study of somnambulism, telepathy and clairvoyance – those latent powers studied by theosophists and apparent in the hypnotic experiments conducted in the medical schools of Paris and Nancy.[111] A society that would provide the space for, and defray the expense of, such experiments seemed the logical solution, but there was debate about what form such a society should take. Central to these discussions was du Prel, whose 1885 book *Philosophie der Mystik* [*Philosophy of Mysticism*] had made him one of Germany's leading writers on both spiritualism and occultism. Du Prel's correspondence with Hübbe-Schleiden made it clear that his involvement was contingent upon the society's divorce from any theosophical taint and its adoption of a programme that mimicked that of the Society for Psychical Research, based in London.[112] The decision to found this new society, the Psychologische Gesellschaft, along the lines insisted upon by du Prel ensured that in its earliest years it acted as a platform for his research agenda and philosophical interests. In practice, this meant that the new society concentrated on hypnotic experiments, which du Prel used to develop his transcendental psychology; a discipline intended to prove the existence of latent mental phenomena such as thought-transference and the reality of a 'transcendental subject'.[113] Over time, however, as the physician Schrenck-Notzing took a leading role in such experiments, it became clear that there were competing agendas within this society. Nonetheless, the Psychologische Gesellschaft represented one of the first venues for psychical research in Germany.

Two years after the foundation of this society in Munich a similar group was formed in Berlin; the so-called Berliner Gesellschaft für Experimental-Psychologie. Like its predecessor, this society also had links with the circle around the periodical *Sphinx*. Max Dessoir, a student of both medicine and philosophy, had become part of this circle through his publications and correspondence and had been involved with the Psychologische Gesellschaft at its inception, presenting papers, attending meetings and conducting experiments whenever he visited Munich. In Berlin, Dessoir's desire to continue his research in 'experimental psychology' saw him help establish the Berliner Gesellschaft für Experimental-Psychologie. In this manner, Dessoir, along with the physician Albert Moll, became one of this new society's central figures. In part this centrality was the result of the dedicated experimentalism of both men. In 1886, for example, Dessoir participated in a series of sittings with the medium Henry Slade – of Zöllner debate fame – which familiarised him with the difficulties of examining mediumistic phenomena, and carried out a series of experiments on thought-transference following the appearance of Preyer's book on muscle-reading, where he concluded that Preyer's theory did not adequately explain all cases.[114] Similarly, Moll began by attending spiritualist séances in Paris and Berlin where he soon became convinced that the phenomena of table-turning and spirit rapping resulted from unconscious muscular pressure on the table, moving on to test the reality of both thought-transference and clairvoyance.[115]

Hoping to add to the research conducted by the Society for Psychical Research in London and the Société de Psychologie Physiologique in Paris, Dessoir, Moll and other members of the Berlin society attempted to explore the latent phenomena of mind through hypnotic and magnetic experimentation and through those spontaneous cases which manifested in spiritualist séances.[116] This willingness to examine the phenomena of spiritualism, however, was quickly diminished when press reports of the society's investigation of a haunting labelled them a spiritualist group.[117] From this point onward, the Berliner Gesellschaft für Experimental-Psychologie narrowed their 'experimental psychology' to concentrate on thought-transference, suggestion and rapport, all of which were analysed within a natural or animist paradigm in terms of fraud, delusion, hallucination, illusion or unconscious mental powers.

Clearly, with its insistence on experiment, its interest in somnambulism, telepathy and clairvoyance, its overlapping personnel, and its use of the periodicals *Psychische Studien* and *Sphinx* as platforms, German psychical research had strong ties to both spiritualism and theosophy. Where it tended to differ from these occult sciences, however, was in its aims, explanatory paradigms and social composition. While the influence of du Prel within the Psychologische Gesellschaft saw at least part of that group pursue a spiritist agenda, the stated aim of both the Munich and Berlin societies was to promote a form of experimental psychology, which would recognise the role of the unconscious. The first statute of the Psychologische Gesellschaft stated in this regard:

> The society intends to facilitate among its members the study of psychology through scientific reports, discussion evenings, experiments and social get-togethers and in particular to foster to the best of its ability the scientific recognition of facts from the transcendental realm.[118]

This new discipline was intended, as Dessoir's neologisms 'parapsychic' and 'parapsychology' suggested, to be an extension of, and complement to, physiological psychology. In keeping with this aim, the explanatory paradigms adopted by those who pursued psychical research tended to be animist. Schrenck-Notzing, for example, who published the findings of his experiments in thought-transference in the *Proceedings of the Society for Psychical Research* in 1891–2, rested his analysis on unknown functions of the brain.

> If it be true that one brain can impress another without the intervention of the known organs of sense, there is no doubt that a discovery of great and far-reaching importance has been made. And if, after the discovery of the chain of physical causation, at present unknown to us, but certainly existing, the centrifugal effects of vivid perceptions extending beyond the limits of our ordinary experience, our knowledge of the functions of the brain would thereby be much enlarged.[119]

While these aims and explanatory paradigms certainly helped distinguish psychical research from spiritualism and theosophy, there were social and economic factors that also differentiated this discipline from its occult peers.

Unlike more egalitarian forms of occultism, such as spiritualism and theosophy, psychical research was a cultural and scientific critique almost exclusive to *bürgerliche* culture. The vast majority of those that engaged in experimentation with mediums were members of the *Bildungsbürgertum,* as evidenced by the large number of artists, philosophers, physicians and psychologists that formed the membership of the psychological societies in Munich and Berlin. Those with aristocratic titles were also a noticeable presence. The 1887 membership list of the Psychologische Gesellschaft, for example, boasted five such honorifics among its ordinary members and two among its associate members.[120] Such lists also reveal the marginal role played by women in such societies. Unlike the spiritualist or theosophical milieu in which women could take a leading role, apart from that of medium, the world of psychical research did not include many women. In both the Munich and Berlin societies, the wives of members could attend or participate in experiments but they never led them.[121] Indeed, it is clear from the statutes of the Psychologische Gesellschaft that women were only eligible to become associate members.[122]

There were two reasons why scientific experimentation in this area was largely restricted to middle- and upper-class men. The first was the level of education required to undertake experimental work and to engage in debate with the representatives of those disciplines, most notably psychology, on which psychical research encroached. An understanding of experimental design, conduct and precautions as well as a familiarity with the literature of psychical research and hypnotic experimentation, much of which was in English and French, was a necessity, and in most cases this meant that psychical researchers were university educated. The second reason that psychical research was restricted to *bürgerliche* culture was the considerable investment of time and money it required.[123] Experimentation of a rigorous kind was expensive because of the equipment required, as was the publication of specialist journals and books. Even for psychical researchers who were employed in the professions such an undertaking was too expensive for any one individual, hence the foundation of societies. Some representatives of this nascent science, however, like the Munich-based Schrenck-Notzing, had aristocratic ties or family money with which they could indulge their passion for psychical research and fund periodicals – a not inconsiderable factor in Schrenck-Notzing's leading role in parapsychological research in Germany from the early twentieth century.[124]

Socio-economic factors were also crucial in deciding the shape and constitution of psychical research in another way. While German psychical researchers were by and large university educated, they did not tend to be academics, existing only on the fringes of the academic world. In the case of du Prel, for instance, his failure to secure a university post saw him take up a form of journalistic activity through which he sought to popularise his scientific and philosophical ideas, and to support himself financially.[125] In so doing, du Prel's work as a scientific populariser and occultist coincided to doubly marginalise him from the academy. In stark contrast to England, where a number of important scientists were financially independent and not reliant on an academic career, scientific research in the German context was carried out almost exclusively in the universities.[126] For German psychical research this signalled the absence of well-known scientists and intellectuals from its clubs and societies, the presence of which had been a significant factor in the success of the Society for Psychical Research, which had been founded in 1882 by the physicist William Fletcher Barrett, the psychologist Edmund Gurney (1847–88), the writer Frederic Myers (1843–1901) and the moral philosopher Henry Sidgwick (1838–1900).[127]

Institutions and publications

Having now described the emergence of psychical research in Germany during the late nineteenth century and its relationship not only to psychology, but also to occult sciences such as spiritualism and theosophy, the following section will examine the material conditions of this nascent discipline, that is, its institutionalisation in societies and its dissemination in journals and books. In so doing, this section will once again demonstrate the difficulty of making absolute distinctions between spiritualism, theosophy and psychical research in the Imperial period. Not only did the psychological societies in Munich and Berlin find it difficult to completely exclude a spiritualist or theosophical element from their membership and their research, but their association with occult journals and publishers also tended to blur the boundaries between their ostensibly scientific approach to the phenomena of somnambulism and mediumship, and that of spiritualism and theosophy. In highlighting this epistemological and disciplinary confusion, which became increasingly frustrating for psychical researchers during the late nineteenth century, this discussion will go some way towards explaining the split of the Psychologische Gesellschaft, which occurred in 1889, and the emergence of 'critical occultism', both of which can be seen as examples of boundary work where the aim was to 'sanitise' psychical research by distancing it from the taint of occultism.

The Psychologische Gesellschaft in Munich and the Berliner Gesellschaft für Experimental-Psychologie were formed during the second half of the 1880s in order to provide a forum for those who wished to experiment with or discuss the strange phenomena associated with hypnotic somnambulism.[128] The men who became members of these groups saw a number of advantages in pursuing their interest in psychical research within the confines of a society. For those who wished to conduct experiments with somnambulists like Lina, a society not only afforded a means of sharing the associated costs, but of lending such experiments the prestige they would lack if conducted by isolated individual researchers.[129] The Psychologische Gesellschaft, for example, asked its members to pay two Marks upon joining and one Mark every month towards costs.[130] It also insisted that its members be educated men with spotless reputations to ensure the society's prestige. In certain circumstances, such psychological societies also provided legal protection for their members. In a context in which German doctors, including a number of psychical researchers, campaigned against the lay use of hypnosis, and in which several states, including Bavaria, retained laws against 'Gaukelei' [charlatanry], these societies avoided legal censure by using their physician-members to conduct their hypnotic experiments. After the dissolution of the Psychologische Gesellschaft in Munich, for example, du Prel's new society found that its lay experimentation with hypnosis and its spiritualism attracted the attention of the authorities.[131] The psychological societies in Munich and Berlin naturally created a forum in which their members could present and discuss their research, but also provided the opportunity for social interaction. In the year 1888–9, for instance, the Psychologische Gesellschaft hosted twenty papers on themes, including mesmerism and hypnotism, occultism and art, somnambulism and the law, poltergeists, and prophetic dreams, as well as seven discussions and eight social gatherings.[132]

In their social composition, regulating statutes, and emphasis on discussion, neither society differed substantially from other contemporary bourgeois clubs and societies, which helped forge bonds of sociability within the middle classes. In their interest in and experiments with somnambulists and mediums, however, these societies had more in common with the spiritualist and theosophical groups, both bourgeois and working class, which populated their cities; numbering in their hundreds by the late nineteenth century. These occult groups offered their members lectures on topical issues and access to lending libraries, as well as the opportunity to attend sittings with famous mediums or somnambulists. Given the scarcity of talented mediums and somnambulists, it was not uncommon for such figures to perform in both spiritualist clubs and psychical research societies. Spiritualist, theosophical and psychical research groups also tended to serve an educative function. In some cases, where adherents sought esoteric knowledge, the club or lodge might offer a finely gradated system of initiation, where senior members or masters were charged with guiding their initiates to enlightenment. In other cases, where experimentation was involved, these groups might need to teach their members the appropriate experimental method and precautionary measures. Individual clubs and societies, however, were not the only means of learning about or participating in the occult and psychical research communities; specialist newspapers, journals and pamphlets also played a significant role.[133]

These publications, some of which were associated with a specific club or society, contained a wide range of material, including editorial comment on current debates and problems, reports on the visits of foreign mediums and experimental findings. Such publications served a proselytising function, but also helped foster ties beyond the local spiritualist club or theosophical lodge, creating an occult community that was national and, in some cases, international. While many of these newspapers and journals were straightforwardly spiritualist or theosophical, there were a number of prominent periodicals where writings on spiritualism, theosophy or occultism sat side by side with those on psychical research. In the *Psychische Studien*, for instance, positive reports of a visiting medium's phenomena might appear in the same issue as a critical article on mediumistic fraud written by a member of one of the psychological societies. Similarly, the theosophical and occult periodical *Sphinx* often contained accounts of Rosicrucianism, spirit photography, and Indian fakirs, alongside the proceedings of the Psychologische Gesellschaft. This lack of distinction between psychical research and other forms of occult practice may have reflected the wide ranging and eclectic interests of both contributors and readers, but may also have resulted from a publishing imperative – a journal dedicated solely to psychical research in Germany was unlikely to have been profitable for its publisher.

The publishing firms which produced such periodicals were a vital part of occult culture.[134] The Leipzig-based firms of Wilhelm Friedrich, Ostwald Mutze and Max Spohr all made something of a speciality of occult works, publishing such periodicals as *Psychische Studien, Zeitschrift für Spiritismus* [*Journal for Spiritualism*] and *Wahre Leben* [*True Life*].[135] Founded in 1878, Wilhelm Friedrich published books and periodicals on theosophy and occultism, while Ostwald Mutze and Max Spohr specialised in the production of spiritualist works. These publishers were attracted to occult themes, not only because of the commercial possibilities presented by the growing audience for such material but also because of their own beliefs. Hermann Ostwald Mutze (b.1841), for example, who founded the family firm in 1865, was quite openly a spiritualist, although he did not frequently attend spiritualist clubs or gatherings.[136] Despite Mutze's absence from such forums his company's publications, like those of Wilhelm Friedrich and Max Spohr, were instrumental in disseminating occultism, at first in Saxony and then throughout Germany. Indeed, these companies formed the basis of what became a vibrant occult press in Germany during the late nineteenth and early twentieth centuries.[137]

The occult press mimicked its mainstream counterpart, catering for every budget and taste. There were, for example, 'Strassenblätter' [boulevard newspapers] that appeared for one or two issues only and depended on rivalry and competition between street vendors for their success, while other periodicals appeared for several decades, their longevity a result of subscriptions.[138] These publications varied greatly in subject matter, presentation and complexity, reflecting the diversity of the occult movement, its membership and their needs. There were, for example, journals such as the *Psychische Studien* that represented the interests of scientific and practical occultists and did not tend to be associated with particular societies or lodges in the way that theosophical and spiritualist journals did.[139] Despite this lack of affiliation many of these publications enjoyed longevity. For example, the *Psychische Studien* began publication in 1874 and ceased only in 1934 under the name *Zeitschrift für Parapsychologie* [*Journal for Parapsychology*]. The *Uebersinnliche Welt* [*Transcendental World*] appeared between 1891 and 1922, the *Zentralblatt für Okkultismus* [*Journal for Occultism*] from 1906 to 1932 and seven other periodicals which began publication between 1909 and 1920 had a life span of five to ten years.[140] The scope of these periodicals was often extremely broad. The *Zentralblatt für Okkultismus,* for example, announced that it was a journal not only for theosophists and spiritualists, but also for occultists of all inclinations, combining Indian mysticism and Buddhism with hypnosis and magnetism.[141] For those whose interest coincided more with the spiritualist movement and whose socio-economic and educational level tended to be lower, there were journals such as the *Neue Spiritualistische Blätter* [*New Spiritualist Papers*]. These journals, which had much in common with theosophical publications, multiplied between 1896 and 1923, in most cases acting as the organ of a spiritualist society.[142] The longest lived of these publications were *Zeitschrift für Spiritismus* and *Wahre Leben,* which appeared between 1896–1931 and 1898–1936 respectively.[143] Despite their success it is difficult to estimate with any precision how many Germans read these publications. While subscription numbers offer some indication members of spiritualist and occult clubs and societies could often access these newspapers and periodicals free of charge.[144] As the historian Sawicki has shown while the estimated readership of the *Neue Spiritualistische Blätter* was around four thousand in 1888 there were only five hundred and twenty subscriptions.[145]

For psychical researchers, as for spiritualists and theosophists, such journals helped foster community. Dessoir, for example, as Adolf Kurzweg has demonstrated, forged strong connections by publishing in both the *Psychische Studien* and *Sphinx*. Through his contributions to *Sphinx,* he became involved in the Munich-based circle that gave rise to the Psychologische Gesellschaft and a group of more empirically minded contributors who resided in Berlin with whom he helped establish the Berliner Gesellschaft für Experimental-Psychologie.[146] Similarly, the publication of the first issue of the *Sphinx* convinced Aksakov to make contact with du Prel. In so doing, he gained an important ally in his campaign to promote spiritualism in Germany. Du Prel, for his part, used the alliance with Aksakov to broaden his connections within the spiritualist community and to finance a series of experiments with mediums.[147] While books did not have the same immediacy as periodicals, which often became forums for on-going debates, they too played an important role in fostering a community of psychical researchers in Germany.

The publishing companies that produced occult periodicals also published books on occult topics. The press of Ostwald Mutze, for example, published works on both spiritualism and psychical research. Wilhelm Friedrich's press, which specialised in theosophical works, was responsible for du Prel's two-part *Studien auf dem Gebiete der Geheimwissenschaften* [*Studies in the Field of the Secret Sciences*] (1890/91) and Karl Kiesewetter's *Geschichte des neueren Occultismus* [*History of Modern Occultism*] (1891).[148] Outside Leipzig there was the Munich-based firm Ernst Reinhardt, which published Albert von Schrenck-Notzing's *Materialisations-Phaenomene* [*Phenomena of Materialisation*] (1914) and in Stuttgart, there was Ferdinand Enke, with whom critical occultists such as Albert Moll, Max Dessoir and Albert Hellwig published.[149] Although the years 1880 to 1900 were marked by a growing audience for occult literature, the financial success of these books and the firms that published them were by no means guaranteed. It is clear, for example, that Ostwald Mutze struggled financially during this period, necessitating a strategic approach to publishing, which assessed the potential of a book based on its relationship to contemporary scandals and debates.[150] Occult publishing became somewhat more successful during the second decade of the twentieth century as a result of a growing audience for such material. While the production of occult literature was by no means small before 1914, the war and immediate post-war period saw an enormous increase in such material. Indeed, the years 1918 to 1935 saw occult publication in Germany reach its peak. According to one Dr Oldenbourg, who published a book on the prestige of German scientific writing, new occult titles numbered around six hundred a year, demonstrating the enormous marketability of such literature and the public's growing enthusiasm for it.[151] The lure of these occult titles was made all the more attractive by their low cost. During the late 1920s and early 1930s, the average price of a book on the topic of occultism remained low despite the economic crisis. In 1929, for example, such a publication cost, on average, 1.59 Reichsmarks and in 1930 only 1.29 Reichsmarks.[152] While the affordability of these texts was a factor, the primary reason for their popularity must be located in the promise of occultism to improve Germans' lives. Indeed, significant numbers of those Germans who became spiritualists or theosophists wedded their interest in occultism to some form of reformist agenda, whether this was the reform of society or the reform of the self.

Modern occultism and reform

Many of those Germans who turned to occultism during the late nineteenth century did so in order to pursue social and political aspirations, that had remained stifled or unfulfilled in other cultural venues. Occultism, sometimes combined with other types of reform, provided a forum in which Germans could experiment with different gender roles, organisational structures, religious beliefs and ways of living, either as individuals or as groups. These experiments were not exclusive to one class or political persuasion, but took place at all levels of society and across the political spectrum, their form reflecting Germans' changing preoccupations. Occultism, as we have seen in the cases of spiritualism and theosophy, was an extraordinarily flexible set of beliefs that changed its outer forms in order to better suit both individual requirements and socio-political exigencies. It was used during the late nineteenth century, for example, to meet the religious needs of Germans through theosophical teachings, and after the First World War to lessen the grief of mothers who had lost sons in the hostilities, through spiritualism.[153] The political heterogeneity that also marked this movement was evident in a number of examples. The small group of nationalist anti-Semitic Germans and Austrians who combined theosophy and race mysticism to become Ariosophists, for example, channelled their disgust with modernity and political liberalism into this occult movement.[154] In contrast, the plebeian spiritualists of Saxony exhibited anti-clerical and socialist tendencies, supported by the discourse of the spirits on themes such as egalitarianism and social reform.[155] Modern occultism enabled Germans to naturalise their worldview and to convey their ideological beliefs in the guise of either scientific laws or religious revelations, in order to convince others of the need for either social and spiritual renewal or political reform.

The practical element of many occult philosophies, which explained how one might contact a dead relative, improve the self through meditation or make investments based on astrological patterns, offered Germans tools with which to deal with modern life, and was undoubtedly a significant factor in their appeal.[156] By setting out guidelines for improving the lives of both individuals and whole communities, occultism also intersected with other contemporary attempts at reform, most notably the 'Lebensreform' [life-reform] movement. This complex of philosophies, which had its roots in early nineteenth-century *Naturheilkunde* – the science of natural health – combined concerns about social justice and reform with a desire to promote temperance, natural health and vegetarianism.[157] Those Germans dedicated to life reform passionately believed that the processes of urbanisation and industrialisation that had accompanied Germany's transformation into a modern nation state were responsible for the degeneration they saw around them. These Germans blamed their illnesses and personal failures on the unnatural manner in which modern people lived. Convinced that a healthy lifestyle could reverse this process of biological and social decline, life reformers recommended exercise, improved diet and natural therapies as a means of reconnecting human beings with nature and creating an ethical and equitable society.[158] Adherents of life reform took up these recommendations to varying degrees, some choosing therapies and health regimes that complemented their otherwise conventional lifestyles, while others adopted a more fundamentalist approach. During the 1880s, for example, a number of German vegetarian groups set about creating communities based on their utopian philosophies, establishing colonies in both North and South America.[159] For these Germans, as well as their less fundamentalist contemporaries, life reform presented a means of reforming modern life and society by reforming the self.

Like clothing reform, vegetarianism and the movement for natural health, modern occultism can be understood as part of the reform impulse that helped characterise both Wilhelmine and Weimar Germany.[160] This was a connection that was acknowledged by contemporaries who understood occultism not just as a substitute for organised religion but as a vehicle for personal growth, health and spiritual fulfilment.[161] It was not uncommon, for instance, for adherents of an occult philosophy such as theosophy or an alternate religious practice like spiritualism to exhibit other types of non-conformist behaviour, including vegetarianism, in this way combining occultism and life reform. The spiritualist club Psyche, for example, whose first members were vegetarians, held their meetings in a vegetarian restaurant in Berlin's Grünstraße.[162] Occult beliefs were also frequently melded with alternative healing practices. Joseph Weißenberg (1855–1941), a Berlin-based healer and prophet, combined prayer healing and magnetism to treat his patients, ascertaining the cause and trajectory of their diseases through clairvoyance.[163] Even universalist occult sciences such as theosophy could be used to gain self knowledge. Significant numbers of German theosophists, for example, concentrated on developing their mental powers or tracing past lives rather than pursuing theosophy's central aim of international brotherhood; in this manner transforming theosophy into a kind of 'cult of the self'.[164]

While many of these occult philosophies and practices were focused on the reform or cultivation of the self, there were others with more ambitious aims. Some of those Germans who dedicated themselves to the study of somnambulism, clairvoyance and thought-transference, for example, believed their experiments capable of transforming scientific and social conditions. For a group of these researchers, who sought to enrich and expand contemporary psychology, the acceptance and empirical analysis of unconscious mental events were the means of achieving scientific reform. For another group, however, the acceptance of such phenomena constituted the first step in overthrowing a materialist worldview and reforming society. In the Psychologische Gesellschaft, these two groups were represented by Schrenck-Notzing, who promoted an 'experimental psychology' intended to expand the mental sciences, and du Prel, who pursued a 'transcendental psychology' in order not only to prove the existence of the soul, but to provide a non-materialist worldview.

Transcendental psychology

For a number of those Germans who became involved in either psychical research or the modern occult movement during the late nineteenth century, the negation of scientific materialism was an important motivation. Based on the supposition that matter alone constitutes reality, this doctrine was a radical materialistic philosophy that emerged in Germany during the 1840s and 1850s under the auspices of the physician Ludwig Büchner (1824–99), the physiologist Jacob Moleschott (1822–93) and the biologist Karl Vogt (1817–95); a group of liberal scientists whose political aspirations had been thwarted in the failed revolutions of 1848–9. The theory of life proposed by these men had a number of far-reaching implications. The first was the demotion of human beings to the status of material entities. Like their fellow creatures, the scientific materialists argued, human beings were a product of nature, which had emerged gradually through a process of natural development and self-education.[165] The second ramification of this theory was the denial of a mind existing independently of the body. In this regard, the scientific materialists contended that the brain was the seat and organ of thought and that cerebration differed little from any other product of the body, including bile and urine.[166] A third implication of this philosophy was the extinction of God and teleology, both of which the scientific materialists argued, were the logical consequence of modern science.[167]

While many Germans felt uneasy with the implications of scientific materialism, their reasons for and responses to this discomfort were by no means monolithic. Given the materialists' use of their theories to promote democracy and anti-clericalism, many of the objections to it rested on political and religious grounds. Materialism's undermining of authority and belief, such critics argued, led inevitably to the social disintegration and philosophical despair that were the hallmarks of modern life. Scientific materialism was also critiqued on an epistemological basis. While Büchner, Moleschott and Vogt contended that a materialist science would enable knowledge of everything, critics argued that the belief that matter and reality coincided completely, was demonstrably false. Psycho-physiological phenomena such as blushing and manifestations of the unconscious, including dreams, were, these critics pointed out, difficult to explain within a materialist paradigm. Such critiques helped fuel a range of responses, including attempts at scientific and cultural reform, which focused variously on the religious, philosophical, political and epistemological consequences of materialism. For one of the leading figures within the Psychologische Gesellschaft, however, the most appropriate response to scientific materialism appeared to be the study of somnambulism.[168]

The belief that experimentation with the somnambulistic phenomena of mind provided a means of compensating for the absences and erasures of a materialistic worldview was central to the 'transcendental psychology' of du Prel.[169] Originally an officer in the Bavarian army, du Prel received a doctorate from the University of Tübingen in 1868 for a thesis on the topic of dreams from the standpoint of transcendental idealism.[170] Influenced by Arthur Schopenhauer (1788–1860) and Eduard von Hartmann, with whom he enjoyed a long correspondence, du Prel began a study of Darwinism during the 1870s in which he applied the concept of the 'Kampf ums Dasein' [struggle for survival] first to astronomy and then to the mind.[171] While his 1874 book *Kampf ums Dasein am Himmel* [*The Struggle for Survival in the Heavens*], was a materialistic and atheistic application of Darwinism to astronomy, his 1885 work *Philosophie der Mystik* described a 'transcendental Darwinism' in which the evolutionary retreat of the psycho-physical threshold revealed not only a range of extraordinary mental abilities, but a 'transcendental subject'.[172]

Du Prel's transition from a materialist understanding of Darwinism to a mystical one had been achieved through the study of the phenomena of abnormal or somnambulistic states, which demonstrated for him the disjuncture between the perceptible and the real.[173] For du Prel, this disparity provided irrefutable proof of the absurdity of scientific materialism's claim to explain all facets of experience.[174] He wrote:

> The materialist is wholly imprisoned in appearance. He holds the eye to be the mere mirror of phenomena, and the world to be just what it is for sense; and so in the investigation of the object is to be found the solution of the world-enigma.... A part of the world having no relation to our senses has no existence for him. Materialism is the offspring of an assumption by which it stands or falls, namely that all that is real is sensuously perceptible.[175]

Du Prel's objections to scientific materialism, however, were more than epistemological. He strongly believed that materialism had extinguished any basis for morality and caused widespread social degeneracy. He complained:

[T]he whole of modern society has been subverted by materialism and thinks far more about political machinations, Peter's pence, legacy hunting and the drafting of brain injuring dogmas than about the imitation of Christ... bald materialism has become the worldview of the educated and Büchner's *Kraft und Stoff* the gospel of the working masses – in such times nothing is to be hoped for.[176]

Through such critiques, du Prel helped articulate many of his contemporaries' fears about modernity, linking the moral and social decay they saw among both Germany's educated elite and working classes to the dominance of a materialistic *Weltanschauung*.

The 'transcendental psychology' that du Prel sought to develop through the Psychologische Gesellschaft represented his response to both the epistemological failings of scientific materialism and its social consequences. This new discipline involved hypnotic experimentation with unconscious mental abilities – called transcendental because they remained latent in the waking state – which pointed to the existence of an intelligent organising principle known as the 'transcendental subject'.[177] The telekinetic and clairvoyant abilities apparent in somnambulism, du Prel argued, were not explicable through reference to the physical organs and must therefore belong to the 'transcendental subject'.[178] That this subject was identical to an organising principle was proven through the ability of somnambulists to explain the inner workings and health of their bodies.[179] The 'transcendental subject's' independence from its corporeal manifestation, however, meant that it was altered neither by bodily change nor death.[180] As the organising principle of life, du Prel explained, this subject was capable of re-embodying or materialising over and over again, allowing for a kind of reincarnation.[181] Given this evidence for the existence of an immortal element within the individual, he argued, the pessimism and moral despair that were the consequence of adopting a materialist worldview could be overthrown and replaced by a new and more optimistic philosophy.[182] For du Prel, then, experiments in somnambulism proved the existence of a 'transcendental subject' and its incorruptibility, thereby undermining materialism both epistemologically and morally.

Beyond its use as an antidote to the moral despair concomitant with a materialist *Weltanschauung*, du Prel's monist philosophy could be used to draw conclusions about the shape and direction of humanity's future evolution; offering those with an interest in the psychical development of the human race a 'transcendental Darwinism'. Combining Darwin's theory with the results of his experimentation in the fields of mesmerism, somnambulism and spiritualism, du Prel maintained that the evolutionary process had erected a barrier between the sensory and the transcendental world.[183] As humankind evolved, he argued, this barrier, the so-called psycho-physical threshold, would recede, revealing humanity's true nature.[184] Du Prel believed that the mystical phenomena associated with somnambulism were anticipations of this biological process; when the barrier between the sensory and the transcendental had been completely removed, everyone would possess these transcendental abilities.

In spite of its claims to constitute a new and better foundation for human life, du Prel's philosophy did not offer any practical solution to problems such as urban squalor or political unrest, to a large extent eschewing the reform of outward conditions.[185] This was demonstrated by du Prel's criticism of both the state's attempt to extend police powers and the social democrats efforts to manipulate social organisation as a means of solving the social and political problems that dominated Imperial Germany's public discourse.[186] The rejection of direct social and political reform by du Prel and his followers was, in part, a result of their political conservatism, although was also a consequence of the way in which they understood social problems. These men imagined social and political organisation, not so much as the products of historical development, but as the outward expression of dominant philosophies and epistemologies. Action and behaviour, according to these men, was contingent upon the way in which one saw the world.[187] The manipulation of political life and the reform of law might elicit positive changes, but they could not deal with the causes of inequality and crime.[188] Such changes could only be achieved by a radical alteration in the way in which people conceived of themselves and the world, that is, through a change in worldview. In Germany, where, according to du Prel, materialism dominated intellectual and cultural life to the detriment of both science and morality, the only hope for reform was the embrace of a complete *Weltanschauung*; a monistic philosophy between materialism and spiritualism that acknowledged the symbiotic relationship of mind and matter. Ultimately, then, du Prel's 'transcendental psychology' was a call for the reform of the self on a massive scale.[189]

The split of the Psychologische Gesellschaft

The 'transcendental psychology' pursued by du Prel and his followers within the Psychologische Gesellschaft was clearly far removed from the 'experimental psychology' promoted by the empirically minded Schrenck-Notzing and his colleagues in both Munich and Berlin. While these men were concerned with the epistemological implications of scientific materialism, and critical of its obstinate blindness to phenomena beyond the threshold of consciousness, they remained uninterested in using such phenomena to develop a mystical *Weltanschauung*. Schrenck-Notzing and those who shared his approach were focussed on the use of hypnotic experimentation to free psychology from its physiological bonds and enable it to explore both conscious and unconscious states. The explanatory paradigms adopted by these researchers were therefore strictly animist. These men saw in the strange phenomena exhibited by somnambulists and spiritualist mediums, neither a 'transcendental subject' nor a possessing spirit, simply the unconscious self. Given this disjuncture between Schrenck-Notzing's approach and that of du Prel it is unsurprising that the Psychologische Gesellschaft divided into two separate groups in the course of 1889.[190]

At the time of its foundation in 1886, the Munich society was dominated by du Prel, who used it as a platform for his ideas and ambitions. Fascinated by the reports of hypnotic experimentation he had read in the French journal *Revue de l'hypnotisme,* he set out to conduct his own experiments in this field.[191] Convinced that German hypnotists, who concentrated on the vasomotor changes brought about by hypnotism, were too materialist, du Prel attempted to use his experiments to make clear the mystical implications of hypnosis.[192] By proving the reality of phenomena such as thought-transference, he believed, he would force these hypnotists to discuss the possibility of spiritism.[193] In constructing the Psychologische Gesellschaft around such hypnotic experimentation, du Prel did attract a number of German physicians and psychologists, including Schrenck-Notzing and Dessoir, who had trained in the hypnotic techniques of the Nancy school. Their participation in the society, however, did not translate to their acceptance of a spiritist analysis of somnambulistic phenomena, instead it led to sustained critique of du Prel's approach. As Tomas Kaiser has shown, du Prel was not really interested in critical exchange about his work and felt that his younger colleagues' criticisms were a divisive force within the society.[194] This belief was particularly apparent in his response to a paper presented before the Psychologische Gesellschaft in 1889 by Dessoir.[195]

In this paper, entitled 'Ueber Arbeitsgebiet und Forschungsweise psychologischer Gesellschaften' ['About the Field of Work and Methodology of Psychological Societies'], Dessoir argued that the study of hypnotism should form the basis of psychological societies' work. While du Prel did not dispute the importance of hypnotism, having himself recommended it as a vehicle for a 'transcendental psychology', he was concerned at the limited scope of the project recommended by his colleague.[196] The narrow parameters Dessoir set for the study of hypnosis, du Prel argued, excluded the mystical phenomena of the mind from the research agenda of the Psychologische Gesellschaft and in so doing left the materialistic explanation of mental life untouched.[197] This disagreement about the purpose of psychological societies and the role of hypnotism within them pointed to an epistemological fissure within the Psychologische Gesellschaft that du Prel ultimately did not feel he could fix.[198] Taking his followers with him, du Prel left the Psychologische Gesellschaft in 1889 to found a Gesellschaft für Experimentalpsychologie [Society for Experimental Psychology], which within a few years changed its name to the Gesellschaft für wissenschaftliche Psychologie [Society for Scientific Psychology]. The aim of this new society, as its programme stated, was the pursuit of a 'transcendental psychology' through the hypnotic exploration of the unconscious.[199]

In the following year Schrenck-Notzing's faction, which retained the name Psychologische Gesellschaft, forged an alliance with their Berlin-based colleagues that became known as the Gesellschaft für Psychologische Forschung [Society for Psychological Research]. This collaboration took on a concrete form in the production of a series of writings contributed by members of both societies and edited by Dessoir, who had taken over the well-known medical publishing concern of Ambrosius Abel in Leipzig.[200] In its programme, which appeared in the *Sphinx* in June 1891, this new society explained that in the first years of its existence the Psychologische Gesellschaft in Munich had in no way deserved its title; its publications reflecting a focus on philosophical questions and metaphysics rather than psychology.[201] The rump of the Munich society and the new Gesellschaft für Psychologische Forschung, however, were committed to a real 'experimental psychology' based on hypnotic research. The programme stated:

> More than two years ago a group of men branched off from the Psychologische Gesellschaft, in order to found a special association. The goal of both societies in Munich (the old Psychologische Gesellschaft and the new Gesellschaft für wissenschaftliche Psychologie) is in part the same; however the paths followed are different. The group of scholars who branched off emphasise more the transcendental–psychological phenomena of the abnormal mental life in the real sense (that is spiritualism, examination of Od and related areas) and go their own way undisturbed. The Psychologische Gesellschaft, however, stands on the positive ground of normal psychology and seeks in close connection with official science to expand the inductive method to anormal psychological phenomena.[202]

The Gesellschaft für Psychologische Forschung, which followed the lead provided here by Schrenck-Notzing's Psychologische Gesellschaft, pursued these aims well into the twentieth century, only ceasing their activities in 1935 under pressure from the Nazi regime.[203]

Conclusion

Just as the emphasis on telepathy as an explanation for all mediumistic phenomena finally forced the spiritualists out of the Society for Psychical Research, so too did the stubborn empiricism of Schrenck-Notzing and his followers oblige du Prel to abandon the society he had help create.[204] In the split of the Psychologische Gesellschaft in 1889 and in the attempts of the Berliner Gesellschaft für Experimental-Psychologie to distance itself from the taint of spiritualism, it is possible to see the efforts of German psychical researchers to establish the boundaries of their new discipline and to force out those who threatened its integrity; a process known as sanitisation. Psychical researchers, as Dessoir's neologism illustrates, strove in the late nineteenth century to portray their discipline as an extension of, or appendix to, psychology, labelling their new science 'experimental psychology' and using an animist paradigm to explain the phenomena of the unconscious sphere. Psychical researchers' critique of physiological psychology and the multiple overlaps between their emergent discipline and modern occultism, however, led to persistent confrontation with academic psychology over the issues of scientific expertise and authority. By the mid-1890s, the desire to divorce their interest in hypnotic experimentation and somnambulistic phenomena from occultism, saw researchers, such as Dessoir and Moll, adopt an approach that became known as 'kritische Okkultismus' [critical occultism]; this allowed paranormal phenomena to be explained naturalistically or as a manifestation of the witness' psychology. This retreat from the 'experimental psychology' of the Psychologische Gesellschaft and the Berliner Gesellschaft für Experimental-Psychologie was related, as the next chapter will show, to German psychical researchers' advocacy of hypnosis as a medical therapy.

Notes

1. A. von Schrenck-Notzing, *Telepathische Experimente des Sonderausschusses der Psychologischen Gesellschaft zu München* (Leipzig: T. Griebens, 1887), 3.
2. A. von Schrenck-Notzing, *Hypnotische Experimente: Comité-Bericht der Psychologischen Gesellschaft in München* (Leipzig: Oswald Mutze, 1888), 1.
3. *Ibid.*, 9–10.
4. *Ibid.*, 6–8.
5. A. von Schrenck-Notzing, 'Übersinnliche Eingebung in der Hypnose', *Sphinx*, 3, 18 (1887), 1.
6. Schrenck-Notzing, *op. cit.* (note 1), 5–6.
7. *Ibid.*, 8; A. von Schrenck-Notzing, 'Albert von Keller als Malerpsychologe und Metapsychiker', *Psychische Studien*, 48 (1921), 193–215.
8. *Ibid.*, 6–10.
9. *Ibid.*, 3–4; 'Programm der psychologischen Gesellschaft in München', *Sphinx*, 2, 1 (1887), 32–4
10. Schrenck-Notzing, *op. cit.* (note 1), 3; 'Programm der psychologischen Gesellschaft', *ibid.*, 32–6.
11. 'Programm der psychologischen Gesellschaft', *ibid.*, 32–6.

12. C. du Prel, 'Über die Bedeutung der transcendentalen Psychologie', *Sphinx,* 5 (1888), 366–76.

13. 'Programm der Gesellschaft für Experimental-Psychologie zu Berlin', *Sphinx,* 5 (1888), 299.

14. *Ibid.,* 297.

15. M. Dessoir, 'Die Parapsychologie', Sphinx, 7 (1889), 342.

16. 'Programm der Gesellschaft für Experimental-Psychologie', *op. cit.* (note 13), 297, 300.

17. A. Kurzweg, 'Die Geschichte der Berliner "Gesellschaft für Experimental-Psychologie" mit besonderer Berücksichtigung ihrer Ausgangssituation und des Wirkens von Max Dessoir' (unpublished PhD dissertation: Free University of Berlin, 1976), 138.

18. 'Programm der psychologischen Gesellschaft', *op. cit.* (note 9), 32.

19. *Ibid.,* 32.

20. 'Programm der Gesellschaft für Experimental-Psychologie', *op. cit.* (note 13), 300.

21. M.G. Ash, *Gestalt Psychology in German Culture, 1890–1967: Holism and the Quest for Objectivity* (Cambridge: Cambridge University Press, 1998), 23.

22. Kurzweg, *op. cit.* (note 17), 11.

23. R. Tischner, *Geschichte der Parapsychologie: Von Mitte des 19. Jahrhundrets bis zum ersten Drittel des 20. Jahrhundrets* (Tittmanig: Walter Pustet, 1960), 121; C. du Prel, 'Es giebt ein transcendentales Subjekt', *Die Entdeckung der Seele durch die Geheimwissenschaften* (Leipzig: Ernst Günthers, 1894), 32.

24. More recent writing on the history of experimental psychology disputes the traditional historiography, arguing that psychology had been understood as a scientific discipline prior to 1879, see G. Hatfield, 'Wundt and Psychology as Science: Disciplinary Transformations', *Perspectives on Science* 5, 3 (1997), 349.

25. D.N. Robinson, *An Intellectual History of Psychology,* 3rd edn (London: Arnold, 1995), 279.

26. Kurzweg, *op. cit.* (note 17), 75.

27. 'Programm der Gesellschaft für Experimental-Psychologie', *op. cit.* (note 13), 297.

28. W. Preyer, *Die Erklärung des Gedankenlesens nebst Beschreibung eines neuen Verfahrens zum Nachweise unwillkürlicher Bewegungen* (Leipzig: Grieben, 1886); F.C.C. Hansen and A. Lehmann 'Über unwillkürliches Flüstern: Eine kritische und experimentelle Untersuchung der sogenannten Gedanken-Übertragung', *Philosophische Studien,* 11 (1895), 471–530.

29. Schrenck-Notzing, *op. cit.* (note 5), 4; Schrenck-Notzing, *op. cit.* (note 2), 3.

30. C. du Prel, 'Übersinnliche Gedankenübertragung', *Sphinx,* 5(1888), 26, 31.

31. D.B. Herrmann, *Karl Friedrich Zöllner* (Leipzig: B. G. Teubner, 1982), 83.

32. Zöllner borrowed heavily here from Helmholtz, who had attempted to make the concept of a fourth dimension comprehensible to a lay audience. Helmholtz's interest in the logical possibility of a fourth dimension was piqued in 1866 while he worked on his *Treatise on Physiological Optics*. While considering space perception, he was led to question the Kantian idea that the axioms of Euclidean geometry are innate and *a priori* conditions of perception. Helmholtz argued in opposition to this theory that our space perceptions could be imagined differently, for example, a fourth dimension could be imagined as could the convergence of two parallel lines, and that therefore, if the ability to imagine something was indeed a criterion for innateness, our spatial perceptions must be learned. He provided a number of examples to illustrate the manner in which we might imagine our space perceptions other than they are. Perhaps the most interesting example was that of his fictional 'surface dwellers', which he stated were in much the same relation to the third dimension as we are to the fourth dimension. See W.H. Stromberg, 'Helmholtz and Zoellner: Nineteenth-Century Empiricism, Spiritism and the Theory of Space Perception', *Journal of the History of the Behavioral Sciences*, 25 (1989), 372–80.

33. Zöllner's introduction to spiritualism came in September 1875 during a trip to London where he became acquainted with William Huggins, a pioneer in astrophysics and a convert to spiritualism. Huggins introduced Zöllner to William Crookes, a physicist and chemist, who described to his guest his experiments with the medium Florence Cook and her materialised control Katie King. This introduction to, and discussion of, the phenomena of mediumship, which included among other things the disappearance and re-appearance of objects, gave Zöllner the opportunity to consider whether such phenomena might be explained by movement into and out of another dimension. See F. Luttenberger, 'Friedrich Zöllner, der Spiritismus und der vierdimensionale Raum', *Zeitschrift für Parapsychologie und Grenzgebiete der Psychologie*, 19 (1977), 200.

34. Luttenberger, *ibid.*, 195–214.

35. J.K.F. Zöllner, *Wissenschaftliche Abhandlungen*, Vol. III (Leipzig: L. Staackman, 1879). This volume was subsequently translated into English by C.C. Massey as *Transcendental Physics* in 1880.

36. Sawicki has argued that Zöllner's interest in spiritualism can be understood as part of an effort by the *Bildungsbürgertum* to establish a humanistic–holistic worldview. His dedication to an holistic science is evidenced by his research on the borders between physics, the psychology of perception and the theory of knowledge. See D. Sawicki, *Leben mit den Toten: Geisterglauben und die Enstehung des Spiritismus in Deutschland, 1770–1900* (Munich: Schöningh, 2002), 303–5.

37. In 1878, Wundt's experimental psychology had not yet consolidated its position as a legitimate science. See M.E. Marshall and R.A. Wendt, 'Wilhelm Wundt, Spiritism, and the Assumptions of Science', in W.G. Bringmann and R.D. Tweney (eds), *Wundt Studies: A Centennial Collection* (Toronto: C.J. Hogrefe, 1980), 165.

38. See W. Wundt, *Der Spiritismus eine sogenannte wissenschaftliche Frage* (Leipzig: Wilhelm Engelmann, 1885); or the English translation by E.D. Mead, 'Spiritualism as a Scientific Question', *Popular Science Monthly,* 15 (1879), 577–93; K.B. Staubermann, 'Tying the Knot: Skill, Judgement and Authority in the 1870s Leipzig Spiritistic Experiments', *British Journal for the History of Science,* 34 (2001), 67–79.

39. E. von Hartmann, *Der Spiritismus* (Leipzig: Wilhelm Friedrich, 1885), 2.

40. E. von Hartmann, 'Geister oder Halluzinationen?', *Sphinx,* 4 (1887), 12–13.

41. A. Aksakov, 'Kritische Bemerkung über Dr Eduard von Hartmann's Werk: "Der Spiritismus"', *Psychische Studien,* 13 (1886), 17–19.

42. *Ibid.,* 162.

43. W. Hübbe-Schleiden, 'Objektivität sogenannter Materialisationen, Alexander Aksakof wider Eduard von Hartmann', *Sphinx,* 4 (1887), 107–26; C. Sellin, 'Eduard von Hartmann und die Materialisationen', *Sphinx,* 1 (1886), 289–304.

44. P. Pytlik, *Okkultismus und Moderne: Ein kulturhistorisches Phänomen und seine Bedeutung für die Literatur um 1900* (Paderborn: Schöningh Verlag, 2005), 47.

45. *Ibid.,* 47–8.

46. R. Hayward, *Resisting History: Religious Transcendence and the Invention of the Unconscious* (Manchester: Manchester University Press), 48–64.

47. 'Programm der psychologischen Gesellschaft', *op. cit.* (note 9), 36.

48. 'Programm der Gesellschaft für Experimental-Psychologie', *op. cit.* (note 13), 298

49. *Ibid.,* 299

50. For an account of this revival which occurred throughout western Europe and the United States, see J. Webb, *The Occult Underground* (La Salle: Open Court, 1974); J. Webb, *The Occult Establishment* (La Salle: Open Court, 1976).

51. A. Owen *The Place of Enchantment: British Occultism and the Culture of the Modern* (Chicago: University of Chicago Press, 2004), 13.

52. *Ibid.,* 12.

53. T. Kaiser, 'Zwischen Philosophie und Spiritismus: Bildwissenschaftliche Quellen zur Leben und Werk des Carl du Prel', (unpublished MPhil dissertation: Universität Lüneburg, 2005), 12.

54. *Ibid.,* 23.

55. C. Treitel, *A Science for the Soul: Occultism and the Genesis of the German Modern* (Baltimore: The Johns Hopkins University Press, 2004), 56–7.

56. *Ibid.*

57. A. Crabtree, *From Mesmer to Freud: Magnetic Sleep and the Roots of Psychological Healing* (New Haven: Yale University Press, 1993), 198–203.

58. *Ibid.*, 175.

59. 'Programm der Gesellschaft für Experimental-Psychologie', *op. cit.* (note 13), 298

60. H. Ellenberger, *The Discovery of the Unconscious: The History and Evolution of Dynamic Psychiatry* (New York: Basic Books, 1970), 58–9.

61. Crabtree, *op. cit.* (note 57), 6–7.

62. Ellenberger, *op. cit.* (note 60), 61–6.

63. Crabtree, *op. cit.* (note 57), 39.

64. Crabtree, *op. cit.* (note 57), 42–3; Ellenberger, *op. cit.* (note 60), 70–2.

65. Somnambulism spread to Germany via Strasbourg. See Sawicki, *op. cit.* (note 36), 136.

66. *Ibid.*, 138–9.

67. *Ibid.*, 132, 138.

68. N. Freytag, *Aberglauben im 19. Jahrhundert: Preußen und seine Rheinprovinz zwischen Tradition und Moderne (1815–1918)* (Berlin: Duncker & Humblot, 2003), 254.

69. Sawicki, *op. cit.* (note 36), 145–6.

70. *Ibid.*, 145.

71. Crabtree, *op. cit.* (note 57), 198–9

72. Ellenberger, *op. cit.* (note 60), 81

73. Crabtree, *op. cit.* (note 57), 201.

74. Crabtree sees Kerner's ideas as the reintroduction of the intrusion paradigm after the introduction of the alternate consciousness paradigm. *Ibid.*, 86, 212.

75. F.X. Charet, *Spiritualism and the Foundations of C.G. Jung's Psychology* (Albany: State University of New York Press, 1993), 31.

76. Treitel, *op. cit.* (note 55), 301, note 20

77. Sawicki, *op. cit.* (note 36), 234

78. Treitel, *op. cit.* (note 55), 39; Sawicki, *op. cit.* (note 36), 240.

79. A. Moll, *Der Rapport in der Hypnose. Untersuchungen über thierischen Magnetismus* (Leipzig: Otto Dürr, 1892).

80. U. Linse, 'Der Spiritismus in Deutschland um 1900', in. M. Bassler and H. Châtellier (eds), *Mystik, Mystizismus und Moderne in Deutschland um 1900* (Strasbourg: Presses Universitaires de Strasbourg, 1998), 98; Sawicki, *op. cit.* (note 36), 10.

81. Linse, *op. cit.* (note 80), 100.

82. *Ibid.*, 99.

83. For a discussion of the problematic nature of female mediumship, see A. Owen, *The Darkened Room: Women, Power and Spiritualism in Late Victorian England* (London: Virago Press, 1989).

84. On occultism and art, see V. Loers (ed.) *Okkultismus und Avantgarde: Von Munch bis Mondrian, 1900–1915* (Frankfurt: Schirn Kunsthalle, 1995).

85. R.L. Moore, *In Search of White Crows: Spiritualism, Parapsychology and American Culture* (New York: Oxford University Press, 1977), 7.

86. The use of such analogies helped underline what its proponents believed was occultism's intimate connection with science and progress. On the use of technological analogies to describe paranormal phenomena in the German context, see L. Bluma, 'Techniken der Kommunikation zwischen Wissen und Spekulation', (Paper presented at Grenzgänge-Wissenschaftliches und okkultes Wissen im 19. und 20. Jahrhundert, Ruhr-Universität Bochum, 11.12.1999). In the British context, see R.J. Noakes, 'Telegraphy is an occult art: Cromwell Fleetwood Varley and the diffusion of electricity to the other world', *British Journal for the History of Science*, 32 (1999), 421–59.

87. Crabtree, *op. cit.* (note 57), 233.

88. Moore, *op. cit.* (note 85), 8.

89. Crabtree, *op. cit.* (note 57),234.

90. *Ibid.*, 236–7.

91. Sawicki, *op. cit.* (note 36), 286.

92. *Ibid.*, 311

93. *Ibid.*, 311–2; U. Linse, 'Das Buch der Wunder und Geheimwissenschaften: Der spiritistische Verlag Oswald Mutze in Leipzig im Rahmen der spiritistischen Bewegung Sachsens', in M. Lehmstedt and A. Herzog (eds), *Das Bewegte Buch: Buchwesen und soziale, nationale und kulturelle Bewegungen um 1900* (Wiesbaden: Harrassowitz, 1999), 223.

94. Sawicki, *op. cit.* (note 36), 312.

95. *Ibid.*, 312.

96. *Ibid.*, 311.

97. Linse, *op. cit.* (note 80), 100; Sawicki, *op. cit.* (note 36), 333–4.

98. Kaiser, *op. cit.* (note 53), 68.

99. For a more detailed discussion of the connections between spiritualism and theosophy, see J. Oppenheim, *The Other World: Spiritualism and Psychical Research in England, 1850–1914* (Cambridge: Cambridge University Press, 1985), 164–74.

100. J. Dixon, *Divine Feminine: Theosophy and Feminism in England* (Baltimore: Johns Hopkins University Press, 2001) , 4.

101. W. Hübbe-Schleiden, 'Aufruf und Vorwort', *Sphinx*, 1, (1886), 4.

102. Kaiser, *op. cit.* (note 53), 59

103. Theosophists denied the possibility of conversing with the spirits of the dead, see Oppenheim, *op. cit.* (note 99), 165.

104. Treitel, *op. cit.* (note 55), 85–6.

105. Dixon, *op. cit.* (note 100), 4.

106. *Ibid.,* 8–10.

107. Treitel analyses the complex relationship between Hübbe-Schleiden's colonialist and theosophical careers, arguing that it is difficult to see him as a proto-Nazi if one considers both his colonial and occult propaganda. She does, however, see continuity between his two positions in his nationalism. Treitel, *op. cit.* (note 55), 86–93.

108. *Ibid.,* 83, 88–9.

109. Hübbe-Schleiden, *op. cit.* (note 101), 2– 3.

110. *Ibid.,* 4.

111. Kaiser, *op. cit.* (note 53), 61–2.

112. *Ibid.,* 62.

113. Pytlik, *op. cit.* (note 44), 50–1.

114. M. Dessoir, 'Mr Henry Slade in Berlin', *Psychische Studien,* 13 (1886), 97–100; M. Dessoir, 'Eine Sitzung mit Herrn Slade in Berlin', *Sphinx,* 1, 1 (1886), 191–4; M. Dessoir, 'Experiments in Muscle-Reading and Thought-Transference', *Proceedings of the Society for Psychical Research,* 4 (1886–1887), 111; M. Dessoir, 'Experiments in Thought-Transference', *Proceedings of the Society for Psychical Research,* 5 (1888–1889), 355–7.

115. A. Moll, *Ein Leben als Arzt der Seele: Erinnerungen* (Dresden: Carl Reissner, 1936), 93; A. Moll, *Hypnotism: Including a Study of the Chief Points of Psycho-therapeutics and Occultism,* A.F. Hopkirk (trans.), 4th edn (London: Walter Scott, 1909), 515.

116. 'Programm der Gesellschaft für Experimental-Psychologie', *op. cit.* (note 13), 297–9.

117. Kurzweg, *op. cit.* (note 17), 202–57.

118. 'Die Gesellschaft bezweckt, unter ihren Mitgliedern das Studium der Psychologie durch wissenschaftliche Vorträge, Diskussionsabende, Experimente und gesellige Zusammenkünfte zu ermöglichen und insbesondere die wissenschaftliche Anerkennung der Thatsachen aus dem transcendentalen Gebiet nach Kräften zu fördern', *Statuten der Psychologischen Gesellschaft in München* (Munich, 1887), 3.

119. A. von Schrenck-Notzing, 'Experimental Studies in Thought-Transference', *Proceedings of the Society for Psychical Research,* 7 (1891–1892), 3.

120. Kaiser, *op. cit.* (note 53), 263–4.

121. Frau du Prel, for example, participated in a series of experiments in thought-transference that took place in her home. Du Prel, *op. cit.* (note 30), 24, 28–31.

122. Kaiser, *op. cit.* (note 53), 255.

123. Linse, *op. cit.* (note 80), 97.

124. Schrenck-Notzing, for example, sponsored the transformation of the *Psychische Studien* into the *Zeitschrift für Parapsychologie.*

125. Kaiser, *op. cit.* (note 53), 12.

126. In the British context, see J.P. Williams, 'The Making of Victorian Psychical Research: An Intellectual Elite's Approach to the Spiritual World' (unpublished PhD dissertation: University of Cambridge, 1984).

127. E. Bauer, 'Spiritismus und Okkultismus', in V. Loers (ed.) *Okkultismus und Avantgarde: Von Munch bis Mondrian, 1900–1915* (Frankfurt: Schirn Kunsthalle, 1995), 71.

128. *Statuten der Psychologischen Gesellschaft, op. cit.* (note 118), 3.

129. Kaiser, *op. cit.* (note 53), 86.

130. *Statuten der Psychologischen Gesellschaft, op. cit.* (note 118), 3.

131. Kaiser, *op. cit.* (note 53), 104.

132. See the schedule of talks given in *Jahresbericht der Psychologischen Gesellschaft in München 1888/1889* (Munich: Knorr & Hirth, 1889), 4–5.

133. Sawicki, *op. cit.* (note 36), 311.

134. Linse, *op. cit.* (note 80), 102.

135. The dominance of Leipzig in occult publishing was due to the predominance of this city in publishing in general up to 1871, and the concentration of Germany's spiritualist movement in Saxony in the last quarter of the nineteenth century. See Linse, *op. cit.* (note 93), 223.

136. *Ibid.,* 239.

137. For information on the Ostwald Mutze Verlag, see *ibid.,* 219–44.

138. I. Besser, 'Presse des neueren Okkultismus in Deutschland von 1875 bis 1933' (unpublished PhD dissertation: University of Leipzig, 1945), 69.

139. There were also a small number of periodicals established during the 1920s that claimed that their content consisted exclusively of scientific papers and descriptions of experiments. Notable were the journals *Zeitschrift für kritischen Okkultismus und Grenzfragen des Seelenlebens,* established by Albert Hellwig and edited by Richard Baerwald and the *Wissenschaftliche Zeitschrift für Okkultismus,* with which the publisher and occultist Ferdinand Maack was involved. These journals, which were not affiliated to any occult organisation, attempted to fill their pages with scientific reports on the phenomena of parapsychology including clairvoyance and the exteriorisation of the senses. *Ibid.,* 24, 69.

140. *Ibid.,* 69.

141. *Ibid.,* 19.

142. Theosophical periodicals followed a similar pattern of evolution as spiritualist publications, experiencing substantial growth in the first two decades of the twentieth century. In the period 1909 to 1923, for example, a new journal appeared every third or fourth year, ten theosophical journals existing alongside one another by 1917. Like spiritualist journals those

theosophical periodicals associated with the large theosophical societies enjoyed longevity often surviving twenty years or more. *Ibid.*, 68.

143. *Ibid.*

144. Linse notes that while spiritualist clubs maintained libraries, their members, who tended to be plebeian, were not particularly interested in reading or studying these texts. In contrast, theosophy, which recruited its members from the aristocracy and middle class, was much more strongly orientated towards reading and study. See Linse, *op. cit.* (note 93), 222.

145. Sawicki, *op. cit.* (note 36), 333.

146. Kurzweg, *op. cit.* (note 17), 96–111.

147. Kaiser, *op. cit.* (note 53), 67–8.

148. Linse, *op. cit.* (note 93), 220.

149. These two publishing houses tended to publish a more rigorous or scientific brand of occult writing. See Treitel, *op. cit.* (note 55)

150. Linse, *op. cit.* (note 93), 243.

151. 'Buchhandel und Okkultismus', *Nachrichtenblatt der Arbeitsgemeinschaft okkulter Verleger,* 1 (1931), 3, in: ADW, CA, AC-S 272 Okkultismus.

152. *Ibid.*

153. Besser, *op. cit.* (note 138), 67.

154. See N. Goodrick-Clarke, *The Occult Roots of Nazism. Secret Aryan Cults and their Influence on Nazi Ideology. The Ariosophists of Austria and Germany, 1890–1935* (New York: New York University Press, 1985); Besser, *ibid.*, 67.

155. While there did develop in Saxony an anti-clerical social reform influenced brand of spiritualism, the strong link that existed between socialism and plebeian spiritualism in England was absent from the German context. See Sawicki, *op. cit.* (note 36), 316–18; U. Linse, *Geisterseher und Wunderwirker,* 59–87. On plebeian spiritualists in England, see L. Barrow, *Independent Spirits. Spiritualism and English Plebeians, 1850–1910* (London: Routledge & Kegan Paul, 1986).

156. Treitel has argued that one of the main attractions of occultism for Germans was this practical element, *op. cit.* (note 55), 83–164.

157. E. Meyer-Renschhausen and A. Wirz, 'Dietetics, Health Reform and Social Order: Vegetarianism as a Moral Physiology: The Example of Maximilian Bircher-Benner (1867–1939)', *Medical History,* 43 (1999), 325.

158. M. Hau, *The Cult of Health and Beauty in Germany: A Social History, 1890–1930* (Chicago: University of Chicago Press, 2003), 10.

159. Meyer-Renschhausen and Wirz, *op. cit.* (note 157), 328.

160. On liberal reform in Germany during the late nineteenth century, see K. Repp, '"More Corporeal, More Concrete": Liberal Humanism, Eugenics, and German Progressives at the Last Fin de Siècle', *Journal of Modern History,* 72, 3 (2000), 683–730.

161. Matthew Jefferies has argued that lifestyle reform was above all the reform of the self, a project with which certain forms of occultism, in particular, theosophy, were completely in tune. See, M. Jefferies, *Imperial Culture in Germany, 1871–1918* (New York: Palgrave Macmillan, 2003), 193.

162. Linse, *op. cit.* (note 80), 101.

163. Linse, *op. cit.* (note 155), 98–9.

164. Treitel, *op. cit.* (note 55), 90, 93–4.

165. L. Büchner, *Kraft und Stoff oder Grundzüge der natürlichen Weltordnung*, 21st edn (Leipzig: Theod. Thomas, 1904), 204.

166. *Ibid.*, 217–18.

167. *Ibid.*, 180–1

168. Du Prel, *op. cit.* (note 12), 371.

169. C. du Prel, 'Okkultismus und Anarchismus', in *Nachgelassene Schriften* (Leipzig: Max Altman, 1911), 107.

170. C. Kiesewetter, *Geschichte des neueren Okkultismus: Geheimwissenschaftliche Systeme von Agrippa von Nettesheim bis zu Karl du Prel* (Leipzig: Wilhelm Friedrich, 1891), 751.

171. Kaiser, *op. cit.* (note 53), 37, 41–4.

172. Sawicki, *op. cit.* (note 36), 306; C. du Prel, *Der Kampf ums Dasein am Himmel: Die Darwin'sche Formel nachgewiesen in der Mechanik der Sternenwelt* (Berlin: n.p. 1874); Kaiser, *op. cit.* (note 53), 41–4; 55–9.

173. C. du Prel, *The Philosophy of Mysticism*, Vol. I, C.C. Massey (trans.), (London: George Redway, 1889), xxiii, 5–7.

174. C. du Prel, *The Philosophy of Mysticism*, Vol. II, C.C. Massey (trans.), (London: George Redway, 1889), 121–2.

175. Du Prel, *op. cit.* (note 173), 6–7.

176. '[D]er ganzen modernen Gesellschaft vom Materialismus zersetzt ist, und weit mehr an politische Umtriebe, Peterspfennig, Erbschleichereien und den Erlaß hirnwütiger Dogmen denkt, als an die Nachfolge Christi… ein platter Materialismus die Weltanschauung der Gebildeten, und Büchners 'Kraft und Stoff' das Evangelium der Arbeitermassen geworden ist, - in solchen Zeiten ist nichts zu hoffen.' C. du Prel, 'Über den Einfluß psychischer Faktoren im Okkultismus', *Sphinx,* (1893), 8–9.

177. Du Prel, *op. cit.* (note 12), 371.

178. *Ibid.*, 371.

179. Pytlik, *op. cit.* (note 44), 50.

180. Du Prel, *op. cit.* (note 12), 371.

181. Pytlik, *op. cit.* (note 44), 51; Du Prel, *ibid.*, 372.

182. Du Prel, *ibid.*, 372.

183. Du Prel, *ibid.*, 31–57.

184. Kiesewetter, *op. cit.* (note 170), 755.

185. Du Prel, *op. cit.* (note 169), 112–13.

186. *Ibid.*, 112.
187. Du Prel, *op. cit.* (note 173), 2.
188. Du Prel, *op. cit.* (note 169), 112–13; Hübbe-Schleiden, *op. cit.* (note 101), 4.
189. *Ibid.*, 4.
190. Bauer, *op. cit.* (note 127), 83.
191. Kaiser, *op. cit.* (note 53), 86.
192. 'Programm der psychologischen Gesellschaft', *op. cit.* (note 9), 33–4.
193. Kaiser, *op. cit.* (note 53), 64.
194. *Ibid.*, 87.
195. *Jahresbericht der Psychologischen Gesellschaft, op. cit.* (note 132), 5.
196. C. du Prel, 'Die praktische Verwertung des Hypnotismus für die transcendentale Psychologie', in *Experimentalpsychologie und Experimentalmetaphysik* (Leipzig: Max Altmann, 1905), 95.
197. C. du Prel, 'Die psychologischen Gesellschaften', in *Nachgelassene Schriften* (Leipzig: Max Altman, 1911), 224.
198. As Kaiser mentions, the immediate cause of this split was unclear. He does bring to light, however, an argument during 1888 between du Prel and Bayersdorfer on one side, and Schrenck-Notzing on the other, that might have contributed to du Prel's decision to leave the Psychologische Gesellschaft. This dispute revolved around Schrenck-Notzing's desire to defend himself against the defamatory comments of a patient he had hypnotised. Du Prel and Bayersdorfer maintained that their new discipline and the society would not withstand the glare of publicity and that Schrenck-Notzing should be forced to leave for bringing both into disrepute. See Kaiser, *op. cit.* (note 53), 65.
199. C. du Prel, 'Programm für experimentellen Okkultismus', *Sphinx*, 18, 95 (1894), 23–33.
200. M. Offner, 'Die deutsche Gesellschaft für psychologische Forschung', *Sphinx*, 11, 66 (1891), 335.
201. *Ibid.*, 333.
202. 'Vor länger als zwei Jahren zweigte sich von der Psychologischen Gesellschaft eine Gruppe von Männern ab, um einen besonderen Verein zu gründen. Das Ziel beider Vereinigungen in München (der älteren Psychologischen Gesellschaft und der jüngeren Gesellschaft für wissenschaftliche Psychologie) ist zum Teil dasselbe; jedoch sind die eingeschlagenen Wege verschiedene. Die abgezweigte Gruppe von Gelehrten betont mehr die transcendentalpsychologischen Erscheinungen des abnormen Seelenlebens im eigentlichen Sinn (also den Spiritismus, die Od-Untersuchungen und verwandte Gebiete) und geht unbeirrt ihren eignen Weg. Die Psychologische Gesellschaft aber steht auf dem positiven Boden der Normal-Psychologie und sucht in engem Anschluss an die offizielle Wissenschaft die induktive

Methode auf anormale psychologische Erscheinungen auszudehnen.' *Ibid.*, 334, n.1.

203. Pytlik, *op. cit.* (note 44), 45.
204. Hayward, *op. cit.* (note 46), 46–7.

2

Hypnotism, Lay Medicine
and Psychical Research at the *Fin de Siècle*

Introduction

In the 1887 programme of the Psychologische Gesellschaft, which advocated an experimental psychology based on hypnotic experimentation, Carl du Prel applauded the work of those medical hypnotists who had helped establish the influence of mind upon body through the manipulation of their patients' vasomotor systems.[1] While such experiments were medically significant, pointing to the possibility of an effective form of psychotherapeutics, they did little to illuminate the philosophical meaning of hypnosis; a question that du Prel and his followers sought to address through a 'transcendental psychology'.[2] Du Prel, as we have seen, had several aims in developing this new discipline, not least of which was to convince the medical hypnotists who joined both the Munich and Berlin societies of the veracity of a spiritist explanatory paradigm.[3] The disintegration of the Psychologische Gesellschaft in 1889, however, appears to have resulted from a disagreement over the purpose of psychological societies and the role of hypnotism within them. In spite of pressure to interpret the somnambulistic feats of Lina Matzinger as signifiers of a 'transcendental subject', these physicians had managed to retain their own research agendas.

This small group of doctors, who attended demonstrations of hypnosis at both the Salpêtrière in Paris and Bernheim's clinic in Nancy, had joined the Psychologische Gesellschaft and the Berlin-based Gesellschaft für Experimental-Psychologie – two of the very few venues in Germany where hypnotic experimentation was undertaken during the 1880s – as a means of fostering their interest and expertise in hypnosis. For these men, the experiments in thought transference and clairvoyance carried out within the psychological societies were significant for revealing the unexplored regions and unimagined capabilities of the human psyche. Such experiments also demonstrated the utility of hypnosis as a means of psychological introspection and as an effective form of therapy for a large number of the physical, psychological and sexual ailments that these doctors encountered in their medical practices. Eager to explore and develop the psychotherapeutic potential they observed here, these physicians, among them Max Dessoir, Albert Moll, and Albert von Schrenck-Notzing, sought, during the closing decades of the nineteenth century, not only to gain jurisdiction over hypnosis – a domain occupied by lay practitioners and occultists – but to have it accepted as a legitimate form of medical therapy.

In order to achieve these goals, however, medical hypnotists had to overcome two major hurdles. The first was the strong association between hypnosis and lay medicine. In the German context, as we will see, medical interest in hypnosis during the 1870s and early 1880s was largely inspired by the spectacular magnetic performances of lay practitioners and itinerant occultists.[4] This proved problematic not only because it appeared to link lay and medical practice but also because it tended to elide the differences between mesmerism and hypnosis. Mesmerism intimated the existence of a mysterious magnetic fluid within the body that could be manipulated via magnetic strokes to create a cathartic crisis; hypnotism depicted the trance-like ambulatory state known as 'somnambulism' as a purely physiological or psychological phenomenon induced through either optical fixation or suggestion. While the experiments conducted by Charcot and Bernheim during the 1880s helped sanitise and legitimise this practice, for the more conservative members of Germany's medical and psychological communities, hypnosis remained a dangerous form of charlatanry. In order to gain acceptance for hypnosis, medical hypnotists were required not only to demarcate their use of suggestion from that of magnetisers and occultists, but to erect a range of epistemological, professional and legal boundaries that would ensure their monopoly of it. The second hurdle to achieving their goals was largely of the medical hypnotists' own making. The pursuit of hypnotic and psychical research by these men within the Munich and Berlin societies blurred the distinctions that they were attempting to draw between their 'legitimate' medical use of hypnosis and the 'illegitimate' lay and occult use of it. While the split of the Psychologische Gesellschaft and the retreat of the Gesellschaft für Experimental-Psychologie from their investigation of spiritualism initially appeared to demarcate psychical research from its occult siblings, the medical hypnotists' campaign to ban all but medical and scientific experiments with hypnosis made even this sanitised stance problematic. In order not to transgress the epistemological, professional and legal boundaries they had helped construct, Dessoir and Moll chose to engage in an act of self-policing; retreating from psychical research with its animist paradigm to take up a position known as 'kritische Okkultismus' [critical occultism] in which paranormal phenomena were largely interpreted within a psychological framework. Schrenck-Notzing, as this chapter will show, refused not only to abandon his animist approach to the paranormal, but in 1904 engaged in a promotion of hypnosis and

84

somnambulistic phenomena, which mimicked that of the itinerant stage mesmerists against whom he had helped campaign. This incident, which alienated him from his colleagues, particularly Dessoir and Moll, represented Schrenck-Notzing's first steps towards an interest in physical mediumship and parapsychology.

The stage mesmerists

During the late 1870s and early 1880s, a number of itinerant stage mesmerists, figures such as Böllert, Donato and Hansen, astounded European audiences with their highly provocative and entertaining demonstrations of animal magnetism. In Germany and Austria, the most significant of these lay mesmerists was the Dane Carl Hansen (1833–97) who had performed in Breslau, Berlin, Leipzig and Vienna during 1879 and 1880. Hansen's demonstrations, like those of his competitors, consisted of both the mesmeric (magnetic strokes) and hypnotic (optical fixation and suggestion) manipulation of audience members, whose loss of volition allowed him to command their performance of a variety of ludicrous acts. The physiologist Rudolf Heidenhain (1834–97), who attended one of Hansen's performances in Breslau, described the mesmerist's routine thus:

> [T]he subjects of his experiments stare fixedly at a faceted and glittering piece of glass. After this preliminary proceeding, he makes a few 'passes' over the face, avoiding actual contact; he then lightly closes the eyes and mouth, at the same time gently stroking the cheeks. The 'media' are now incapable of opening their eyes or mouth; and after a few more passes over the forehead, fall into a sleep-like condition. In this state they are exhibited by Mr Hansen as will-less automata, who, at his command, assume all kinds of positions, and perform the most unreasonable and ridiculous actions, such as eating a raw potato, under the impression that it is a pear; riding cross-legged on a chair, with the idea they are riding in a horse-race....[5]

While Hansen's repertoire and technique differed little from those of other stage mesmerists active in Germany and Austria at the time, it was complaints that his demonstrations had a deleterious effect on audiences which forced German-speaking legislators and physicians to take a serious interest in mesmerism.

Public performances of animal magnetism during the 1870s and 1880s, while undoubtedly popular, were regarded in some quarters as a serious threat to mental, physical and moral health. In Vienna during February 1880, for example, the police brought a halt to Hansen's performances after consultation with the Viennese medical faculty suggested that mesmerism posed a health risk in the hands of amateurs.[6] The matter was investigated subsequently by Richard Krafft von Ebing (1840–1902), on behalf of Das

Gesundheitsamt [the Sanitary Board], and revealed a long history of concern in Austria about the unregulated use of animal magnetism.[7] In Berlin in 1881, the Wissenschaftlichen Deputation für das Medizinalwesen [Scientific Committee on Medical Affairs], as part of the Preußische Kultusministerium [Prussian Ministry of Arts and Culture], banned demonstrations of mesmerism after Hansen was held responsible for awakening dormant hysterical tendencies in his audiences.[8] The Prussian authorities were concerned furthermore that public displays of mesmerism might disturb the peace and promote superstition.[9] Heidenhain's pamphlet, from which the minister for education and the arts had drawn evidence to justify this ban, reiterated this concern. Reminding his readers of the recent Zöllner controversy, Heidenhain expressed anxiety that, 'In an age in which this is possible, there is imminent danger that phenomena such as Mr Hansen displays may lead to a new form of superstition.'[10] The loss of volition attendant on mesmeric performances and the weak mental and moral constitutions of audiences, largely comprising of the working classes, made both civil unrest and psychic epidemics a possibility in the minds of German legislators and physicians.

The suspension of the will achieved in the mesmeric state was of particular concern to commissions, such as those held in Vienna and Berlin. Such a loss of volition was considered dangerous, not only because of evidence that it weakened the nerves and stimulated mental disorder but also because it allowed for the sexual or criminal exploitation of mesmerised subjects. Crimes against individuals in non-volitional states naturally had their precedent in the abuse of chemical anaesthetics, such as chloroform and laughing gas, but mesmerism provoked fears not only that crimes might be committed against people in a magnetic trance but that such persons might be induced to commit offences against others.[11] This titillating combination of sex, danger and suggestibility made crime and animal magnetism a preoccupation of the sensational press and numerous medical treatises, which called for the practice of mesmerism to be restricted to licensed physicians.[12] These calls were repeated throughout the 1880s and 1890s as the German medical community became increasingly interested in mesmerism and hypnosis and as their desire to professionalise and monopolise healthcare in a newly unified Germany prompted them to launch a series of bitter and protracted campaigns against lay practitioners. Legislation for the restriction of mesmerism and hypnosis, however, was to prove a frustrating and largely ineffective endeavour as lay practitioners moved their performances from public venues to private societies and domiciles to avoid prosecution.[13]

Hansen's magnetic demonstrations, although the subject of intense public criticism, introduced many German-speaking physicians to mesmerism for the first time, initiating the so-called 'Hansen phase' in hypnotic research (*c.*1879 to 1884).[14] While careful not to legitimate the activities of contemporary stage mesmerists, Albert Moll acknowledged, during the late 1880s, the pivotal role of itinerant performers like Hansen in bringing hypnosis to the attention of German-speaking scientists, such as Heidenhain, Krafft-Ebing, Preyer, Weinhold and Wundt. He wrote:

> Just as I refuse to join in the general condemnation of Mesmer, I try and recommend others to try, to judge such men as Hansen, Böllert, and Donato, fairly. Their motives may have been selfish, but they have certainly been of great service to science.... To the honour of those mentioned, it should be expressly stated that all three of them were invariably ready to help representatives of science in the most straightforward way.[15]

Cognisant of the role which Hansen had played in fostering his interest in animal magnetism, Heidenhain told the Schlesische Gesellschaft für Vaterländische Kultur [Silesian Society for Home Culture] in January 1880 that:

> I myself, when I first read reports of Hansen's representations, came to the first of the above-mentioned conclusions [that the whole affair was nonsense].... But I entirely changed my opinion after I had seen Mr Hansen in this town before an assemblage of physicians who had hitherto been absolute disbelievers on the subject, perform his experiments with success on several of these very men. I soon found an opportunity of more closely investigating the phenomena I had witnessed, as I myself succeeded in inducing the same condition observed in Hansen's media in a number of medical men and students – including a student brother of my own – persons whose credibility is beyond question, and who are capable of giving an intelligent description of their own perceptions.[16]

Those physicians, like Heidenhain, who attempted to recreate the range of mesmeric phenomena produced by Hansen, were soon convinced that they dealt, not with a magnetic fluid or a mysterious rapport, but with certain predictable and well-known physiological changes. Wilhelm Wundt wrote in this regard that, 'of a mysterious rapport between the magnetiser and magnetised there appears no trace, just as the ability to magnetise seems in no way connected with certain special people.'[17]

With these findings in mind, German scientists began to speculate along somatic lines, for example, suggesting as Heidenhain did:

> [T]hat the cause of the phenomena of hypnotism lies in the inhibition of the activity of the ganglion-cells of the cerebral cortex... the inhibition being

87

brought about by gentle prolonged stimulation of the sensory nerves of the face, or of the auditory or optic nerve.[18]

Another popular physiological explanation for the magnetic state was changes in cerebral blood supply.[19] Wundt speculated that the peculiar phenomena of sleep, dreams and mesmerism might result from an inhibition of activity in certain parts of the cerebral cortex and an increase in the activity of other parts, due to the simultaneous contraction and dilation of capillaries in certain regions of the brain.[20] The physiological focus adopted by physicians such as Heidenhain, Weinhold, Preyer, Wundt and Krafft-Ebing was accompanied also by a change in nomenclature. Adopting the terminology suggested by the British physician James Braid (1795–1860), the term 'magnetic state' was replaced by the term 'hypnotic condition'.[21] While the investigations undertaken by these scientists marked the beginnings of scientific and medical interest in this field, their focus on the academic and theoretical questions posed by hypnosis and their concentration on physiological causes saw the therapeutic potential evident in the work of lay mesmerists neglected.[22]

The Salpêtrière and Nancy schools

Despite German efforts to render hypnosis a legitimate object of scientific investigation, the European scientific and medical communities remained largely hostile to hypnotism during the 1870s and early 1880s. Associated with animal magnetism, whose scientific pretensions had been rejected by two Royal Commissions in France, and with the sensational and potentially harmful performances of contemporary stage mesmerists, hypnotism was dismissed by many European scientists as an elaborate form of charlatanry. Furthermore, for those scientists and physicians who acknowledged the reality of hypnosis, there were epistemological barriers to its use. The study of hypnosis and allied states appeared illegitimate within those emergent professions such as neurology and psychiatry, whose authority was founded on a materialist concept of mind and body. In this view, psychological phenomena, such as those demonstrated in hypnosis, were simply the reflection of brain function, interesting only in as far as they indicated the underlying action of that organ.[23] In 1882, however, this epistemological objection to the study of hypnosis was overturned when the eminent French neurologist Jean-Martin Charcot (1825–93) presented a paper on hypnotism before the Parisian Académie des Sciences.[24] Charcot's examination of hypnotism, which he had arrived at through an investigation of metallotherapy, purported to show that hypnosis was a modification of the nervous system inducible only in hysterics and consisting of three distinct stages: catalepsy, lethargy and somnambulism.[25] By arguing that hypnosis was a pathological state symptomatic of hysteria and accompanied by discernible and predictable physiological change, Charcot brought hypnosis in line with the scientific community's somatic *Weltanschauung*, in this way legitimising scientific engagement with it.

Charcot's desire to rehabilitate hypnosis sprang from a concern to bring clinical observations closer to experimental medicine as well as to illuminate and obliterate, in accordance with his broader political agenda, ignorance and superstition.[26] Charcot's efforts to establish the immutability of his three-stage model of hysterical attacks, for example, had led him to consider the existence of hysteria among men and to turn his positivist gaze on historical phenomena, such as demoniac possession and mystical ecstasy.[27] By comparing the stages of the hysterical attack with visual and descriptive representations of possession and ecstasy, Charcot argued for the retrospective diagnosis of hysteria, not only attempting to prove the universal applicability of his laws, and the medical profession's exclusive competency to deal with hysteria, but also establishing, in line with the secularising project of the Third Republic, the moral and intellectual inferiority of the clerical worldview.[28] In a similar manner, Charcot's pathologisation of hypnotism was intended to establish doctors as the only legitimate practitioners of hypnosis and to exclude from its use the lay healers, performers and spiritualists who represented alternative sources of ideological, religious and spiritual authority.[29] In Germany also, a contest took place between these groups and the medical community to control the meaning and application of hypnosis in the latter part of the 1880s.

While Charcot's pathologisation of hypnosis succeeded in making the scientific study of hypnotism respectable, his theory did not remain unchallenged. Predating Charcot's theatrical displays of hypnotism and hysteria in Paris, a country doctor in Nancy had come to his own conclusions about the hypnotic state. A.A. Liébeault (1823–1904) began to use hypnosis in his practice during the 1860s, offering hypnotic treatment at no charge to his patients as a way of extending his empirical knowledge of hypnotism and suggestion and providing a largely peasant clientèle with affordable non-heroic amelioration of pain and disease. Liébeault, who had experimented extensively with both magnetism and Braidism, was convinced that suggestion alone, rather than a mysterious fluid or pathological modification of physiology, was responsible for the phenomena of hypnotism.[30] He published his findings and musings on this topic in 1864 in a book entitled *Du sommeil et des états analogues*. This work received little attention until 1882 when Liébeault's therapeutic procedures were discovered by Hippolyte Bernheim (1840–1919), professor of medicine at Nancy, who incorporated hypnosis and suggestion in his medical arsenal.[31] In 1884, Bernheim, who like Liébeault was of the opinion that hypnosis was neither pathological nor a close relative of neuroses such as hysteria, published his findings, creating a stir among those at the Salpêtrière in Paris. Bernheim's work and that of others attached to the Nancy school argued not only that hypnosis and hysteria were unrelated, but that Charcot's three hypnotic stages had been manufactured through suggestion and therefore possessed no objective reality. Bernheim wrote:

> I have never been able to induce in any cases, the three phases of the Salpêtrière School, and it is not for want of trial.... Once only did I see a subject who exhibited perfectly the three periods of lethargy, catalepsy and somnambulism. It was a young girl who had been at the Salpêtrière for three years, and... subjected to a special training by manipulations, imitating the phenomena which she saw produced in other somnambulists of the same school, taught by imitation to exhibit reflex phenomena in a certain typical order, the case was no longer one of natural hypnotism, but a product of false training, a true *suggestive hypnotic neurosis*.[32]

The debate which followed consisted of a barrage of scientific pamphlets between the two schools and entered the public realm through Charcot's lectures, coverage in the scientific and popular press, and the engagement of both schools in a number of sensational legal trials which involved the criminal misuse of hypnosis.[33] By 1887, however, it had become apparent that the views of the Salpêtrière school could no longer compete with those of Nancy and the debate slowly petered out. The teachings of the Nancy school now began to spread throughout Europe, carried primarily by physicians who had visited Bernheim's clinic and were enthusiastic about the system of psychotherapeutics developed there.[34] In German-speaking countries this dissemination was carried out by a small group of physicians including Auguste Forel, Albert Moll and Albert von Schrenck-Notzing.

The birth of medical hypnotism in Germany

While not well received by its audience, 'Hypnotismus in der Therapie' ['Hypnotism in Therapy'], the paper presented by Moll to the Berliner medizinische Gesellschaft [Berlin Medical Society] on 26 October 1887, was one of the first expositions of the methods of the Nancy school in the German context.[35] Moll's paper, based on both his clinical observations and his experiences in Paris and Nancy, described the conflict between the Salpêtrière and Nancy schools and argued for the efficacy of both waking and hypnotic suggestion for a range of afflictions including alcoholism, bed-wetting, chorea and anomalies of menstruation. Moll's 1886 sojourn in Paris, part of a lengthy European tour, coincided with the heated debate between the Salpêtrière and Nancy schools.[36] This afforded the young physician the opportunity to observe and compare both theories first hand. Moll informed the Berliner medizinische Gesellschaft that although attendance at Charcot's clinics and lectures had provided him with the opportunity to witness some outstanding examples of lethargy, catalepsy and somnambulism among Parisian hysterics, he had remained unconvinced that the possibility of suggestion had been completely excluded from these performances.[37] Arriving at Bernheim's clinic in Nancy towards the end of 1886, Moll was quickly convinced that the three stages Charcot had identified as part of the hypnotic state were a result of suggestion and expectation. In the course of his visit, he was also persuaded of the efficacy of both waking and hypnotic suggestion in the amelioration of pain and disease.[38] On this point he assured his listeners that while 'hypnotic treatment certainly does not offer us a panacea. The results are, however, already very encouraging.'[39] Moll concluded his paper by recommending that his audience conduct further experimentation along Nancian lines and incorporate hypnosis and suggestion in their medical practice.

Despite Moll's obvious enthusiasm for the medical use of hypnosis and suggestion, and the extraordinary examples he provided of their ability to produce physiological change, his paper met with both ridicule and criticism from members of the Berliner medizinische Gesellschaft.[40] Moll noted that 'particularly when I spoke of experiments, in which the suggestion of a blister plaster actually produces blisters, general laughter went through the salon.'[41] This opposition, on the part of the medical society, to Moll's promotion of hypnotic therapy, was articulated not only through sniggers, but also through Mendel's and Ewald's diatribes. The psychiatrist Emanuel Mendel (1839–1907) opposed the therapeutic use of hypnosis, claiming that it was inherently dangerous.[42] Basing his argument on the pathological theory of hypnosis posited by Charcot, and on the widely held belief that hypnosis weakened the nervous system, he claimed that hypnotic treatment provoked nerves in those with no prior history of nervous affliction and caused an exacerbation in those who already laboured under such a condition.[43] Carl Anton Ewald (1845–1915), the editor of the *Berliner klinische Wochenschrift* [*Berlin Clinical Weekly*], was also resistant to the inclusion of hypnosis within the medical arsenal on the basis that it could not be considered a medical treatment.[44] According to Moll, Ewald pronounced:

[A] medical treatment it is not; a medical treatment requires medical skill and medical knowledge, but something that every shepherd, that every shoemaker and tailor can do, if only he possesses the necessary self confidence... one cannot call a medical treatment.[45]

Mendel's and Ewald's hostility to the therapeutic use of hypnosis and suggestion betrayed the medical community's concern with the safety of medical hypnosis and its widespread use by lay practitioners – issues which were to become bugbears for both medical hypnotists and their opponents throughout the 1880s and 1890s. Ewald's evocation of technical skill and knowledge was also indicative of an increasing concern on the part of the German medical profession to clearly delineate and defend the borders of medicine in order to exclude lay competition and to monopolise healthcare for themselves.

Despite his disappointment at the response of his peers, Moll continued to utilise hypnosis and suggestion in his medical practice and in a number of hospitals around Berlin. He also began to host private functions during which he introduced small groups of physicians to the techniques of the Nancy school.[46] He wrote in this regard:

> I invited every week about seven or eight doctors to an evening with me, held a talk and demonstrated the phenomena of hypnotism for them. I also showed them in particular the difference between Charcot's theory and that of Nancy…. Barely one German knew anything about the teachings of Liébeault and Bernheim.[47]

In 1889, Moll presented to the medical society findings from the numerous hypnotic experiments he had conducted since 1887 in a second paper titled, 'Therapeutische Erfahrungen auf dem Gebiete des Hypnotismus' ['Therapeutic Experiences in the Field of Hypnotism']. This time his reception was slightly more enthusiastic. Mendel, as in Moll's first presentation, voiced objections to the therapeutic use of hypnosis and presented a number of case studies to prove its inherent danger.[48] However, Ewald did not dismiss hypnosis on this occasion, and was gracious in recognising it as a legitimate field of research, but reminded his audience, much to Moll's dismay, that 'we must be conscious, that through its application, and I myself have applied it, we step over the field of medical skill and treatment and into that of psychology.'[49] Moll, whose prime concern was to establish hypnosis as a legitimate form of therapeutics, responded to Ewald by arguing that medicine had the responsibility to use the advancements of other sciences, like physics, chemistry and psychology, as part of its therapeutic regime.[50]

The more tolerant atmosphere which greeted Moll during his second presentation in April 1889 was, in part, the result of the propaganda and education campaign he had conducted within Berlin's medical community in the interlude between his two talks, but was also attributable to Auguste Forel's (1848–1931) publications in the field during 1887 and 1889.[51]

Forel's first works on the therapeutic use of hypnosis, the article 'Einige therapeutische Versuche mit dem Hypnotismus (Braidismus) bei Geisteskranken' ['Some Therapeutic Tests with Hypnotism (Braidism) on Mentally Ill People'] (1887) and the pamphlet *Der Hypnotismus: seine Bedeutung und seine Handhabung* [*Hypnotism: Its Meaning and its Implementation*] (1889) had a more immediate and more resounding impact on the German speaking medical community than Moll's early attempts to promote hypnosis through academic papers and small scale demonstrations. Forel's success was due to his position as a renowned and respected psychiatrist at the University of Zurich and as director of the Burghölzli asylum. In contrast, Moll's struggle to find a receptive audience was a product of his relative obscurity before the publication of his influential work *Der Hypnotismus* in 1889.[52] Nevertheless, both men played a crucial role in the early promotion of hypnosis, suggestion and psychotherapy in German speaking countries, and were in part responsible for the gain in momentum experienced by the hypnotic movement in Germany during 1888 and 1889.

The therapeutic application of hypnosis and suggestion

The growth in Germans' enthusiasm for the teachings of the Nancy school and for the experimental and therapeutic application of hypnosis, which occurred during the late 1880s and early 1890s, was evident in the number of prominent physicians, including E. Baierlacher of Nürnberg, J.G. Sallis of Baden-Baden, and Albert von Schrenck-Notzing of Munich who now began openly to practise and experiment with hypnotic therapy.[53] This evolving interest in psychotherapeutics was also apparent in the appearance of a number of noteworthy publications. In 1888, for example, the young physician Max Dessoir published a two-volume work entitled *Bibliographie des modernen Hypnotismus* [*Bibliography of Modern Hypnotism*].[54] This exhaustive publication demonstrated the widespread and increasing interest in Germany and throughout Europe in hypnotism and suggestion. The results of Moll's investigations in the field of hypnosis were published in *Der Hypnotismus*. This book, which investigated the range of phenomena associated with animal magnetism and hypnotism, went through numerous editions and printings and became a classic in the field. In 1892, a periodical dedicated exclusively to hypnosis was founded in Berlin. Entitled *Zeitschrift für Hypnotismus* [*Journal for Hypnotism*], and established by the psychiatrist J. Grossmann, this journal attracted and maintained a high level of scholarship in four languages and represented the transition of serious hypnotic research from France to Germany.[55]

This new-found enthusiasm for the study and application of hypnosis saw Berlin and Munich in particular become centres of hypnotic endeavour.

In Berlin, for instance, hypnotic suggestion became a fashionable treatment for a range of ailments, including writers' cramp, stuttering, bed-wetting, rheumatic pain and sleep disorders, and was often used in combination with other therapies, such as faradic treatment, massages and baths.[56] The Prussian capital also became a centre for hypnotic research with the Berliner Gesellschaft für Experimental-Psychologie conducting a large number of experiments in this field.[57] In Munich, the promotion of hypnotism as both therapy and experimental method was spearheaded by Schrenck-Notzing, who used hypnotic suggestion on a large number of his patients.[58] As one of the first physicians in Germany's south to take an interest in hypnosis, his promotional efforts included presentations such as a paper of nearly four-hours duration, given in January 1889 to a room of three hundred of Munich's most respected citizens, and another in October 1889 to a businessmen's club on the practical application of hypnosis.[59] Like Moll, Schrenck-Notzing recommended the use of hypnotism and suggestion for a wide range of ailments and addictions, including hysteria, neurasthenia, alcoholism and morphine addiction. He was particularly enthusiastic, however, about its application in the field of sex research, announcing that 'suggestion therapy it appears to me is of ground-breaking significance for the different forms of sexual pathology, particularly contrary sexual feeling [homosexuality].'[60]

One of the main sources of interest in the therapeutic use of hypnosis and suggestion during the 1880s and 1890s was the nascent field of sexology. Indeed, beside the hypnotism movement itself, sexology was the greatest promoter and populariser of hypnosis during the late nineteenth century.[61] The pioneers in this field, including Krafft-Ebing, Moll and Schrenck-Notzing, were followers of the Nancy school, who were active in the campaign to have hypnosis recognised as a medical therapy and were psychiatrists whose empirical experience had convinced them of hypnosis' potential for the alteration of undesirable sexual behaviour.[62] The most influential work in this respect was that of Schrenck-Notzing entitled *Die Suggestions-Therapie bei krankhaften Erscheinungen des Geschlechtsinnes* [*Suggestion-Therapy with the Pathological Phenomena of the Sexual Sense*] (1892) in which he advocated the use of hypnotic suggestion in cases of both male impotence and female frigidity. The success of hypnotic therapy in cases of sexual pathology was demonstrated for Schrenck-Notzing not only by the large proportion of patients who experienced some improvement of their condition, but also by the large numbers of those who did not suffer a relapse. In the thirty-two cases of sexual insensitivity he treated, for example, Schrenck-Notzing reported complete failure in only five cases, with improvement or cure in twenty-seven cases, ten of which appeared to be permanent in the light of subsequent observation.[63]

The success of hypnotic suggestion in cases of functional impotence, masturbation and sexual hypersensitivity was even better at between sixty and sixty-five per cent and also presented low rates of relapse.[64] Another 'disorder' of the sex instinct that Schrenck-Notzing and his contemporaries believed to be susceptible to hypnotic manipulation was homosexuality. In cases of sexual inversion or homosexuality, Moll had found that post-hypnotic suggestion could be used to eliminate or decrease a desire for men in his homosexual patients.[65] While he obtained good results by inculcating his patients with heterosexual ideas, he noted that the physician should not expect such treatment to be easy, given the deep roots of such inclinations.[66] That such therapy was not always successful was illustrated by Schrenck-Notzing, who related a case in which a man, who had undergone hypnotic therapy after his prosecution for homosexual sex, could not be rid of either his disgust for women or his desire for men, despite fifty-five inductions of hypnosis.[67] Schrenck-Notzing presented this case in the context of a larger paper on sexual psychopathology and the law, in which he, convinced like many of his colleagues that homosexuality was a medical rather than criminal problem, advocated the alteration of §175 of the German legal code, which criminalised sexual conduct between men.[68]

While such uses of suggestion indicated growing interest in hypnosis as a form of therapeutics, its application by German physicians remained limited even at the turn of the century. In 1902, the Kultus- und Erzeihung-Ministerium [Ministry for Culture and Education] launched an inquiry into the therapeutic potential of hypnosis, asking state medical councils to make submissions based on the experiences of physicians within their districts. A number of these regulatory bodies sent their members questionnaires, posing questions such as:

1. Have you ever applied hypnosis therapeutically?
2. What number and type of illnesses have you treated in this manner?
3. What experiences have you had with reference to the applicability of this therapy?
4. What have been your therapeutic successes?
5. Have you observed any injury of your patients as a result of the application of hypnosis?

The Aerztekammer für die Provinz Ostpreussen [State Medical Council for East Prussia] conducted a survey of this kind receiving 292 responses to the 682 questionnaires they had sent to doctors in their region.[69] A mere eighteen of these practitioners claimed to have used hypnosis therapeutically, the majority having done so on just one or two occasions, for the treatment of nervous disorders such as hysteria, neurasthenia and hypochondria, and complaints such as headache and toothache.[70] According to the respondents, they achieved good results with their patients, ameliorating their pain and discomfort without injury to their mental or physical health. Comparable results were recorded for the Rhine provinces and the Hohenzollern lands, where 106 of the 2,570 doctors questioned had applied hypnosis therapeutically.[71] In these regions, hypnosis was overwhelmingly utilised in the treatment of psychoses and nervous disorders, but had also gained favour in the treatment of impotence and substance abuse.

While this inquiry revealed the therapeutic potential of hypnosis, particularly in the treatment of nervous disorders, it demonstrated also, in the small number of practitioners who claimed to have made use of hypnosis or suggestion, German doctors' continued ignorance about and indifference to hypnotism.[72] Nearly twenty years after Moll's paper on the therapeutic use of hypnosis, universities appeared no closer to including this technique in their medical curricula than they had during the 1880s. Indeed, opposition to hypnosis as a medical therapy remained strong, as demonstrated by the commission of inquiry conducted by the Berlin–Brandenburg Aerztekammer [Berlin–Brandenburg Medical Council] into the matter. Auguste Forel noted that this commission, comprised of the physicians Aschenborn, Gock, Mendel and Munter had come to the conclusion that hypnosis was incapable of curing illnesses, arguing that it affected no organic change in diseases such as tuberculosis or cancer. While Forel did not dispute the inability of hypnosis to combat such afflictions, he pointed to the fact that academic medicine was equally incapable of defeating these diseases. Hypnosis, he argued, could at least offer the patient relief from pain and restful sleep.[73] The commission concluded their report with the recommendation that hypnosis be left on the stage, where they were in no doubt it belonged, and out of the consulting room.[74] The belief that hypnosis was a form of entertainment best suited to the theatre or cabaret was in direct contrast to the conviction of medical hypnotists such as Forel that hypnotism and suggestion were highly effective forms of therapy over which the medical community must achieve a monopoly.

Hypnotism and experimental psychology

While medical hypnotists continued throughout the 1880s and 1890s to promote the therapeutic use of hypnotic suggestion, their interest in hypnosis did not remain restricted to this potential to heal. A number of physicians and psychologists, for instance, became interested in hypnosis for the insights it promised into the human mind. Schrenck-Notzing, in particular, enthusiastically promoted hypnosis not only as an effective form of therapy for functional and behavioural problems, but also as the basis of a truly experimental psychology.[75] He told an audience in Munich on 16 January 1889 that:

> Through the methodical examination of hypnotic phenomena, through the positive and definite results attained thus far, which have yielded an interesting contribution to the problems of psychological and physiological life, we have now for the first time made the important field of experimental psychology possible and placed it on an even footing with every other type of scientific endeavour.[76]

A number of medical hypnotists, including Dessoir, Moll and Schrenck-Notzing, argued that the experimental use of hypnosis offered psychologists access to aspects of mental life, including sleep, dreams and the unconscious, which had previously been closed to them.[77] Indeed, enthusiasm for the use of hypnosis as a means of psychological introspection led some psychologists to declare that hypnotism was to the psychologist what vivisection was to the physiologist.[78] Of particular interest to these practitioners was the dynamic unconscious revealed by hypnosis. Moll wrote in this regard:

> That there *are* subconscious mental acts was known long before the advent of modern hypnotism. But what we owe to hypnotism is a new, almost ideal method of putting such acts to the test of experiment. In this connection hypnotism has proved most fruitful. Post-hypnotic suggestion shows us how delicate the workings of the secondary consciousness sometimes are....[79]

Experiments in both post-hypnotic suggestion and automatic writing allowed psychologists to probe this secondary consciousness and enabled speculation as to whether consciousness was essentially a unitary or fragmentary entity.

In Germany, as elsewhere during the late 1880s and 1890s, a number of psychologists utilised hypnotism and suggestion to engage with and study the phenomena of double consciousness. The best known of these studies in the German context was that of Max Dessoir, entitled *Das Doppel-Ich* [*The Double-Ego*] (1889).[80] Dessoir argued in this book that:

> We carry in us, as it were, a hidden sphere of consciousness, that, gifted with reason, feeling and will, is capable of determining a series of actions. The simultaneity of both spheres I call double consciousness.... It follows from this that our personality is composed from two operating conscious halves, more or less independent from one another, that one could figuratively call over- and under- consciousness.[81]

Dessoir's study of this phenomenon, like that of F.W.H. Myers of the Society for Psychical Research, was significant for its use of healthy rather than hysterical subjects on the basis of the belief that everyone, mentally sound or unsound, possessed at least two levels of consciousness held together by discrete chains of memory. Dessoir attempted to prove these contentions with a series of examples drawn from everyday life, psychopathology and the hypnotic state. In everyday life, Dessoir pointed to activities such as dressing oneself or walking a familiar route as examples of subconscious acts; in the field of psychopathology, he argued that dreams and spontaneous cases of double personality were indicative of another layer of consciousness; and in deep hypnotic, states he contended a preponderance of the secondary personality could be induced. The notion of a divided self, and of consciousness as something labile and fragmentary, changed the way that people understood the relationship between mind and body and allowed for speculation about the possibility of still more spheres of consciousness and about the existence of certain hidden powers of mind. Despite the excitement caused by these discoveries, there remained a number of physicians and psychologists who rejected hypnosis as a suitable tool for psychological introspection and remained suspicious of suggestion's therapeutic qualities.

Wundt, for example, proved himself a vocal critic of both the therapeutic and experimental use of hypnosis during the 1880s and 1890s. Placing hypnosis on a continuum with sleep and dreams, Wundt saw the hypnotic state primarily in terms of a loss of volition, which when frequently induced diminished a subject's power of resistance to suggestion. Convinced of the dangers of repeated hypnotisation, Wundt declared the therapeutic use of hypnosis two-edged. He wrote:

> It cannot be disputed that a cautious and intelligent use of suggestion may be of avail for the temporary, perhaps even for the permanent, removal of diseases due to functional derangement of the nervous system, or to harmful practices, like alcoholism or the morphine-habit…. [But] if its effects are strongest when the patient is predisposed to it in body and mind, or when suggestion has become a settled mode of treatment, it may obviously be employed to intensify or actually induce a pathological disposition. It must be looked upon, not as a remedy of universal serviceability, but as a poison whose effect may be beneficial under certain circumstances.[82]

Wundt was also convinced that hypnotic experiments were easily contaminated by unintentional suggestions on the part of the experimenter and others and that the loss of memory associated with hypnotic sleep made psychological introspection and observation of this state impossible.[83] The difficulty Wundt envisioned in performing accurate hypnotic experiments led him to conclude that the great majority of such experiments possessed no scientific value at all or led only to the discovery of interesting, but isolated phenomena of uncertain value to psychology.[84] Wundt also rejected the existence of double consciousness on the evidence of continuous memory from one hypnotic sleep to another saying that, 'it is wholly unnecessary to assume the existence of a mysterious mental double, the "other self" or second personality, or to set up any other fanciful hypotheses so plentiful in this field.'[85]

The therapeutic application of hypnosis was not, however, Wundt's primary concern. Responsible for the introduction of psychology to a laboratory setting and dedicated to establishing psychology as a scientific rather than a philosophical discipline, Wundt was angered by the way in which the term 'experimental psychology' had become associated almost exclusively with the experiments of so-called psychological societies; a reference to the Psychologische Gesellschaft in Munich and the Gesellschaft für Experimental-Psychologie in Berlin.[86] The interest of both occultists and medical hypnotists in thought transference and clairvoyance and their use of the label 'experimental psychology' to describe their endeavours threatened the academic respectability of Wundt's nascent science.[87] In this regard, Wundt was particularly critical of medical hypnotists, such as Dessoir, Forel and Moll, who combined an interest in hypnotic therapy with experimental studies of thought transference and clairvoyance. Such experiments, Wundt contended, blurred the boundaries between science, philosophy and mysticism.[88] On this point he declared:

> Most hypnotic investigators are either physicians, who employ suggestion for therapeutic purposes, or philosophers, who think that they have discovered in hypnotism a basis for new metaphysical systems, and who, instead of examining the phenomena in the light of well-established psychological laws, reverse the matter and erect their psychological superstructure upon hypnotic foundations.... Though there are found observers who have remained sane enough to hold aloof from all these absurdities, many even of them evince the fatal effect of the influence under which they have fallen by declaring these superstitions to be after all 'open questions', which deserve, if they do not demand, a closer examination.[89]

Moll, who held the impartial investigation of such matters to be legitimate, maintained that Wundt's *a priori* rejection of the study of the phenomena of hypnotic sleep was misguided.[90] Similarly, Schrenck-Notzing declared, 'The problem of mental suggestion is for us an open question; we have no prejudice in favour of any hypothesis, and are accessible to any information that may throw light on the subject.'[91] Wundt, however, argued that research into thought transference put scientific law in question, intimating the existence of two worlds; one governed by immutable universal laws and the other in which such laws were malleable.[92] He also maintained that the legitimisation of 'hypnotic mysticism' and its practice in societies for psychical research posed a threat to public health.

> The great danger is, that persons of insufficient medical training, working not for therapeutic ends, but 'in the interests of science' – though there is absolutely no guarantee of the real existence of their scientific devotion, – may exert an influence upon the mental and bodily life of their fellow-men such as, if continued for any length of time together, cannot fail to be injurious.[93]

The risk to mental health envisaged by Wundt was reminiscent of campaigns against lay practitioners such as Hansen in the preceding decades; his belief that hypnosis inevitably led to a weakening of the nervous system was similar to that of Charcot. He warned Dessoir on this point that the study of mediumship, telepathy and clairvoyance was a dubious scientific endeavour given the massive amateur interest in the topic.[94] These were criticisms which medical hypnotists could not ignore and which they attempted to deal with in the course of their campaign against the lay use of hypnosis.

The medical campaign against quackery

For those physicians determined to establish hypnosis and suggestion as legitimate and scientific forms of medical therapy, their use by lay healers and performers posed a number of pressing problems. If, for example, as Ewald had suggested during Moll's 1886 lecture to the Berliner medizinische Gesellschaft, any shepherd, shoemaker or tailor could induce hypnosis, what particular claim could medical hypnotists have to expertise in this field? How was hypnosis as practised by physicians different from that which astounded audiences during stage performances and spiritualist séances? In order to answer these questions, to dissociate medical hypnosis from the practices of stage mesmerists, lay healers and spiritualists, and to ensure a medical monopoly of hypnotism and suggestion, medical hypnotists conducted an aggressive campaign against the non-medical use of hypnosis. Their primary concern was to push for legislation that would guarantee their monopoly and criminalise or pathologise the use of hypnosis by those without medical qualifications. These efforts reflected the precarious grasp that medicine had on a recently appropriated domain and the broader concern of the German medical community, which had emerged with national unification, to exclude lay practitioners from the medical marketplace and to gain for themselves a monopoly over all aspects of health.[95] Medical hypnotists' attempts to address these problems can thus be understood in the context of a specific debate over the use of hypnotism and suggestion, and in the context of the medical community's campaign to obliterate quackery.[96]

During the closing decades of the nineteenth century, representatives of 'Schulmedizin' [academic medicine] in Germany felt their scientific prestige and social position threatened by lay practitioners, whose promotion of natural or folk medicine put them in direct competition with doctors. This perceived vulnerability was due to a number of cultural and political factors. Despite tangible advances – breakthroughs in areas such as aseptic surgery and bacteriology – and increases in both the standard of living and life expectancy, many Germans were disillusioned with official medicine because of the apparent inability of doctors to combat illness and disease.[97] This disillusionment was a result not just of a belief in medicine's impotence, but also of concern about the effects of modern life, as epitomised by industrialisation and urbanisation, on health. In their search for alternatives, a considerable number of Germans turned to natural medicine and lifestyle reform, while others resorted to hypnotic treatment, prayer healing and patented cure-alls. These services and medicines were available from a host of lay practitioners who had developed a lucrative niche alongside official medicine during the mid-nineteenth century, catering to the popular demand for healthcare.[98] Although, under the elaborate medical hierarchies operating in the German states prior to Unification, lay medicine was technically illegal, lay practitioners were considered a necessary part of the medical infrastructure and seldom faced prosecution.[99] With the foundation of the Reich and the collapse of this finely gradated system in favour of the 'Gewerbeordnung' [trading regulations] that began operation in the North German League in 1869 and in the German Reich in 1871, doctors found themselves having to compete with lay healers on an equal basis.[100] As a result, forms of popular self-help and lay medical practice that had been tolerated by doctors during the mid-nineteenth century were condemned as public health hazards during the 1880s and 1890s as the medical profession sought to regain and consolidate their power through an aggressive campaign to monopolise healthcare and stigmatise lay medicine.[101]

The medical community's opposition to 'Kurpfuscherei' [quackery] took the form of letters and petitions, often from 'Ärztekammern' [local medical councils], demanding the imposition of fines or jail sentences for those who practised medicine without the appropriate qualifications.[102] In 1903, this opposition was formalised with the foundation of a Deutsche Gesellschaft zur Bekämpfung des Kurpfuschertums [German Society for the Combat of Quackery], the purpose of this society was to convince the public of the danger that lay practitioners posed to both health and finance and to instruct

101

them in the most effective means of dealing with illness.[103] This attempt to educate Germans about quackery was not restricted to the publication of health warnings in the popular press, but extended to the public exhibition of, and exhortation against, the dubious, even dangerous, methods utilised by unqualified practitioners. An exhibition sponsored by the Deutsche Gesellschaft zur Bekämpfung des Kurpfuschertums in Breslau during 1904, for example, featured electro-homeopathy, magnetism, and exorbitantly priced cure-alls, as well as displays intended to document both the legal status of quackery within the German Reich and the attempts of private citizens and the state to combat it.[104] The society was also active as a lobbying body, petitioning lawmakers to impose heavy penalties on those quacks who courted the public in newspapers and magazines with promises of miraculous remedies for every kind of affliction.

While the majority of doctors were of the opinion that the threat posed by lay practitioners to their professional ambitions and public health required some kind of solution, not all were convinced that the imposition of legislation against such practices would be either beneficial or effective. In March 1899, for example, the *Berliner Tagesblatt*, noting the efforts of the medical community to eradicate quackery, quoted an elderly physician who suggested that a 'Kurpfuschereiverbot' [ban on quackery] might prove counter-productive. Such a prohibition, he argued, would impede the exchange between doctors and lay practitioners from which medicine had benefited in the past and was likely to result in a public backlash given its interference with the right to self-determination.[105] Similar concerns were voiced by representatives of the Berliner Heilgehülfen Verein [Berlin Medical Assistance Society] who reminded the Minister of the Interior that should doctors succeed in banning either the remuneration of non-medical healing practices, including massage and baths, or the freedom to advertise such services, the Reich would lose the revenue produced by around twenty-thousand tax-payers.[106] Despite such misgivings, the prohibition of lay medicine was formalised in 1902 with legislation that made the public advertisement of remedies and cures punishable by fines of up to sixty Marks.[107] These penalties were levied not only against lay practitioners like Max Sonnenmann, whose advertisements in two Berlin newspapers guaranteed the cure of all skin, urine, bladder, kidney and female complaints, but also against the publications in which they appeared.[108] In 1904, the Interior Ministry's commission to combat quackery discussed drafts of a far more punitive law. This draft legislation provided for the prosecution of those unqualified individuals who treated people and animals from afar ['Fernbehandlung' or distant treatment], provided treatment for sexually transmitted diseases or attempted cures with hypnosis and suggestion. Under this new law anyone caught publicly advertising or extolling the virtues of these treatments was to face up to one year in prison and a three-thousand Mark fine.[109] The inability of such legal measures to adequately deal with the problem of lay medicine, however, was reflected in the drafting of numerous laws against *Kurpfuscherei* in the decades that followed. In no other area, however, was this failure as explicit as in the medical community's struggle to combat lay hypnosis and suggestion.

Medical hypnotists and lay practitioners

The campaign against the practice of hypnotism and suggestion by lay healers and occultists, which took place in a series of books, pamphlets, governmental reports and lectures, acknowledged that the work of stage mesmerists and lay healers had played a crucial role in introducing German physicians to hypnosis, but argued that contemporary lay hypnotists' performances were now not only superfluous, but detrimental to advances in the field.[110] On this point, Moll stated:

> It is perfectly true that at one time such public exhibitions served to draw the attention of scientists to hypnotism, but nowadays they are more calculated to repel people from the scientific study of that question, since they degrade hypnosis into an object of vulgar curiosity, instead of elevating it to one of research.[111]

In the same vein, Schrenck-Notzing wrote that, 'the purpose of such performances, namely to direct the attention of science towards hypnotic phenomena, has been today without a doubt accomplished.'[112] Medical hypnotists, while cognisant of the pivotal role played by itinerant mesmerists such as Donato and Hansen, feared that a connection with the sensational performances of lay hypnotists might further threaten the possibility of establishing hypnosis as both a legitimate form of medical therapy and as a tool of psychological investigation.[113] This seemed a strong possibility in the existing climate of hostility, on the part of a number of physicians and psychologists, towards the medical use of hypnotism and suggestion. In order to dissociate themselves from the theatrics of stage mesmerists and spiritualists, medical hypnotists began to charge lay hypnotists with both ignorance and the endangerment of their patients' health.

Medical hypnotists attempted to portray hypnosis practised by amateurs as inherently dangerous, a technique that threatened to compromise the physical, psychological and moral health of both individuals and entire populations. They argued that the incompetence of lay hypnotists led inevitably to physical or psychological injury and that unscrupulous lay hypnotists possessed the means both to render their victims helpless against sexual attack and to induce them to commit crimes against others. Lay hypnotists' ignorance of contra-indications and their inability to establish whether their patients suffered pre-existing conditions was utilised by medical hypnotists to prove that lay practitioners could not be trusted to induce hypnosis safely. Schrenck-Notzing argued that:

> [T]he amateur hypnotist can not know how things stand in relation to his victim's health, that perhaps he has a heart condition, that perhaps as the result of an inherited burden he carries within him a propensity to epileptic fits, to mental illness or to hysteria....[114]

He made a similar point referring to the lay hypnotist's lack of technical skill, stating that 'through incorrect manipulation of the experimental subject latent dispositions to sicknesses, hysteria, epilepsy, psychopathological attacks and the like, could be awoken.'[115] Even Moll, who had argued that medical hypnosis did not have any detrimental effects, stated that:

> [W]e should never think of denying the possibility of mental disorders being caused by the unscientific use of hypnotism; such cases have repeatedly been reported, especially after some public hypnotiser has made his appearance – for example, by Finkelnberg in connection with Hansen's public experiments, by Lombroso in connection with Donato's....[116]

In order to prove this point Moll, Schrenck-Notzing and others, provided the details of numerous cases in which dormant tendencies to conditions such as hysteria had been awoken by the so-called 'unscientific' use of hypnotism. These examples were of two varieties. The first concerned individuals who had been injured in the course of amateur hypnotic experiments and pointed to provisions within the existing legal codes of European countries to punish such offences. The second involved the injury of groups of people, and pushed for legislation to ban lay performances of hypnosis in both public and private.

Schrenck-Notzing claimed to have treated a large number of individuals who had suffered injury to their health as a result of having been hypnotised by amateurs.[117] He wrote:

> We ourselves have had the opportunity during the last year to observe no less than six people in Munich whose health had been injured by serving as mediums at the spiritualist experiments of amateurs. One of these cases concerned a journeyman tailor, a second concerned an agent and the third concerned a sculptor. All three people displayed marked signs of male hysteria, that had been artificially provoked for the first time as a result of these experiments....[118]

For some of these unfortunates, Schrenck-Notzing warned, the prognosis was bleak – they would end their days in asylums – but further abuses could be prevented by the apprehension and prosecution of lay hypnotists.[119] There already existed within the German legal code, as Moll and Schrenck-Notzing demonstrated, provisions for the prosecution of similar crimes, which could be used to litigate against lay hypnotists in cases of injury or criminal conduct under hypnosis. For example, injury as a result of negligence, particularly if the negligent party was a so-called 'charlatan', was punishable under German law by two years in jail.[120] A precedent also existed for the punishment of crimes committed against hypnotised subjects in the law covering offences against individuals in non-volitional states induced by chloroform, narcotics or spirits.[121] These laws, however, were not so readily applicable in instances in which lay hypnotists caused psychological or moral harm to communities or groups. For this reason, medical hypnotists were concerned to provide examples of mass injury caused by hypnosis and to stress the necessity of police bans on public displays of hypnotism similar to those instigated in Italy, Belgium and Switzerland.

The danger posed not only to individuals, but to whole communities, by amateur demonstrations of mesmerism and hypnotism in public places as well as in homes and clubs, was stressed in Schrenck-Notzing's claim that:

> A great danger, today as always, is presented by unsystematic hypnotic experiments, which are carried out to gratify spectacle hungry crowds in public locales, or as is often the case in Germany, in closed societies, spiritualist clubs, somnambule cabinets or in salons. It is well known that such stimuli have given rise to hypnotic epidemics (e.g. in Breslau, Pforzheim, Milan, in barracks, boys' schools, guesthouses etc.).[122]

Such epidemics were not without precedent, according to Schrenck-Notzing, who saw mass suggestion at work in many facets of social life, including religion, fashion, politics and the press, with fanaticism and superstition being particularly contagious.[123] There was no doubt in Schrenck-Notzing's mind that psychic epidemics of this type had led to the commission of crimes, an example of which was anarchism. These epidemics, instances of mass suggestion, were believed also to have implications for civil unrest. In Germany, just as in Italy, the debate over the lay use of hypnosis impacted on questions about the inherent suggestibility of women and the masses and entered into the new science of crowds.[124] Government interest in hypnosis and suggestion was not, however, restricted to concern about their implications for civil unrest, but turned, thanks to medical hypnotists' efforts, to the possibility of using them as a form of mass education. In 1902, the Prussian government commissioned a report on the medical uses of hypnosis, with a particular focus on the use of mass suggestion in efforts to educate populations about tuberculosis and venereal diseases.[125]

Whether the threat imagined by medical hypnotists was real, or the number of lay hypnotists as great as was purported, remains unclear. A survey conducted by the Reich government between 1902 and 1903, however, suggests that medical hypnotists' claims were probably exaggerated. To the question of whether they knew of any cases in which hypnosis had been utilised by unqualified persons for therapeutic purposes and whether these had resulted in injury, officials from Aurich, Hanover, Königsberg, and Merseburg overwhelmingly answered in the negative. Respondents from Merseburg, for example, noted four cases of lay hypnosis, but remained unclear as to whether this treatment had been helpful or harmful.[126] Nevertheless, in July 1903, the Minister der geistlichen Unterrichts- und Medizinalan-gelegenheiten [Minister for Religious Instruction and Medical Affairs], chose to remind police departments throughout the country of a decree, dated 12 May 1881, in which the public performance of so-called magnetism had been banned because of the potential harm to those people used as mediums during such displays. As a result of a case in which severe injury had resulted, he wanted to remind the police that magnetism, suggestion and hypnosis should be considered synonymous and treated accordingly.

Medical hypnotists' attempts to discredit lay hypnosis were not limited to warnings about its dangers, but included efforts to impugn the moral and mental health of unlicensed practitioners.[127] In an article on magnetic healing that appeared in 1907, Moll mentioned an exhibition on charlatanism held at the Reichstag, in which statistics on the prosecution of charlatans appeared under the heading, 'The Moral Inferiority of Charlatans'. Moll's years of experience with such dubious characters had convinced him, he wrote, not only of the propensity to criminality that such statistics illustrated, but also of the mental abnormality of charlatans, particularly magnetists and lay hypnotists.[128] The majority of these people, Moll maintained, were psychopaths, a fact that he believed might deter the public's consultation of lay practitioners, more than exorbitant fines.[129] Accusations of mental illness served to undermine lay hypnotists' claims to expertise and efficacy in a particularly effective manner, pathologising both the practice and the practitioners. The use of the pathology metaphor was a strategy that Moll and others were to employ to great effect during the Weimar Republic in their campaign against a number of prominent parapsychologists.[130]

The final task of the medical hypnotists' campaign to criminalise the use of hypnosis by amateurs was to 'sanitise' their own use of it by proving that in the capable hands of physicians, hypnotism and suggestion were not only benign, but beneficial. By analogy with other branches of medicine and with established means of treatment, medical hypnotists suggested that their superior medical skill and knowledge were protection against hypnotic injury and that their respectability guaranteed against the criminal or sexual exploitation of patients during the hypnotic state. Comparing a number of other therapies with hypnosis in order to establish the necessity of its application by a physician, Schrenck-Notzing wrote:

> No medicine of lasting effect on our bodies, regardless of whether one thinks about surgery, about pharmacology, electricity or hydrotherapy, can be said to be absolutely without danger – just as psychotherapy in the guise of hypnotic suggestion is not. As in all other branches of medicine, the measure of hypnosis' danger depends on the technical (here psychological) certainty, the knowledge and experience of the doctor.[131]

While not denying that there existed certain dangers even with the medical use of hypnosis, medical hypnotists argued, often by constructing analogies between hypnotism and certain labile drugs, that the safety of the procedure depended almost exclusively upon the skill and expertise of the practitioner. Schrenck-Notzing stressed that:

> Hypnotism must only be applied by doctors, in the hands of empirics and charlatans it presents the same dangers as the application of deadly substances, like the application of morphine and digitalis by people that do not have adequate previous expertise at their disposal.[132]

Playing on fears inspired by the obsession of both the sensational and medical press with crime and hypnosis, medical hypnotists used an analogy between the loss of volition experienced in hypnosis and that induced by chemical anaesthetics to indicate the necessity of a trustworthy experimenter in the course of any application of hypnosis. Moll wrote:

> The temporary loss of the will can hardly be considered an objection to hypnotic therapeutics from the ethical standpoint, though it has occasionally been brought forward. If it were, we should have to give up all administration of chloroform, for there is a loss of will in chloroform narcosis. The main point is to choose a trustworthy experimenter. We only take chloroform from a person we can trust to administer the anaesthetic without danger, and whom we believe will take no advantage of the loss of will induced.[133]

The concerns highlighted by this campaign were not exclusive to German medical hypnotists, but were instead common to medical hypnotists from a number of countries. This was demonstrated by the declaration of over one hundred doctors in Paris during the 1888 conference of the International Association for Hypnotism that:

1) All public demonstrations of hypnosis are to be forbidden by the authorities;
2) The practical application of hypnotism for therapeutic and scientific purposes is to be regulated by law;
3) It is desirable that the study and the application of hypnotism be considered in medical instruction.[134]

In Germany, while these aims were pursued, they were compromised not only by the activities of lay hypnotists, who evaded surveillance and prosecution by performing in homes and private clubs, but also by those medical hypnotists whose interest in the ostensibly paranormal phenomena of hypnosis blurred the boundaries they were trying to establish between the medical and lay use of hypnosis.

The retreat from psychical research

During the 1880s, Dessoir, Moll and Schrenck-Notzing had indulged their interest in hypnosis both in their private clinics and in the psychological societies of Munich and Berlin where somnambulists, such as Lina Matzinger, demonstrated feats of thought-transference and clairvoyance. While none of these men had sought to establish a system of metaphysics based on these phenomena, the distinction they had drawn between their 'experimental psychology' and the 'transcendental psychology' of du Prel seemed less than adequate in the face of their campaign to eradicate lay hypnosis. The difficulty was that the experiments conducted with somnambulists and mediums bore a striking resemblance to the domestic séances and stage performances they so roundly condemned; even though the paradigms with which they attempted to explain paranormal phenomena were vastly different from those utilised by occultists and mesmerists. The open-minded attitude with which these medical hypnotists approached paranormal phenomena also posed a problem if they wanted to be taken seriously within Germany's medical and scientific communities. As Wundt had pointed out, to accept the reality of thought-transference and clairvoyance was to accept the malleability of scientific laws.[135] In this context, an animist approach, which tended to view the physical phenomena experienced in spiritualist séances as the result of hallucination or fraud, but admitted the possibility that psychical phenomena such as thought-transference and clairvoyance might constitute real mental abilities, was professionally dangerous to maintain. For Dessoir and Moll the answer appeared to be to retreat from psychical research and to take up a new position known as 'critical occultism'.

Critical occultism, which interpreted both physical and psychical phenomena naturalistically, allowed its proponents to retain an interest in paranormal research without fear of the pseudo-scientific taint that had become attached to psychical research. Unlike the animist explanatory paradigm in which the possibility of thought-transference and clairvoyance remained open, this new approach attributed all apparent cases of these phenomena to fraud, unconscious physical cues, errors in perception or the psychological problems of those who witnessed them. This approach allowed Dessoir and Moll to secure their reputations as scientists and to dismiss the competing knowledge claims of the mesmerists, spiritualists and psychical researchers with whom they competed for epistemic authority over hypnosis.[136] Ultimately, then, this new paradigm dealt with the epistemological and professional threat posed by the paranormal and those who studied it by psychologising them.[137]

Taking up critical occultism during the 1890s, Dessoir and Moll published works in which ostensibly paranormal phenomena were explained naturalistically, primarily as the products of suggestion. In this manner, these medical hypnotists were able to demystify hypnosis, demonstrating that mesmerism did not involve an invisible magnetic fluid and deconstruct spiritualism, showing that the two or more distinct personalities manifested by mediums during somnambulistic trance were not a result of spirit possession. The appearance of such tracts reflected medical hypnotists' desire to monopolise the therapeutic and psychological use of hypnosis and the increasingly public profile of lay hypnotists and healers whose presence in both the courtroom and the press became more frequent during this era. In the hands of men such as Dessoir and Moll, hypnosis and suggestion therefore became powerful weapons of scientific enlightenment and explanation, wielded against the moral, mental and professional threat of lay medicine and its bedfellow occultism.[138]

The use of magnetism by lay practitioners for therapeutic purposes represented a direct challenge to medical hypnotists, who saw in 'Heilmagnetismusa' [therapeutic magnetism] needless mystification of hypnosis and a threat to their monopoly over its use. In a work intended for medical witnesses, who were increasingly faced in Berlin's courtrooms with cases of an occult kind, Moll attempted to demystify magnetism, explain its relationship to hypnosis and outline the dangers associated with its therapeutic use by amateurs. Magnetism, Moll explained, differed from hypnosis in that it was understood to involve the influence of one person on another by means of an invisible fluid, focused by the magnetist's will and transmitted by magnetic strokes, rather than by suggestion.[139] All of magnetism's wondrous effects could be explained, according to Moll, through recourse either to suggestion or simple physical explanation. The cataleptic rigidity and analgesia frequently induced by magnetists in their patients as proof of magnetic power, for example, could be explained through suggestion rather than a mysterious fluid capable of paralysing and anaesthetising the body.[140] While suggestion explained many such magnetic effects, some ostensibly paranormal events associated with mesmerism appeared to be the result of physical causes. The ability of people to tell the difference between magnetised water and non-magnetised water, for example, was due, Moll argued, to the movement of the magnetist's hands above the water. This allowed chemical material, dust and other particles from the skin to mix with the water, subtly altering its flavour.[141]

Magnetism's use by lay people as both palliative and curative, however, was Moll's main concern. He attempted to list here the most common sources of error leading to a belief in the efficacy of therapeutic magnetism. Autosuggestion or expectation, he wrote, often accounted for a patient's improvement or recovery after visiting a magnetist, as did the spontaneous improvement or remission typical of diseases, such as cancer.[142] It was also common for magnetists to prescribe dietary changes, baths or pills, which might account for any improvement in a patient's health. Perhaps more significant, however, was the fact that many magnetists wrongly diagnosed their patients' illnesses. False diagnosis accounted for those cases in which people recovered from incurable aliments or diseases in the wake of a visit to a magnetist. This point was demonstrated in another work also in which Moll attempted to demystify Christian Science. According to Moll, the healing powers of Mary Baker-Eddy (1821–1910) and her followers were a result of faulty diagnosis and suggestion. He wrote:

> The belief of a patient, that he will be healed by the use of this or that
> medicine, works in a suggestive manner. And in this respect we can explain
> it through suggestion, when people, who trust in Christian Science, become
> better through this treatment.[143]

The dangers of this mixture of misdiagnosis and belief were serious. While faith healing might seem a harmless, if ludicrous, fashion, its rejection of academic medicine, Moll argued, could prove dangerous if not fatal.

Such critiques were not limited to magnetism, but were used to account for occult phenomena. Dessoir, in his work *Der Doppel-Ich*, utilised his theory of a secondary consciousness to explain the phenomena of spiritualism, including automatic writing and trance speech.

> Thoughts, which slumber in the deepest depths of the soul and therefore
> appear foreign to the individual, show themselves in the remarkable

movements of automatic writing and trance speech. No wonder that such messages of a second sphere of consciousness on which the personality fully synthesises as messages from the realm of ghosts.[144]

These analyses were attempts to provide naturalistic explanations for ostensibly paranormal phenomena and to provide psychological explanations, ranging from lapses in concentration and errors of perception to neurotic fantasies, for belief in the occult. Dessoir, for example, made a study of the psychology of conjuring, reflecting on the fallible nature of the senses and the manner in which conjurers took advantage of such sensory weaknesses.[145]

The exigencies of their campaign to have hypnosis accepted as a medical therapy and to ensure a medical monopoly of this form of psychotherapeutics necessitated self-policing on the part of Dessoir and Moll, who moved away from their early advocacy of psychical research – a position predicated on an open-minded attitude toward paranormal phenomena – to a new stance on the occult known as critical occultism. The epistemological lens offered by this new approach allowed nearly every instance of the paranormal to be seen in terms of suggestion, fraud or delusion. The desire of Dessoir and Moll to claim hypnosis and suggestion for medicine, to regulate its use and meaning, forced them largely to abandon their interest in the phenomena of mediumship and to posit naturalistic explanations for the unusual phenomena concomitant with hypnotic trance. Their colleague, Schrenck-Notzing, however, chose a different path. He did not abandon his interest in the phenomena of somnambulism and mediumship or his open-mindedness about the reality and significance of such phenomena. Furthermore, he continued to present his findings in forums that blurred the borders between science, entertainment and spiritualism, creating an irrevocable split between him and his former colleagues.

Schrenck-Notzing and the *Traumtänzerin*

The theatrical vulgarisation of hypnosis, with which medical hypnotists had charged stage hypnotists and spiritualists during the 1880s and 1890s, had not been entirely absent from their own demonstrations of hypnotism and suggestion. Experiments in hypnosis and post-hypnotic suggestion, conducted by Schrenck-Notzing in a crowded auditorium in Munich during 1889, had caused widespread amusement when one somnambule, convinced he was an African adventurer, attempted to solicit members of the audience for his colonial army in South Africa, and when another somnambule, in the belief he was Bismarck, had addressed the audience as members of the Reichstag.[146] As we have seen, medical hypnotists, including

Dessoir, Moll and Schrenck-Notzing, campaigned throughout the last two decades of the nineteenth century to criminalise similar demonstrations on the part of non-medical hypnotists and to dissociate and sanitise their use of hypnosis in both therapeutics and psychological investigation from any connection with what they saw as the vulgar and unscientific performances of stage mesmerists and spiritualists. In 1904, however, Schrenck-Notzing embarked on a course, which would alienate him from his peers, sponsoring and promoting the kind of public performances against which he and other medical hypnotists had fought so vigorously throughout the 1880s and 1890s. His fascination with a young French woman by the name of Magdeleine G., a so-called 'Traumtänzerin' [dream- or sleep-dancer], and his conviction that her performances were of both scientific and artistic significance, signified his entrenchment within psychical research with its animist explanatory paradigm and his distance from the critical–psychological approach to occult phenomena adopted by Dessoir and Moll. This episode also marked his first steps towards becoming Germany's foremost propagandist of parapsychological research.

Schrenck-Notzing, who met the sleep-dancer Magdeleine G. in Paris during 1903, engaged her to perform for a number of Munich-based clubs and societies, members of which were interested in the scientific and artistic possibilities of her somnambulistic demonstrations of dance and pantomime. Sponsored and hosted by the Psychologische Gesellschaft, these performances enabled Munich's artistic and medical élite to investigate this fascinating and potentially significant phenomenon. Under the tutelage of her impresario and magnetist Magnin, Magdeleine was paraded in front of close to four thousand people during private demonstrations in the Bavarian capital, performing a host of hypnotically inspired waltzes, marches and pavanes to the music of Chopin and Wagner. The sensation caused by her lithe movements and classically clad form created demand for a series of public performances in Munich, Stuttgart and Berlin, which titillated the German public in a manner that did little to promote the scientific or therapeutic potential of hypnosis, but which did inspire a host of imitators in cabarets and variétés throughout Germany.[147] While Magdeleine's supporters touted the scientific and artistic significance of her somnambulistic performances, comparing them to those of contemporary actresses and dancers such as Sarah Bernhardt and Isadora Duncan, critics argued that they served only to strengthen the connection between hypnotism and the theatrics of stage mesmerists, rendering them of negligible scientific value. The debate that Schrenck-Notzing's promotion of the *Traumtänzerin* inspired, highlighted not only the fact that there existed enormous interest in the artistic possibilities of unconscious states, but that the separation that medical hypnotists desired to achieve between medical hypnosis, occultism and lay practitioners was by no means complete.

Magdeleine G., a Parisian woman of around thirty years of age, married with two small children, had gone to the magnetist Magnin during the winter of 1902/3 in the hope that he might be able to cure the severe headaches from which she suffered.[148] After a small number of mesmeric treatments, Magnin noticed that while in trance his patient exhibited an extraordinary artistic sensitivity to music, dancing in a highly expressive and technically sophisticated manner, in spite of a lack of formal training in dance. In the wake of this discovery, Magnin began to exhibit Magdeleine in venues throughout the French capital, where Schrenck-Notzing first saw her in 1903. The performances that so impressed Schrenck-Notzing and which he exported to Munich involved an induction of trance by Magnin, followed by instrumental music or verse to which the somnambulist responded immediately with impassioned dance or mime. Depending on the mood of the piece played or recited, Magdeleine's movements could take on a religious solemnity or a Dionysian fervour, that her supporters believed was worthy of the greatest actresses of the day. Her rendition of Salomé, for example, impressed her audience for its resemblance to performances of Oscar Wilde's play of the same name.[149] These demonstrations, the prelude to which was often a short talk on both Magdeleine's medical history and hypnotic theory, also afforded audiences an opportunity to witness and in some cases to test for themselves the phenomena associated with hypnosis and suggestion. Physicians who attended these performances, for example, were encouraged to manipulate the sleep-dancer's limbs in order to ascertain the presence of catalepsy, a reliable indicator of the hypnotic state.[150] According to Schrenck-Notzing, who first introduced Magdeleine and Magnin to a Munich audience in February 1904, the sleep-dancer's debut marked an important event in both the history of psychology and of theatre; her peculiar form of somnambulistic phenomena being of great psychological and artistic significance.[151]

The psychological value of these demonstrations, according to Schrenck-Notzing, was the manner in which they showcased hypnosis as a means of freeing the consciousness from social and cultural inhibitions, thereby unleashing innate talents and primal inspiration.[152] In Magdeleine's case, hypnosis appeared to promote a dramatic and choreographic talent typical of the eastern European folk improvisation that formed her Romanian heritage, a talent to which she did not have access in the waking state.[153] The sleep-dancer's somnambulistic pantomime also helped elucidate the problematic relationship between hysteria and artistic talent. The physicians who examined Magdeleine during her time in Germany diagnosed her with a mild form of hysteria, which rendered her particularly susceptible to

Image 2.1

The Traumtänzerin Magdeleine G. at the Munich Schauspielhaus, 1904.
Reproduced with permission from the Institut für Grenzgebiete der Psychologie
und Psychohygiene e. V., Freiburg im Breisgau (private collection).

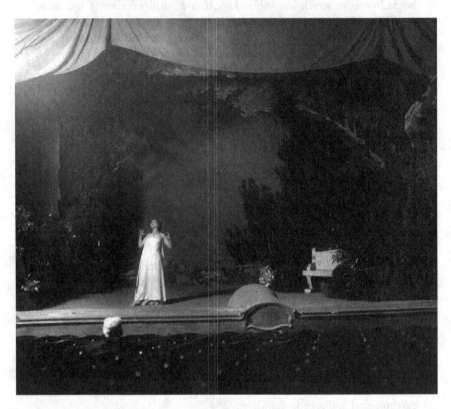

suggestion and which manifested itself most spectacularly when it combined with her innate genius for movement in the hypnotic state. Schrenck-Notzing speculated that the hysterical temperament which lent Magdeleine's performances their passion was present in all great actresses, as witnessed by the tears produced by Sarah Bernhardt and Eleonora Duse in tragic roles.[154] The interest in, and popularity of, Magdeleine's somnambulistic dance was a result, not only of this widespread fascination with hypnosis as a mechanism by which to access the creative recesses of the mind, but also of certain artistic currents evident in Munich during the *fin de siècle*.

The modernist movement in Munich emerged during the 1890s as a response to moribund liberalism, censorious political Catholicism and official neo-classicism, interacting with both the new commercial mass-culture and traditional popular culture.[155] In the theatre this translated into a rejection of those forms that privileged the spoken word and an embrace of physical performance, including clowning, acrobatics, dance and pantomime, which allowed modernist playwrights not only to escape the problematic bonds of language, but to flout a sensuality that was at once transgressive of Catholic mores and appealing to a mass market.[156] Expressionist actors attempted to approximate the properties of dance, mime and sculpture in order to embody a range of human spiritual conditions and to physically express abstract ideas, rather than to play out mimetic images which exemplified these conditions.[157] In its focus on poetic image, as opposed to psychological insight, modern theatre began increasingly to resemble vaudeville, a form of amusement that combined songs, acrobatic stunts, magic tricks and animal acts to become the most dominant form of urban entertainment in Imperial Germany.[158] In this context, Magdeleine's appearance at Munich's Schauspielhaus, home of modernist theatre in the Bavarian capital, the repertoire of which included Max Halbe's *Jugend,* Oscar Wilde's *Salomé,* and Gerhart Hauptmann's *Biberpelz,* begins to make sense (see Image 2.1).[159]

A modernist approach was apparent in the plastic and visual arts also, where a revolt against the official salon occurred, the impetus for which came from a group known as the Munich Secession who encouraged the exploration of new artistic directions, including naturalism and impressionism.[160] The rejection by Munich's avant-garde of official art, politics and religion also helped explain their interest in occultism, which informed the thinking and the art of a number of Munich based artists and writers including Fidus (Hugo Höppener) (1868–1948), Stefan George (1868–1933), Ludwig Klages (1872–1956), and Wassily Kandinsky (1866–1944).[161] As a result of both pragmatic and aesthetic concerns some of these artists employed mediumship and mysticism as forms of artistic inspiration. The artists Adolf Bayersdorfer, Albert von Keller, Gabriel von Max and Wilhelm Trübner, all of whom were members of the Psychologische Gesellschaft, composed a series of sketches and paintings during the 1880s and 1890s on occult and mystical themes using somnambulists and mediums as artistic models.[162] This community's embrace of a range of occult philosophies was noted by a Stuttgart newspaper, which wrote that members of the Munich Secession, had been almost as interested in occultism during the 1890s as they were in art.[163] Magdeleine's Munich triumph thus occurred in a context where not only her dance and pantomime were met by appreciative audiences, but where the occult elements of her performance were guaranteed to pique the interest of artists and art theorists.

Image 2.2

The Traumtänzerin Magdeleine G., Munich, 1904.
Reproduced with permission from the Institut für Grenzgebiete der Psychologie
und Psychohygiene e. V., Freiburg im Breisgau (private collection).

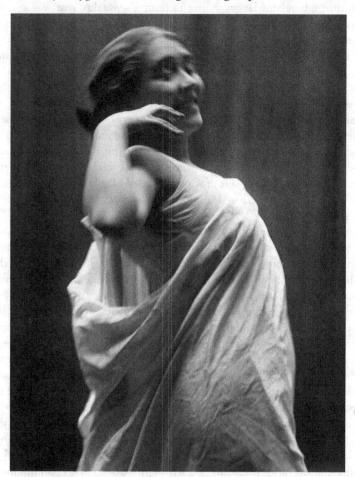

The questions that emerged from Magdeleine's demonstrations overwhelmingly concerned the connection between creative acts and somnambulism, the significance of which was debated both in the theatres and auditoriums in which she performed and in the press. Reviews of the sleep-dancer's somnambulistic feats, which appeared in newspapers in Munich and Stuttgart, suggested that dramatic expression in its highest form existed on a continuum with somnambulism, drawing its power from the unconscious rather than from the conscious mind or reason.[164] Indeed, the ecstatic highs attained by actresses such as Charlotte Wolter in her role as Medea, and Eleonora Duse as Magda in Hermann Sudermann's *Heimat* could be understood as approaching this state. The artists, art theorists and critics who attended the sleep-dancer's performances also asked themselves what art in the widest sense – that is, mime, dance, painting and plastic – could learn, and usefully adapt, from Magdeleine's somnambulism?[165] Schrenck-Notzing, in his book on the *Traumtänzerin*, argued that her principal value to the artist was as a type of human still life, from which he or she could work in cases where an impression of the subject matter would otherwise be difficult to attain.[166] Albert von Keller, one of the founders of the Munich Secession and a leader of the Munich avant-garde had used hypnotised models like Lina, whose poses and gestures he could manipulate either manually or by placing them in front of a painting to suggest a certain emotional or psychological expression, since the 1880s.[167] Excited by Charcot and Richer's study of demonic possession in art, which had revealed Andrea del Sarto's and Philippino Lippi's use of hysterics and ecstatics as models, Keller began to use somnambulistic mediums to achieve psychological and spiritual depth in his paintings.[168] From the numerous photographs taken of Magdeleine he painted no less than twenty portraits, many of which featured the *Traumtänzerin* as Cassandra.[169]

According to Schrenck-Notzing, Magdeleine's performances also offered a curative for the dramatic arts, where training and convention often inhibited artistic inspiration.[170] The raw passion and spontaneity that was a feature of the sleep-dancer's somnambulistic pantomime, would, if they could be harnessed, prove an enormous asset to both the actor and the dancer. Choreography, informed by the unconscious, he argued, would utilise gesticulation and mime to express emotional experience in the most complete way possible.[171] The uninhibited naturalness of somnambulistic dancers would suffuse ballet, in particular, with a passion that was often absent due to the constraints of tradition and imagination. This was just the sort of expressive power that Isadora Duncan exhibited during her 1904 performances in Berlin, where her inspired improvisational interpretations of the music of Gluck, Beethoven and Chopin captivated the stage designer Gordon Craig.[172] The ecstatic quality of Duncan's dance, Schrenck-Notzing maintained, was similar to that exhibited in Magdeleine's somnambulistic waltzes and pavanes. Indeed, Duncan's performances, with their reference to Hellenistic dance, demonstrated for him, that significant steps had already been taken towards incorporating the lessons learned from the study of the *Traumtänzerin* into the performing arts (see Image 2.2).[173]

The instinctive feel that Magdeleine demonstrated for music during the somnambulistic state transformed her choreography from a meaningless movement of limbs into a rhythmic representation of the inner life of the soul. Dance and pantomime were the physical expression of her inner creative energies, a projection of her dreams and ideas. According to Schrenck-Notzing, Magdeleine's body had become an ideoplastic instrument through which every emotional stirring found its appropriate expression.[174] This conceptualisation of the Parisian's somnambulistic dance as an ideoplastic manifestation, that is, as a projection of psychic energies outside the body in material form, was perhaps the first step towards Schrenck-Notzing's interest in and acceptance of physical mediumship, which he was also to theorise in terms of ideoplastic powers. While Magdeleine's true significance may have been her role as the link between Schrenck-Notzing's interest in hypnotism and his eventual advocacy of physical mediumship, to his contemporaries he maintained her importance in terms of her contributions to drama, art, dance and hypnosis.

Not everyone, however, was so convinced of the significance or the veracity of Magdeleine's stage exploits. The *Stuttgarter Neues Tageblatt* [*Stuttgart Daily News*], for example, noted that a war of words had broken out in both Munich and Stuttgart over the reality of the dream-dancer's trance. The combatants argued over whether Magdeleine's artistic feats were carried out in a veridical hypnotic state, or whether they were part of a deception perpetrated in full consciousness? Many of those critics who regarded the dream-dancing phenomenon as a clear-cut case of fraud saw the Psychologische Gesellschaft's promotion of Magdeleine as an unscrupulous attempt to create a sensation among Munich's élite and to generate debate about hypnosis.[175] One commentator despaired that the heroes of Munich liberalism, the artists, dramatists and physicians who attended Magdeleine's performances, appeared to have become as credulous as the Bavarian peasantry.[176] There was concern also that Schrenck-Notzing's study and promotion of this case, which blurred the boundaries between experiment and entertainment, constituted a gross misuse of science. Moll wrote in this regard:

> The way in which he intervened in the case of Mme Magdeleine G., the sleep-dancer, was calculated to make the public think there was something occultistic about her performances, and was very reprehensible. I am referring to his unjustifiable assertion that, in the first experiment, the effect of the music on the somnambulistic lady was such, that she developed a power of dramatic expression 'far beyond the possibilities of the actor's art'. Still more reprehensible was the way in which he foisted this lady, whose performance contributed nothing new to science, upon an unsuspicious public. In my opinion, the way he stage-managed the lady's performances in

118

the presence of large audiences was an insult to science, and such methods should be rigidly excluded from the laboratory psychologist.[177]

The sleep-dancer's performances, the appeal of which was their mixture of sensation and occultism, were more closely related to the demonstrations of stage hypnotists than they were to the experiments of medical hypnotists, whose aim it was to divorce hypnosis and suggestion from occultism and secure a medical monopoly over them. Schrenck-Notzing's promotion of Magdeleine, which intimated the paranormal nature of her talent and enabled their public exhibition, retarded this project.

Moll was convinced that the problems embodied in Magdeleine's somnambulistic performances, if any, were of an artistic rather than a scientific kind. When invited by Schrenck-Notzing to investigate the phenomena exhibited by the Parisian in a Berlin theatre, he refused, protesting that he was not an expert in the arts and that he was uninterested in demonstrations of such dubious scientific merit. He wrote, 'We know that people can dance, likewise we know that people in hypnosis can dance. I therefore see no scientific problem in the fact that Miss M. dances in hypnosis.'[178] Moll also refuted Schrenck-Notzing's claims that Magdeleine had received no training in either drama or dance and that her profound talent had emerged only with the induction of a hypnotic trance. Far from having had no training in dance, Moll argued, the dream-dancer was derived from a family of dancers, her uncle, a dance master, having provided her with instruction. Even if she was genuinely unable to perform in the waking state, consciously oblivious of the subtleties of the art, it was possible that she had been trained in the hypnotic state, a possibility that, while interesting, did not, according to Moll, render the case worthy of scientific attention.

The consequence of Schrenck-Notzing's promotion of Magdeleine was, according to Moll, a veritable psychic epidemic in Germany. Somnambulistic performers of all kinds, including sleep-singers, sleep-flautists and sleep-riders, emerged out of obscurity to inflict on the public their variety numbers.[179] Investigation of these somnambules, some of whom presented themselves to Moll, nearly always revealed training in dancing, singing or riding and little evidence to suggest that they were incapable of the same artistic feats in the waking state.[180] Derelict in his duty to promote hypnosis as a means of medical therapy and psychological introspection, rather than a spectacle or fairground attraction, Schrenck-Notzing, through his promotion of Magdeleine G., gained Moll's eternal ire. His transformation in the years that followed into Germany's premier propagandist for parapsychology ensured that he had found his nemesis in Moll.

Conclusion

The study of the paranormal in Germany during the late nineteenth and early twentieth centuries was intimately linked with scientific interest in hypnotism and suggestion. The engagement of medical hypnotists – physicians who had adopted the methods of the Nancy school – with the paranormal phenomena of hypnotic sleep represented some of the first experiments in the German context in the field of psychical research and provided the basis for an 'experimental psychology' freed from the bonds of physiology. The interest of these physicians in paranormal phenomena, however, compromised their promotion of hypnosis as a legitimate form of medical therapy because of the lack of distinction between their explorations of thought-transference and clairvoyance and those of lay people and occultists. This awkward intersection of medicine, lay therapy and occultism, forced medical hypnotists, such as Dessoir and Moll, to engage in boundary-work to protect their professional and epistemological interests from lay practitioners and occultists, and in self-policing to ensure that their campaign was not undermined by their own interest in the paranormal. The retreat of Dessoir and Moll from psychical research led to the construction of a new stance on the paranormal known as critical occultism, the explanatory paradigm of which psychologised both the paranormal and those who maintained its objective reality.

In spite of the risks to his reputation and the medical hypnotists' campaign, Schrenck-Notzing refused to abandon psychical research and its animist paradigm. In part, this stubborn dedication to psychical research was a result of epistemological conviction, but it can also be seen as a consequence of the new-found financial independence afforded by his marriage.[181] The security provided by his wife's money allowed the Baron to abandon his medical practice and to follow his interests wherever they might lead, including the controversial terrain across which the *Traumtänzerin* pranced and pirouetted. In the decades that followed, this money allowed Schrenck-Notzing to build a laboratory in his home for research with physical mediums, to back a number of journals in the field of parapsychology, and to promote the scientific study of the paranormal among both the scientific community and the public. The case of the sleep-dancer, however, marked more than just the Baron's financial independence. It also formed the transition between Schrenck-Notzing's studies of hypnosis and his interest in mediumship, particularly of a physical kind. The appearance of the somnambulistic Parisian on the German stage marked furthermore the juncture at which Dessoir and Moll, who remained dedicated to the promotion of hypnosis and suggestion as medical therapies and to their use as weapons of scientific enlightenment, embraced critical occultism. Indeed, Schrenck-Notzing's sponsorship of Magdeleine G. helped demarcate the terrain over which parapsychologists and critical occultists would do battle during the decades that followed.

Notes

1. 'Programm der Psychologischen Gesellschaft in München', *Sphinx,* 2, 1 (1887), 33.
2. *Ibid,* 33–4.
3. T. Kaiser, 'Zwischen Philosophie und Spiritismus: Bildwissenschaftliche Quellen zur Leben und Werk des Carl du Prel (unpublished MPhil dissertation: Universität Lüneburg, 2005), 64.
4. N. Freytag, *Aberglauben im 19. Jahrhundert: Preußen und seine Rheinprovinz zwischen Tradition und Moderne (1815–1918)* (Berlin: Duncker & Humblot, 2003), 282.
5. R. Heidenhain, *Hypnotism or Animal Magnetism: Physiological Observations,* L.C. Woolridge (trans.), 4th edn (London: Kegan Paul, Trench & Co, 1888), 4.
6. J.R. Laurence and C. Perry, *Hypnosis, Will and Memory: A Psycho-legal History* (New York: Guilford Press, 1988), 217–18.
7. A. Moll, *Hypnotism: Including a Study of the Chief Points of Psycho-Therapeutics and Occultism,* A.F. Hopkirk (trans.), 4th edn (London: Walter Scott, 1909), 441.
8. B. Wolf-Braun, 'Mesmerismus, Hypnotismus und die parapsychologische Forschung: Rapport und Mentalsuggestion als Gegenstand der Wissenschaft im ausgehenden 19. und frühen 20. Jahrhundert', (Final report for the Institut der Grenzgebiete der Psychologie und Psychohygiene, University of Bonn, 1999), 72.
9. *Ibid.,* 72.
10. Heidenhain, *op. cit.* (note 5), 4.
11. Laurence and Perry, *op. cit.* (note 6), 185.
12. On these concerns in the French context, see Ruth Harris, *Murders and Madness: Medicine, Law, and Society in the Fin de Siècle* (Oxford: Clarendon Press, 1989), 155–207.
13. Moll, *op. cit.* (note 7), 440.
14. A. Gauld, *A History of Hypnotism* (Cambridge: Cambridge University Press, 1992), 302–6; Freytag, *op. cit.* (note 4), 282–90.
15. Moll, *op. cit.* (note 7), 442.
16. Heidenhain, *op. cit.* (note 5), 5.
17. 'Von einem geheimnisvollen Rapport zwischen dem Behandelnden und dem Behandelten zeigt sich aber keine Spur, wie denn auch die Fähigkeit zu magnetisieren keineswegs an bestimmte Personen gebunden ist.' W. Wundt,

'Der Aberglaube in der Wissenschaft', in *Essays*, 2nd edn (Leipzig: Wilhelm Engelmann, 1906), 379.

18. Heidenhain, *op. cit.* (note 5), 46.

19. Gauld, *op. cit.* (note 14), 303–5.

20. W. Wundt, *Outlines of Psychology*, C.H. Judd (trans.), 3rd edn (London: Williams & Norgate, 1907), 312–13.

21. Heidenhain, *op. cit.* (note 5), 6.

22. Gauld, *op. cit.* (note 14), 305.

23. See, M.J. Clark, 'The Rejection of Psychological Approaches to Mental Disorder in Late Nineteenth-Century British Psychiatry', in A. Scull (ed.), *Madhouses, Mad-Doctors and Madmen: The Social History of Psychiatry in the Victorian Era* (London: The Athlone Press, 1981), 271–312.

24. A. Harrington, 'Hysteria, Hypnosis, and the Lure of the Invisible: The Rise of Neo-Mesmerism in *Fin-de-Siècle* French Psychiatry', in W.F. Bynum, R. Porter and M. Shepherd (eds), *The Anatomy of Madness: Essays in the History of Psychiatry, Volume III*, (London: Routledge, 1988), 226.

25. *Ibid.*, 226.

26. Harris, *op. cit.* (note 12), 166.

27. J. Goldstein, *Console and Classify: The French Psychiatric Profession in the Nineteenth Century* (Cambridge: Cambridge University Press, 1987), 369–70.

28. *Ibid.*, 370–73.

29. Harris, *op. cit.* (note 12), 194

30. H. Bernheim, *Suggestive Therapeutics: A Treatise on the Nature and Uses of Hypnotism*, C. Herter (trans.), 2nd edn (Edinburgh: Young J. Pentland, 1890), 207.

31. *Ibid.*

32. *Ibid.*, 91.

33. For an account of the press coverage given to this debate see R. Hillman, 'A Scientific Study of Mystery: The Role of the Medical and Popular Press in the Nancy-Salpêtrière Controversy on Hypnotism', *Bulletin of the History of Medicine*, 39, 2 (1965), 163–82. For the role of crime and hypnosis in this debate, see Harris, *op. cit.* (note 12), 155–207.

34. On the manner in which the teachings of the Nancy school spread across Europe, see Gauld, *op. cit.* (note 14), 336–53.

35. A. Moll, *Ein Leben als Arzt der Seele: Erinnerungen* (Dresden: Carl Reissner, 1936), 30.

36. *Ibid.*, 20–30.

37. *Ibid.*, 26.

38. *Ibid.*, 29.

39. '[J]a gewiß die hypnotische Behandlung uns eine Panacee nicht bietet. Indessen sind doch die Resultate… bereits recht ermutigend.' Quoted in O.

Winkelmann, 'Albert Moll (1862–1939) als Wegbereiter der Schule von Nancy in Deutschland', *Praxis Psychotherapie*, 10, 1 (1965), 4.

40. Moll, *op. cit.* (note 35), 31.
41. 'Besonders als ich von den Versuchen sprach, durch Suggerieren eines Blasenpflasters tatsächlich Blasen zu erzeugen, ging ein allgemeines Lachen durch den Saal.' *Ibid.*
42. Moll, *op. cit.* (note 7), 23.
43. Moll, *op. cit.* (note 35), 42.
44. *Ibid.*, 31.
45. 'Eine ärztliche Behandlung ist das nicht; zu einer ärztlichen Behandlung gehört ärztliche Kunst und ärztliches Wissen, aber etwas, was jeder Schäferknecht, was jeder Schuster und Schneider machen kann, wenn er nur das nötige Selbstvertrauen besitzt... das kann man doch nicht mit dem Namen ärztliche Behandlung belegen.' *Ibid.*
46. Winkelmann, *op. cit.* (note 39), 5.
47. 'Ich lud jede Woche etwa sieben, acht Ärzte an einem Abend zu mir ein, hielt ihnen einen Vortrag und demonstrierte die Phänomene des Hypnotismus. Auch zeigte ich ihnen besonders den Unterschied zwischen Charcots Lehre und der von Nancy. [...] Kaum ein Deutscher wußte etwas von den Lehren Liébeaults, Bernheims usw.' Moll, *op. cit.* (note 35), 33.
48. Winkelmann, *op. cit.* (note 39), 5.
49. 'Aber wir müssen uns bewußt sein, daß wir bei ihrer Anwendung, und ich selbst habe sie angewendet, aus dem Gebiete der ärztlichen Kunst und Behandlung heraus in das der Psychologie hinübertreten.' Moll, *op. cit.* (note 35), 32
50. *Ibid.*
51. Moll, *op. cit.* (note 7), 23; Gauld, *op. cit.* (note 14), 341–2.
52. Gauld, *ibid.*, 341.
53. Moll, *op. cit.* (note 7), 23–4.
54. M. Dessoir, *Bibliographie des modernen Hypnotismus* (Berlin: C. Duncker, 1888).
55. Gauld, *op. cit.* (note 14), 344–5.
56. Moll, *op. cit.* (note 35), 37–9; P. Weindling, 'Medical Practice in Imperial Berlin: The Casebook of Alfred Grotjahn', *Bulletin of the History of Medicine*, 61 (1987), 407.
57. M. Dessoir, *Buch der Erinnerung*, 2nd edn (Stuttgart: Ferdinand Enke, 1947), 126–7.
58. Moll said of Schrenck-Notzing that, 'He was the first medical psychotherapist in South Germany....' A. Moll, *Psychologie und Charakterologie der Okkultisten* (Stuttgart: Ferdinand Enke, 1929), 20.
59. A. von Schrenck-Notzing, *Über die praktische Bedeutung des Hypnotismus* (Augsburg: Wirthschen, 1889).

60. 'Von bahnbrechender Wichtigkeit erscheint mir die Suggestivbehandlung für die verschiedenen Erscheinungsformen der sexuellen Parästhesie, besonders bei der conträren Sexualempfindung.' A. von Schrenck-Notzing, *Die Bedeutung der hypnotischen Suggestion als Heilmittel* (Berlin: Bong & Co., 1895), 105.

61. Gauld, *op. cit.* (note 14), 298.

62. Moll, *op. cit.* (note 7), 24.

63. Schrenck-Notzing, *op. cit.* (note 60), 105.

64. *Ibid.,* 104–5.

65. A. Moll, *Perversions of the Sex Instinct: A Study of Sexual Inversion*, M. Popkin (trans.), (Newark: Julian Press, 1931), 198.

66. *Ibid.,* 198–9.

67. A. von Schrenck-Notzing, 'Beiträge zur forensischen Beurtheilung von Sittlichkeitsvergehen mit besonderer Berücksichtigung der Pathogenese psychosexualler Anomalien', *Archiv für Kriminalanthropologie*, 1 (1898), 140–1.

68. *Ibid.,* 5–25; Moll, *op. cit.* (note 65), 207.

69. 'Bericht über die Enquête betreffend den Heilwerth der Hypnose', *Aerztekammer für die Provinz Ostpreussen*, 28 (V. Periode 1900–1902: 6) Sitzung zu Königsberg im Landhause am 18. Oktober 1902, in: GStA PK, I. HA Rep. 76 Nr. 1324.

70. *Ibid.*

71. 'Erlass des Herrn Ministers vom 5. April 1902 betreffend die Hypnose', Aerztekammer der Rheinprovinz und der Hohenzollern'schen Lande. Sitzung der V. Wahlperiode, 12 November 1902, in: GStA PK, I. HA Rep. 76 Nr. 1324.

72. A. Forel, *Die Hypnose vor der Aertzekammer*. Separatabdruck aus der *Münchener medizinischen Wochenschrift*, 32 (1902), in: GStA PK, I. HA Rep. 76 Nr. 1324; Freytag has argued that the emphasis on nervous disorder was in part a result of medical hypnotists' efforts to distance their practice from magnetism, which was applied as a 'cure-all' by lay practitioners. Freytag, *op. cit.* (note 4), 286–7.

73. Forel, *ibid.*

74. *Ibid.*

75. A. von Schrenck-Notzing, *Über Hypnotismus und Suggestion* (Augsburg: Wirthschen, 1889), 38.

76. 'Durch die methodische Untersuchung der hypnotischen Phänomene, durch die bis jetzt erlangten positiven und feststehenden Resultate, welche einen interessanten Beitrag liefern zur Lösung der psychologischen und physiologischen Lebenserscheinungen, ist erst eigentlich in neuerer Zeit der wichtige Forschungszweig einer Experimental-Pychologie möglich geworden

und jeder anderen naturwissenschaftlichen Untersuchungsart als ebenbürtig zur Seite gestellt.' *Ibid.*, 3.

77. Schrenck-Notzing, *op. cit.* (note 59), 7.
78. Moll, *op. cit.* (note 7), 446.
79. *Ibid.*, 450.
80. *Ibid.*, 445–6.
81. 'Wir tragen gleichsam eine verborgene Bewusstseinssphäre in uns, die, mit Verstand, Empfindung und Willen begabt, eine Reihe von Handlungen zu bestimmen fähig ist. Das gleichzeitige Zusammensein beider Sphären nenne ich Doppelbewusstsein…. Es folgt m. E. aus ihnen die Zusammengesetztheit unserer Persönlichkeit aus zwei mehr oder minder unabhängig voneinander operienden Bewusstseinshälften, die man bildlich als Ober- und Unterbewusstsein bezeichnen könnte.' M. Dessoir, *Das Doppel-Ich*, 2nd edn (Leipzig: Ernst Günther, 1896),11, 13.
82. W. Wundt, 'Lecture Twenty-Second', in *Lectures on Human and Animal Psychology*, J.E. Creighton and E.B. Titchener (trans.), 2nd edn (London: Swan Sonnenschein & Co., 1894), 333–5. Originally published as W. Wundt, *Vorlesung über die Menschen- und Tierseele* (Leipzig: Wilhelm Engelmann, 1894).
83. W. Wundt, *Outlines of Psychology*, C.H. Judd (trans.), 7th edn (London: Williams & Norgate, 1907), 313. Originally published as W. Wundt, *Grundzüge der physiologischen Psychologie* (Leipzig: Wilhelm Engelmann, 1896); Wundt, *op. cit.* (note 82), 335–6.
84. W. Wundt, *Principles of Physiological Psychology*, E. Titchener (trans.), 5th edn (London: Swan Sonnenschein & Co., 1910), 11.
85. Wundt, 'Lecture Twenty-Second', *op. cit.* (note 82), 331.
86. Wundt, *op. cit.* (note 84), 11.
87. Wolf-Braun, *op. cit.* (note 8), 75.
88. W. Wundt, *Hypnotismus und Suggestion*, 2nd edn (Leipzig: Wilhelm Engelmann, 1911), 7.
89. Wundt, 'Lecture Twenty-Second', *op. cit.* (note 82), 336.
90. Moll, *op. cit.* (note 7), 485.
91. A. von Schrenck-Notzing, 'Experimental Studies in Thought-Transference', *Proceedings of the Society for Psychical Research*, 7 (1891–2), 6.
92. Wundt, *op. cit.* (note 88), 8–9.
93. Wundt, 'Lecture Twenty-Second', *op. cit.* (note 82), 336.
94. Dessoir, *op. cit.* (note 54), 127.
95. P. Weindling, *Health, Race and German Politics between National Unification and Nazism, 1870–1945*, (Cambridge: Cambridge University Press, 1989), 21.
96. *Ibid.*

97. M. Hau, *The Cult of Health and Beauty in Germany: A Social History,*
1890–1930 (Chicago: University of Chicago Press, 2003), 1.

98. Weindling, *op. cit.* (note 95), 21.

99. J.U. Teichler, '"Der Charlatan strebt nicht nach Wahrheit, er verlangt nur
nach Geld." Zur Auseinandersetzung zwischen naturwissenschaftlicher
Medizin und Laienmedizin im deutschen Kaiserreich am Beispiel von
Hypnotismus und Heilmagnetismus', (unpublished PhD dissertation:
University of Leipzig, 1999), 6.

100. A. Labisch, 'From Traditional Individualism to Collective Professionalism:
State, Patient, Compulsory Health Insurance, and the Panel Doctor
Question in Germany, 1883–1931', in M. Berg and G. Cocks (eds),
Medicine and Modernity: Public Health and Medical Care in Nineteenth- and
Twentieth-Century Germany (Cambridge: Cambridge University Press, 1997),
36.

101. Weindling, *op. cit.* (note 95), 21.

102. On the role of *Ärztekammer* as a form of professional representation, see
Labisch, *op. cit.* (note 100), 37.

103. See *Berliner Lokal-Anzeiger,* 1 March 1903 and 5 March 1903, in: GStA PK,
I. HA Rep. 76 Nr. 1329.

104. 'Ausstellung der deutschen Gesellschaft zur Bekämpfung des
Kurpfuschertums, Breslau 1904', in GStA PK, I. HA Rep. 76 Nr. 1330.

105. *Berliner Tagesblatt,* 30 March 1899, in GStA PK, I. HA Rep. 76 Nr. 1328r.

106. Letter: Der Berliner Heilgehülfen Verein – Das kaiserliche Ministerium des
Innern für das deutsche Reich. 2 December 1898, in GStA PK, I. HA Rep.
76 Nr. 1328.

107. 'Bekanntmachung betreffend öffentliche Anzeigen von Heilmitteln und
Heilmethoden', *Berliner medizinische Wochenschrift,* 3 (June 1902), in GStA
PK, I. HA Rep. 76 Nr. 1329.

108. 'Zur Bekämpfung der Kurpfuscherei', *Aerztliches Correspondenzblatt für*
Niedersachsen, 1, 18 (1902), 143, in GStA PK, I. HA Rep. 76 nr. 1329.

109. 'Entwurf eines Gesetzes, betreffend die Bekämpfung der Kurpfuscherei. 12.
Dezember 1904 im Reichsamte des Innern geplogenen kommissarischen
Verhandlung über die Gründzüge eines Gesetzes, betreffend die Bekämpfung
der Kurpfuscherei', in GStA PK, I. HA Rep. 76, Nr. 1331, III B 4280.

110. For a more exhaustive account of the conflict between the medical
community and lay hypnotists, see Teichler, *op. cit.* (note 99).

111. Moll, *op. cit.* (note 7), 440.

112. 'Der Zweck solcher Schaustellungen, nämlich die Aufmerksamkeit der
Wissenschaft auf die hypnotischen Phänomene zu lenken, ist ja ohnehin
heute längst erfüllt.' A. von Schrenck-Notzing, *Die gerichtlich medicinische*
Bedeutung der Suggestion: Vortrag gehalten gelegentlich des zweiten

internationalen Congresses für experimentellen und therapeutischen Hypnotismus in Paris (August 1900), (Leipzig: F.C.W. Vogel, 1900), 24.

113. Freytag, *op. cit.* (note 4), 285.
114. 'Der hypnotisirende Laie kann nicht wissen, wie es mit den gesundheitlichen Verhältnissen seines Opfers steht, das vielleicht ein Herzleiden besitzt, vielleicht auf Grund erblicher Belastung den Keim zu epileptischen Anfällen, zu Geistkrankheit oder Hysterie in sich trägt....' Schrenck-Notzing, *op. cit.* (note 112), 28.
115. '[D]urch unrichtiges Manipuliren in den Versuchspersonen latente Dispositionen zu Erkrankungen, hysterischen, epileptischen, psychopathtischen Anfällen u. dergl. geweckt werden können.' *Ibid.*, 8.
116. Moll, *op. cit.* (note 7), 293.
117. Ironically, Schrenck-Notzing found himself accused of harming one of his patients through hypnotic therapy in 1888, an accusation he tried to counter by taking his patient to court. See Kaiser, *op. cit.* (note 3), 65.
118. 'So hatten wir selbst Gelegenheit, während des letzten Jahres an nicht weniger als 6 Personen in München, welche als Medien bei den spiritistischen Versuchen von Laien gedient hatten, Gesundheitsbeschädigungen zu beobachten. In einem dieser Fälle handelte es sich um einen Schneidergesellen, in einem zweiten um einen Agenten, in einem dritten um einen Bildhauer. Alle drei Personen zeigten Erscheinungen ausgesprochener männlicher Hysterie, die jedoch erst durch die Versuche künstlich erzeugt... wurden.' A. Schrenck-Notzing, 'Die gerichtliche Bedeutung und mißbräuchliche Anwendung des Hypnotismus', *Psychologische Gesellschaft zu München,* (November 1889), 13.
119. Schrenck-Notzing, *op. cit.* (note 75), 38.
120. Schrenck-Notzing, *op. cit.* (note 112), 7.
121. *Ibid.*, 3.
122. 'Eine grosse Gefahr bieten heute noch immer die planlosen hypnotischen Experimente, welche zur Befriedigung einer schaulustigen Menge in öffentlichen Localen, oder wie vielfach in Deutschland üblich, in geschlossenen Gesellschaften, spiritistischen Vereinen, Somnambulencabinets oder auch in Salons vorgenommen werden. Hinreichend bekannt sind auf solche Anregung hin entstandene hypnotische Epidemieen (z.B. in Breslau, Pforzheim, Mailand, in Kasernen, Knabenschulen, Pensionaten etc.', *ibid.*, 7.
123. *Ibid.*, 12.
124. D. Pick, *Faces of Degeneration: A European Disorder, c.1848– c.1918* (Cambridge: Cambridge University Press, 1989), 150.
125. Weindling, *op. cit.* (note 95), 23.
126. Der königliche Regierungs-Präsident, No. Id. 2631. An den Herrn Minister der geistlichen Unterrichts- und Medizinalangelegenheiten in Berlin. Betrifft Anwendung der Hypnose von nicht approbierten Heilpersonen. Erlass vom

5. April v. Js. No. 491 M. Berichterstatter: Regierungs und Geheimer Medizinalrat Dr Penkert. Merseburg, 26 März 1903. GStA Pk, I. HA Rep. 76 Nr. 1325.

127. Moll's attempt at boundary-work here provides one of many examples apparent in debates over lay medicine and parapsychology of what D.J.Hess has called the pathology metaphor. See D.J. Hess, *Science in the New Age: The Paranormal, Its Defenders and Debunkers, and American Culture* (Madison: University of Wisconsin Press, 1993), 30.

128. A. Moll, 'Ueber Heilmagnetismus und Heilmagnetiseure in forensischer Beziehung', *Vierteljahrsschrift für gerichtliche Medizin und öffentliches Sanitatswesen*, 35 (1907), 16–17.

129. *Ibid.*, 19.

130. I explore the attempt to pathologise parapsychologists further in Chapter 6.

131. 'Kein Mittel von nachhaltiger Wirkung auf unseren Körper, gleichgiltig ob man dabei an die Chirurgie, an die Pharmacope, die Elektricität oder Hydrotherapie denkt, lässt sich als absolut ungefährlich bezeichnen, - also auch nicht die Psychotherapie im Gewande der hypnotischen Suggestion.. Wie in allen anderen Zweigen der Heilkunde, hängt auch bei hypnotischen Massnahmen die Gefährlichkeit ab von der technischen (hier psychologischen) Sicherheit, den Kenntissen und Erfahrungen des Ärztes.' Schrenck-Notzing, *op. cit.* (note 60), 100–1.

132. 'Der Hypnotismus darf also nur durch Aerzte angewendet werden, in den Händen der Empiriker und Charlatans bietet er dieselben Gefahren, wie die Anwendung von Morphium und Digitalis durch Personen, die nicht über ausreichende Vorkenntnisse verfügen.' Schrenck-Notzing, *op. cit.* (note 75), 39.

133. Moll, *op. cit.* (note 7), 287.

134. '1. Alle öffentlichen hypnotischen Schaustellungen durch die Behörden zu verbieten seien; daß 2. Die praktische Anwendung des Hypnotismus zu therapeutischen und wissenschaftlichen Zwecken gesetzlich geregelt werde; daß 3. Es wünschenswerth sei, das Studium und die Anwendung des Hypnotismus im medizinischen Unterricht zu berücksichtigen.' Schrenck-Notzing, *op. cit.* (note 59), 8.

135. Wundt, *op. cit.* (note 88), 8–9.

136. S. Lachapelle has documented a similar phenomenon in France, where psychiatrists and psychologists studied mediumship in pathological terms in order to negate the threat it posed to physiological models of mind. See S. Lachapelle, 'A World Outside Science: French Attitudes Towards Mediumistic Phenomena, 1853–1931', (unpublished PhD dissertation: University of Notre Dame, 2002), 154.

137. R. Hayward, *Resisting History: Religious Transcendence and the Invention of the Unconscious* (Manchester: Manchester University Press), 44–64.

138. B. Wolf-Braun, '"Was jeder Schäferknecht macht, ist eines Ärztes unwürdig": Zur Geschichte der Hypnose im wilhelminischen Kaiserreich und in der Weimarer Republik (1888–1932)', *Hypnose und Kognition,* 17 (2000), 144.

139. Moll, *op. cit.* (note 128), 2–4.

140. *Ibid.,* 7.

141. *Ibid.,* 4.

142. *Ibid.,* 14.

143. 'Der Glaube eines Patienten, dass ihm dieses oder jenes Heilmittel nützen würde, wirkt in solcher Weise suggestiv. Und insofern können wir es durch die Suggestion erklären, wenn Leute, die zu der Christian Science Vertrauen haben, durch diese Behandlung gebessert werden.' A. Moll, *Gesundbeten: Medizin und Okkultismus* (Berlin: Hermann Walther, 1902), 24.

144. 'Gedanken, die in der untersten Seelentiefe schlummern und daher dem Individuum als fremde erscheinen, äussern sich in den ihm bemerkbaren, wenngleich unverständlichen Bewegungen des automatischen Schreibens und des Trancesprechens. Kein Wunder, dass solche Mitteilungen einer zweiten Bewusstseinssphäre an die Persönlichkeit ausfüllende Synthese als Botschaften aus der Geisterwelt gedeutet werden....' Dessoir, *op. cit.* (note 81), 60.

145. M. Dessoir, 'Zur Psychologie der Taschenspielerkunst', *Nord und Süd,* 52 (1890), 194–221.

146. Schrenck-Notzing, *op. cit.* (note 75), 7–13.

147. On variety and cabaret in the German context, see P. Jelavich, *Berlin Cabaret* (Cambridge: Harvard University Press, 1993), 20–8.

148. A. von Schrenck-Notzing, *Die Trauntänzerin Magdeleine G.: Eine psychologische Studie über Hypnose und dramatische Kunst* (Stuttgart: Ferdinand Enke, 1904), 22.

149. F. Maier, 'Die "Schlaftänzerin" Madeleine G. in München', *Psychische Studien,* 31, 5 (1904), 245.

150. *Ibid.,* 237, 239.

151. Schrenck-Notzing, *op. cit.* (note 148), 9; P. Pytlik, *Okkultismus und Moderne: Ein kulturhistorisches Phänomen und seine Bedeutung für die Literatur um 1900* (Munich: Schöningh Verlag, 2005), 63–8.

152. Schrenck-Notzing, *op. cit.* (note 148), 121.

153. *Ibid.,* 63.

154. *Ibid.,* 71.

155. P. Jelavich, *Munich and Theatrical Modernism: Politics, Playwriting, and Performance, 1890–1914* (Cambridge: Harvard University Press, 1985), 9.

156. *Ibid.,* 1–10.

157. D.F. Kuhns, *German Expressionist Theatre: The Actor and the Stage* (Cambridge: Cambridge University Press, 1997), 175.

158. Jelavich, *op. cit.* (note 147), 20–1.

159. A. von Schrenck-Notzing, 'Albert von Keller als Malerpsychologe und Metapsychiker', *Psychische Studien*, 48 (1921), 208; On Munich's Schauspielhaus see, Jelavich, *op. cit.* (note 155), 151–60.

160. Jelavich, *ibid.*, 188.

161. On the relationship between Munich's avant-garde and occultism see, V. Loers and P. Witzmann, 'Münchens okkultistisches Netzwerk', in V. Loers (ed.), *Okkultismus und Avantgarde: von Munch bis Mondrian, 1900–1915* (Frankfurt: Schirn Kunsthalle, 1995), 238–41.

162. Schrenck-Notzing, *op. cit.* (note 159), 193–215.

163. Maier, *op. cit.* (note 149), 239–41.

164. *Ibid.*, 247.

165. F. Maier, 'Neues von der Schlaftänzerin', *Psychische Studien*, 31, 5 (1904), 313.

166. Schrenck-Notzing, *op. cit.* (note 148), 116.

167. Schrenck-Notzing, *op. cit.* (note 159), 199.

168. The book Keller studied was, J. Charcot and P. Richer, *Les Démoniaques dans l'art* (Paris: Delahaye et Lecrosnier,1887); Schrenck-Notzing, *op. cit.* (note 159), 198.

169. *Ibid.*, 210.

170. Schrenck-Notzing, *op. cit.* (note 148), 118.

171. *Ibid.*, 116

172. Kuhns, *op. cit.* (note 157), 67–8.

173. Schrenck-Notzing, *op. cit.* (note 148), 116.

174. '[M]uss der Körper zu einem ideoplastischen Instrument geworden sein, in welchem jede seelische Regung ihren adäquaten Ausdruck findet.' *Ibid.,*121.

175. Maier, *op. cit.* (note 165), 311.

176. *Ibid.*, 315.

177. Moll, *op. cit.* (note 7), 533–4.

178. Moll, *op. cit.* (note 58), 20.

179. *Ibid.*

180. *Ibid.*

181. Schrenck-Notzing married Gabriele Siegle whose family money derived from I.G. Farben.

3

In the Laboratory of the *Geisterbaron*:
Experimental Parapsychology in Germany

Introduction

During the late nineteenth and early twentieth centuries, psychical researchers converted hotel rooms, clubrooms and private residences into experimental spaces. Using those props available, a card or dining table, a piece of dark cloth strung up to act as a medium cabinet, the physical environment in which psychical researchers examined mediums did not differ significantly from those domestic spaces adapted for spiritualist séances. While other nascent sciences, including experimental psychology, had established themselves in laboratories and universities by the dawn of the twentieth century, psychical research's experimental setting had remained largely indistinguishable from that of spiritualism. In order to differentiate themselves from the spiritualists, psychical researchers, like their contemporaries in the emergent human sciences, engaged in a process of sanitisation.[1] By mimicking the methodologies and principles of established sciences, including physics, biology and psychology, psychical researchers were able to distance themselves from spiritualism and promote their discipline as a new experimental science. This boundary-work, the purpose of which was to bolster the scientific credentials of psychical research and ultimately to gain it a place within the German university system, was manifest in three significant changes that occurred during the first decades of the twentieth century. First, was the retirement of terms such as 'psychical research' and 'scientific occultism' in favour of the word 'parapsychology', second was a new concentration on the physical phenomena of mediumship, and third was the transfer of this enterprise from the clubrooms and parlours in which the study of the paranormal had undergone its genesis, into purpose-built laboratories.

The similarity between the venues utilised by psychical researchers and spiritualists was not the only difficulty faced by those with a scientific interest in the paranormal; a problem of differentiation existed also in terms of their experimental material. Psychical researchers were dependent for their supply of experimental subjects, that is, mediums, upon spiritualist home circles where psychic talent tended to be fostered and developed. The maturation of mediums within the spiritualist paradigm, however, proved problematic for those researchers eager to institute rigid scientific controls during experiments. Mediums, more familiar with the informal and religious atmosphere of domestic séances, often seemed unable to perform without the props of spiritualism: including the circle, created by participants joining hands; music, provided either by a music box or instrumentalist; and the medium cabinet, a curtain or more permanent structure erected in a corner of the séance room in order to shelter the entranced medium.[2] Mediums also frequently complained that the sceptical stance and invasive methods adopted by psychical researchers inhibited their production of paranormal phenomena, the generation of which they contended were dependent on an atmosphere of trust and belief. The difficulties presented by mediums as experimental subjects, their insistence on certain physical conditions and props and their reticence about the rigorous application of the scientific method, served to further distance psychical researchers from the ideal represented by laboratories in the physical and psychological sciences. The inability of these researchers to modify mediums' behaviour aligned them once again with the spiritualists and occultists from whom they strove consistently to divorce themselves. It was apparent in this situation, as one observer complained, that so long as the study of mediumship continued to develop outside of a laboratory environment, psychical researchers would be forced to live with their mediums' spiritualist baggage.[3]

The laboratory erected by Albert von Schrenck-Notzing in his palatial Munich residence was an attempt to resolve those methodological problems arising from the scientific study of mediumship. The transfer of this enterprise into purpose-built laboratories, the design of which paid homage to laboratories in both the physical and psychological sciences, differentiated psychical research from experimentation in the spiritualist context. For Schrenck-Notzing it also signified an important step in psychical research's evolution from a pseudo-science, indistinguishable from spiritualism, into a legitimate scientific endeavour. He wrote in this regard, 'modern spiritism has the same relation to the future science of mediumistic process as astrology did to astronomy or alchemy to chemistry.'[4] Experimentation in this context enabled psychical researchers to manipulate and control mediums in a manner that was not possible in the séance room. Schrenck-Notzing's laboratory, replete with stereoscopic cameras, sphygmograph and specialist lighting, as well as a medium cabinet, was a hybridisation of spiritualist and scientific space that posed less of a threat to its psychologically fragile subjects than those laboratories found in the hard sciences. Situated on Munich's Karolinenplatz, it was host to hundreds of experiments and witness to numerous materialisations and telekinetic manifestations in the period just prior to and following the First World War.

This laboratory was important and unique from another point of view also: it contained mediums who were tied to Schrenck-Notzing on a long-term contractual basis, his intention being to wean them of their spiritualist training and to slowly acclimatise them to the more rigid conditions of the laboratory. In his four years of experimentation with the French medium Eva C., (Marthe Béraud) (b. 1887), for example, he had gradually decreased the medium's reliance on spiritualist ritual, including séance circles, trance personalities and singing, and increased the amount of light to which the medium and her phenomena were exposed. By 1913, he noted, Eva could tolerate a six-lamp chandelier of more than one hundred candle-power.[5] The laboratory, as Schrenck-Notzing's experience illustrated, helped regulate and control psychical researchers' interactions with mediums and denuded the phenomena they produced of their religious significance. Stripped of their spiritual role, assessed in psychopathological or biological terms and restrained by an economic bond to their employer, those mediums studied by Schrenck-Notzing were moulded, through their training and re-education in a laboratory environment, into more suitable experimental subjects.

The *Geisterbaron*, as one Munich newspaper dubbed the owner of this impressive facility, managed with the aid of his wife's fortune, not only to monopolise some of Germany's best mediumistic talent, but also to exert substantial control over the leading periodical in this field, the *Psychische Studien*, which was reissued in 1925 as the *Zeitschrift für Parapsychologie*.[6] Schrenck-Notzing's virtual monopoly of the means of both production and publication in this field, as well as his focus on and advocacy of the physical phenomena of mediumship, served to make him Germany's best known and most controversial parapsychologist during the early twentieth century. His dominant position within the parapsychological community, however, became a source of resentment during the mid- to late 1920s, particularly among a younger generation of researchers who believed that Schrenck-Notzing's 'dictatorship' was detrimental to the field.[7] The publication of the Baron's research with the physical mediums Eva C. and Willy Schneider also fostered conflict. This was manifested in a series of ongoing debates between Schrenck-Notzing and his critics over the reality of the phenomena produced in his laboratory and more fundamental issues including the nature of scientific knowledge and authority. Schrenck-Notzing's laboratory, which attracted Europe's best physical mediums and a host of illustrious séance participants, including Hans Driesch, Ludwig Klages, Thomas Mann and Gustav Meyrink, was the undoubted centre of parapsychological research in Germany from the First World War up until the Baron's death in

1929.[8] Indeed, the laboratory of the *Geisterbaron* offers the most advantageous vantage point from which to observe the attempt to create an experimental parapsychology during the pre- and inter-war period in Germany.

This chapter examines the parapsychology of the 1910s and 1920s from within the confines of Schrenck-Notzing's laboratory in order to gain insight into the paranormal experiences which formed the raw material of parapsychology, an understanding of the volatile power relations that existed between parapsychologists and mediums, and an awareness of the manner in which parapsychology, assuming the trappings of scientific endeavour, fought to become a legitimate new science. Through an examination of the experimental records produced in the Baron's home, this chapter will argue that the study of mediumship in a laboratory environment altered the meaning attributed to paranormal phenomena, imbuing it with psychopathological or biological significance.[9] The reinterpretation of these phenomena within a scientific paradigm allowed parapsychologists to diminish, although by no means totally extinguish, the power that mediums enjoyed in the spiritualist context. This chapter will contend furthermore that Schrenck-Notzing's laboratory, with its eclectic mix of both spiritualist and scientific paraphernalia, was symbolic of an irresolvable paradox at the heart of this emerging science. This was the apparently inimical relationship between scientific investigation, with its demands for rigour, objectivity and repeatability, and mediumistic phenomena, manifestations of a spontaneous and unpredictable nature dependent on trust, but mixed with both conscious and unconscious fraud. The effort to divorce this nascent discipline from spiritualism and occultism and to mimic both the physical and psychological sciences, thus served only to highlight parapsychology's border status.

From the séance room to the laboratory

The adoption during the 1920s of the term 'parapsychology' [Parapsychologie], coined in 1889 by Max Dessoir, in preference to 'psychical research' or 'scientific occultism', provided strong semantic and epistemological links between experimental psychology and the scientific study of the paranormal. With its reference to those phenomena which occur alongside normal mental events, this word also made explicit parapsychologists' dedication to expanding the frontiers of science. T.K. Oesterreich, in his 1920 book *Der Okkultismus in modernen Weltbild* [*Occultism in the Modern Conception of the World*], was one of the first to advocate the use of this term, recognising its potential to signify both psychical research's distance from spiritualism and its intimate connection with psychology. The use of Dessoir's neologism was not, however, intended to deny the contribution of physics and biology to this field. Rather, as Oesterreich argued, it was meant to encourage researchers to take a psycho-physical or psycho-biological approach to the phenomena of mediumship.[10] Oesterreich, like many of his contemporaries, believed that the phenomena of mediumship consisted of the exteriorisation and materialisation of psychological processes. In this context, then, the science of mediumship was understood as an amalgam and extension of physical, biological and psychological theories and methodologies; a disciplinary conception that was better connoted by the term 'parapsychology' than its precursors. This change in nomenclature not only provided a more accurate description of the scientific study of mediumship, but also reflected the belief that this discipline had successfully evolved from a pseudo- or proto-science into a legitimate field of scientific endeavour. The title of Schrenck-Notzing's posthumously published article series, 'The Development of Occultism into Parapsychology in Germany', for example, illustrated vividly the manner in which parapsychologists imagined themselves in the final stages of an evolutionary process that began with superstition and ended with science.[11] This putative transformation had been achieved, according to Schrenck-Notzing, through a concentration on the physical phenomena of mediumship and the design and construction of a small number of purpose-built parapsychological laboratories.

Following the *fin de siècle*, psychical researchers both in Germany and abroad became increasingly focused on the physical phenomena of mediumship. Schrenck-Notzing's 1904 investigation of the *Traumtänzerin*, Magdeleine G., for example, marked the transition of his interest from the psychical phenomena native to somnambulistic states, to the physical phenomena associated with mediumship. By 1909, Schrenck-Notzing had begun a series of experiments with the French medium Eva C. whose particular talent was materialisation. This process involved the appearance of misshaped bodies, heads and limbs, which often seemed to issue from the medium's orifices (see Image 3.1 overleaf). In the early twentieth century, psychical researchers, following the physiologist Charles Richet's lead, argued that the materialised arms and hands they witnessed in the presence of physical mediums were constructed from ectoplasm; an amorphous organic substance or form of energy, which mediums were able to exteriorise and mould.[12] Richet's neologism proved versatile enough not only to fashion disembodied heads, but also to help explain telekinesis, another common form of physical phenomena. The term 'telekinesis' had been coined in 1890 by Aleksandr Aksakov, editor of the *Psychische Studien*, who used it to describe the movement of objects at a distance, most probably by spirits.[13] By the 1920s, however, many psychical researchers believed that the household objects that swayed and levitated in the presence of physical

135

Image 3.1

Eva C. with materialisation, 1913.
Reproduced with permission from the Institut für Grenzgebiete der Psychologie
und Psychohygiene e. V., Freiburg im Breisgau (IGPP collection).

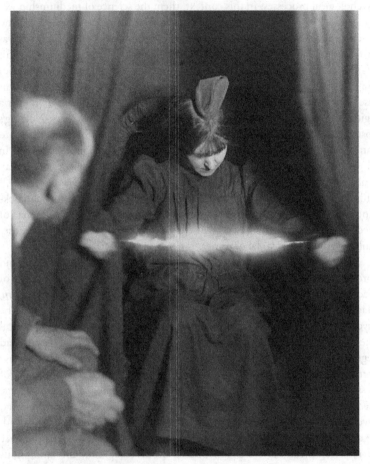

mediums such as Willy Schneider were moved not by spirits, but by invisible ectoplasmic threads.

The emphasis on, and interest in, the physical phenomena of mediumship that emerged during the early decades of the twentieth century was the result both of epistemic and methodological exigencies and changes within the contemporary psychological sciences. In the 1910s and 1920s, psychical researchers strove to develop and promote their discipline as an experimental science. In so doing, it became clear that their claims to scientific status needed to be based on phenomena that, at least in principle, were objective and accessible to the methods of the physical sciences.[14] While telepathy and clairvoyance – phenomena of a largely subjective and invisible nature – appeared unsuited to this kind of experimentation, it seemed possible that materialisation and telekinesis might be successfully transferred to the laboratory where they could be examined, measured and photographed. In the field of psychology during the early twentieth century, stress on objectivity and materiality saw a decline in interest in those phenomena, including hypnosis and hysteria, related to unconscious processes, leading to both a renewed emphasis on laboratory psychology and the emergence of applied psychology.[15] The study of these subjective phenomena had linked psychical research to psychology during the nineteenth century and offered a form of scientific legitimacy by proxy. As psychologists became more concerned with objective measurable phenomena, transferring their research into the laboratory or the field, it is perhaps unsurprising that psychical researchers sought to mimic their more legitimate sibling.

Schrenck-Notzing's construction of a laboratory on the ground floor of his Munich villa made concrete the English physicist and psychical researcher Sir Oliver Lodge's (1851–1940) vision of a parapsychological laboratory equipped with apparatus, similar to those used in the physical sciences, for measuring and registering the physical phenomena of mediumship.[16] Lodge had written in 1902 that the question of the physical phenomena appeared:

> [C]apable of answer, with sufficient trouble, in an organised psychical laboratory: such a laboratory as does not, I suppose, yet exist, but which might exist, and which will exist in the future, if the physical aspect of experimental psychology is ever to become recognised as a branch of physics.[17]

Schrenck-Notzing's laboratory, modelled on that of the Berlin-based engineer Fritz Grunewald (1885–1925), was designed to enable the rigorous application of the scientific method to mediumistic phenomena and to render independent the perceptive capabilities of the sense organs, which were subject to deception, by transferring them to physical apparatus, such as self-registering balances, cameras and thermometers.[18] Borrowed from medical, psychological and physical laboratories, such instruments were intended to monitor changes in the medium's body mass during levitation, capture telekinetic or ectoplasmic activity on photographic plates, and measure the medium's body temperature and vital signs. The foundation of this laboratory and others like it also inspired a number of noteworthy innovations. The Munich-based laboratory of the animal psychologist and parapsychologist Karl Krall (1863–1929), for example, was the birthplace of the electrical medium control, a device designed to monitor mediums' movements by connecting their limbs and those of their controls to an electrical circuit.[19] If the red, dark yellow, green or light yellow light bulbs that the circuit illuminated, flickered or went out, this informed the experimenter that the medium had escaped his or her restraints.[20]

Determined to subject the phenomena produced in his laboratory to the most stringent scientific analysis, Schrenck-Notzing also made use of some of Munich's independent medical facilities. In February 1916, for example, he sent a small quantity of ectoplasm to the Öffentliches Laboratorium für chemische, mikroskopische und bakteriologische Untersuchungen zu medizinisch-diagnostichen und technischen Zwecken [Public Laboratory for Chemical, Microscopic and Bacteriological Examination for Medical-Diagnostic and Technical Purposes], whose report stated:

> The material was initially observed in water and glycerine; after further treatment with iodine and aniline dye material solution in glycerine-gelatine.
> The preparation shows large epithelial groups and some different epithelium, whose multiple cores are clearly recognisable. As pollutants are found strands of cotton, grains of starch and fungus spores. Bacteria (bar forms) were observed in a lesser quantity.[21]

The inclusion in the Baron's arsenal of instruments borrowed from medicine, psychology and physics and the use of external facilities, such as the Public Laboratory, demonstrated his dedication to a scientific approach and the kinship that he hoped to foster between parapsychology and more established sciences.

The attempt of Schrenck-Notzing and others to establish parapsychology as an experimental and laboratory science during the early twentieth century was in part a response to late nineteenth-century critiques of the scientific study of mediumship. Wundt's appraisal of Zöllner's experiments with Henry Slade, for example, had outlined the crucial differences between mediumistic and psychological experiments – indeed, the rules that Wundt established for experimentation in his Leipzig laboratory can be seen as a response to the problems and inconsistencies he witnessed in the Slade experiments.[22] Wundt, as we have seen, had several concerns about what he had witnessed in the presence of Slade: including the tripartite role of the medium as experimenter, subject and interpreter; the apparent lack of causality in the experiment; the lackadaisical recording and measurement of events; and the interaction of the medium and the experimenter.[23] As a result of these concerns, Wundt ensured that the following rules were observed in his laboratory: only the experimenter had the authority to interpret results; experiments followed strict action and reaction schemes; subjects were known and trusted by the experimenter; subjects did not know the purpose of the experiment; careful, quantifiable measurements of phenomena were taken; and strict separation between experimenter and subject was maintained.[24] Schrenck-Notzing's laboratory was an attempt to address such critiques and to bring parapsychology closer to the ideal embodied by experimental psychology. The laboratory's design, however, which continued to incorporate a number of spiritualist props, including an enclosed medium cabinet, ensured that this experimental space continued to distinguish the scientific study of the paranormal from those sciences it wished to emulate.

Schrenck-Notzing's decision to construct his laboratory in a domestic setting, however, was not without precedent. In the first half of the nineteenth century, physicists such as Heinrich Gustav Magnus (1802–70) and Franz Neumann (1798–1895), built laboratories in their homes, funding them, as did Schrenck-Notzing, out of their own pockets.[25] The presence of these physical cabinets, large collections of instruments housed in glass-enclosed cases, in domestic spaces reflected the emphasis within German universities on teaching rather than experimentation prior to 1848, a situation that had altered dramatically by the last quarter of the nineteenth century.[26] The new emphasis on experimentation that emerged after 1850 helped foster an atmosphere conducive to the emergence of an experimental psychology, a discipline that abandoned the philosophical approach to the mind favoured within German universities in the first half of the nineteenth century, in order to apply physiological apparatus and procedures.[27] The psychological laboratory founded in Leipzig by Wundt, like the physical cabinets maintained by Magnus and Neumann, contained a vast array of instruments intended to measure and record physical responses. These apparatus included electromagnetic devices for measuring the duration of phenomena, dynamometers and sphygmographs borrowed from the physiological context, and self-registering balances used to detect movement.[28] Believing the physical phenomena of mediumship to be of psycho-physical origin, as Sir Oliver Lodge had maintained, German parapsychologists furnished their laboratories with the same apparatus. In so doing, they imagined that the development of parapsychology would mimic that of physics and experimental psychology; experimentation in private laboratories eventually leading to the establishment of parapsychological laboratories within German universities.

The parapsychological laboratories erected by Grunewald and Schrenck-Notzing featured blackout curtains identical to those used in physics laboratories, allowing sunlight to be quickly and completely eliminated from the room.[29] In the parapsychological context, darkness was necessitated by mediums' sensitivity to light and the use of photographic equipment, which also found its way into Germany's physics institutes during the late nineteenth century.[30] Grunewald's laboratory also contained a 'Federwaage' [spring balance] on which the medium's chair was placed, its movements registered electrically on a galvanometer.[31] This device and a host of other electromagnetic apparatus designed by Grunewald bore some resemblance to those instruments used in Wundt's laboratory to record the reaction time of participants subjected to luminous or sonorous stimuli.[32] Other items adapted by Grunewald and Schrenck-Notzing for use in their laboratories, included a sink with tap and water pump, an analytical scale enclosed in a glass case, and an electrically illuminated clock used to time the appearance and duration of mediumistic phenomena.[33] While these experimental spaces resembled physical and psychological laboratories in some particulars, the extent of this resemblance was limited not only by the inclusion within the parapsychological laboratory of a range of spiritualist paraphernalia, but also by the lackadaisical application of those physical apparatus and methodologies imported from physics and psychology.

Spiritualist additions, including the medium cabinet, a gauze-covered medium cage and the séance circle, tended to differentiate the parapsychological laboratory from those in the psychological and physical sciences. The prominence of such spiritualist props, however, was not the only way in which these experimental spaces differed from those in established sciences. While parapsychologists strove to adapt measuring devices and registering apparatus derived from physics and psychology, their intention being to replace the senses with a more objective and less flawed means of observation, their efforts often proved futile. Mediums, upon whom parapsychologists were reliant for the production of the phenomena they wished to study, frequently claimed that the use of such apparatus, a galvanometer or an electrical control, for example, inhibited their ability to produce telekinetic movement or ectoplasm. Their complaints about the discomfort caused by these apparatus or the disturbing influence that electrical currents and bright lights had on the phenomena convinced many parapsychologists to limit the use of such instruments or to modify their methodology to better suit their temperamental subjects. Schrenck-Notzing, for example, was unable to apply a device he had designed during a series of experiments with Willy Schneider at the University of Munich during 1922. The medium announced his dislike of this instrument, a box-like construction that Schrenck-Notzing called a 'Zeigeapparat', and generated no phenomena until its removal.[34] In contrast, Willy's younger brother Rudi (1908–57) managed, after a brief period during which he got used to the device, to produce telekinetic phenomena, even while shackled to an electrical medium control.[35] The Baron concluded from these experiences that not all mediums could be subjected to experimentation of such an exacting kind, a conclusion that led to the inconsistent application of such checks and controls.[36]

The experimental spaces constructed by parapsychologists, intended to mimic the layout and adapt the instruments utilised in laboratories for the psychological or physical sciences, lent the emerging field of parapsychology a scientific air and allowed parapsychologists to modify the conditions under which such experiments were performed. The transference of the scientific study of mediumship to this new environment also enabled parapsychologists to establish themselves as the legitimate authorities and interpreters in this field, denuding mediumistic phenomena of their spiritualist meaning. While such laboratories had been established in response to the critiques of psychical research made by Wundt and others, the actual resemblance between these spaces and those psychological and physical laboratories attached to universities in cities such as Leipzig and Berlin remained minimal. Parapsychologists' application of the apparatus and the use of those methods employed in psychology and physics continued to be flawed and uneven as a result of mediums' insistence on the use of spiritualist props, their reluctance to submit to rigid scientific control, and the struggle between experimenters and mediums over meaning and authority. The apparent incommensurability between the scientific method and the production of mediumistic phenomena – reflected in the compromises that parapsychologists made between the séance room and the laboratory in their construction of experimental spaces – remained a central problem for German parapsychology in its struggle to become an experimental science. This uneasy juxtaposition of science and spiritualism also helped define the experience of those that attended sittings in Schrenck-Notzing's laboratory.

The laboratory experience

The Karolinenplatz laboratory, while in many respects unique, had a precursor in the experimental space designed and furnished by Fritz Grunewald, who had become convinced as early as 1908 that an understanding of the physical phenomena would emerge only through the application of those methods utilised by the physical sciences.[37] The realisation of this project, however, proved both technically and financially prohibitive. Grunewald wrote in this regard:

> From the beginning of my laboratory-moderated experiments, it was for me just simply about working to penetrate ever deeper the nature of the peculiar phenomena. I also recognised very soon, that an extensive physical apparatus

was necessary, in the form of a well fitted-out laboratory. The ideal, which I already had in mind in the years 1908 and 1909, is, temporarily mind you, not yet achieved. For that the accompanying circumstances were too difficult and the means too insufficient.[38]

Grunewald's 1920 book on this topic provided a template for laboratory research in the field of parapsychology, listing the precautions, equipment and methodology that had proved productive in his own experimental work with mediums.[39] This model was adopted by Schrenck-Notzing who possessed the financial means to construct an experimental space, equipped with the necessary physical apparatus, which would allow for the rigorous testing of mediumistic powers in an atmosphere conducive to such phenomena. The Baron's money and social status also enabled him to promote parapsychology and its findings, by way of frequent and well-publicised experiments, among Germany's intellectual and scientific élites.

Those men and women who assembled in the Baron's laboratory, many of whom played prominent roles in both Munich's and Germany's social, cultural and political life, did so for a variety of reasons. Many felt compelled to witness and investigate the potentially significant phenomena of mediumship for scientific reasons. Numerous physicists, psychologists and biologists attended sittings with Schrenck-Notzing in order to ascertain the reality and ramifications of mediumistic phenomena. In a milieu in which there occurred a series of revolutionary epistemological changes in the physical, psychological and biological sciences, it seemed possible that the strange forms and fluids emitted from mediums' bodies might be of scientific or philosophic significance.[40] As Schrenck-Notzing noted:

> Modern physics regards matter as a form of motion, and is dominated by the idea of energy. Psychology also is gradually emancipating itself from the purely physiological conception of mental life; and under the leadership of the philosopher Bergson, it tends to acknowledge the superiority of the psychical over the physical. Thus the circumstances are much more favourable to the investigation of great new problems and facts than they were some decades ago.[41]

Many of those who explored the phenomena of mediumship for this reason found succour in them for a non-materialist or vitalist worldview.

Other participants in parapsychological experiments craved reassurance that the self survived death in some manner. In the aftermath of the First World War, séances in Germany, as elsewhere, acted as a means of both contacting and memorialising the war dead.[42] While the public and scientific response to Schrenck-Notzing's advocacy of physical mediumship had been one of amused incredulity before the Great War, by 1918 there had developed a distinct sympathy for and interest in the Baron's research, a change fostered by the catastrophic events of the previous four years.[43] In contrast, a not-insignificant number of those that attended Schrenck-Notzing's experiments regarded a night with the *Geisterbaron* as an amusing diversion or fashionable form of entertainment. Indeed, these gatherings often took on a festive atmosphere with chatter and music actively encouraged among the participants. Such evenings were, as Albert Hellwig, a fervent critic of Schrenck-Notzing, put it, a synthesis of theatre and salon, an observation that highlighted the difficulty of distinguishing this hybrid space, not only from the spiritualist séance room, but also from those venues, including the stage and the street, that played host to similar spectacles.[44]

Regardless of their individual motivations, every participant in the Baron's experimental evenings was compelled by their host, as a condition of their attendance, to provide an experimental protocol.[45] These testimonials recorded the participant's impressions of the sitting, noting the medium's disposition, the precautions taken to prevent fraud, and the appearance of any phenomena. Dr Hans Winterstein, professor of physiology at the University of Rostock, for example, who attended a séance at the Karolinenplatz laboratory in 1922, provided a report in which he thanked the Baron for allowing him to attend, described the telekinetic movement of both a music box and wastepaper basket, and stressed what he saw as the great importance of continued experimentation in this field.[46] Schrenck-Notzing's laboratory was responsible for the production of hundreds, if not thousands, of such reports, a collection that was drawn on by the Baron throughout the 1910s and 1920s in order to compile books, which acted as hagiographies of certain mediums and as proofs of the contested phenomena of mediumship.[47] The list of authoritative names from all fields and the sheer volume of positive reports that appeared in such volumes combined to create evidence for the reality of paranormal phenomena that was difficult to dismiss out of hand.

The experimental protocols collected by Schrenck-Notzing, many of which were published as evidence of the existence of phenomena such as materialisation and telekinesis, provided an account of the environment in which parapsychological experimentation took place: the preconditions for these experiments; details of the checks and controls used to prevent both conscious and unconscious fraud; and anecdotes about the labile and socially subversive behaviour of mediums. Such reports provided descriptions of the phenomena of mediumship, that is, the trance personalities of mediums, the materialised limbs and heads that protruded from their bodies and the household objects that appeared to move of their own accord in the presence of such paraphysically endowed individuals, hinting also at the social, political and epistemological milieu in which these manifestations took place. The protocols produced in the Baron's laboratory not only acted as evidence of the paranormal, but also offered their reader access to the experiential nature of experimental parapsychology in the German context.

Schrenck-Notzing's laboratory, which, like that of the engineer Grunewald, boasted a medium cabinet, comfortable furnishings, and an array of apparatus for measuring the medium's movements and paraphysical emissions, represented a merger of spiritualist and scientific space. Descriptions of the room, such as that provided by Thomas Mann, noted this hybridisation in the congenial arrangement of the participants' chairs, often in a semi-circle facing the medium cabinet, in the presence of household items, which included wastepaper baskets, typewriters and bells, as well as slightly more unusual objects, such as luminous pieces of felt, which were attached to the medium's clothing, electrical medium controls and stereoscopic cameras.[48] A protocol provided by the philosopher and psychologist T.K. Oesterreich, following his June 1922 sitting with Willy Schneider, also noted the inclusion of spiritualist paraphernalia in this scientific space.

> In the first part of the sitting a gauze cage was located in the middle of the participants' semi-circle, which, with the exception of the slit, was closed. In it stood a table, on this a music box, which was bound with a double wax-sealed string.[49]

These items, transferred directly from the spiritualist context, stood in stark contrast with the galvanometers and dynamometers imported from laboratories in the physical and psychological sciences.

Oesterreich's protocol also made mention of the manner in which the room was illuminated, hinting at the progress Schrenck-Notzing had made in getting his medium to accept more light. He stated that 'the lighting was considerably brighter than the beginning of April' when he had last attended an experiment with the Baron.[50] The sittings attended by Mann were perhaps more typical, distinguished as they were by the feeble red light exuded by lamps and ceiling fixtures swathed in red and black cloth.[51] The report provided by the writer Gustav Meyrink, author of *Der Golem*, noted both the means of illumination and its impact on the senses. He wrote, 'the sitting took place in a darkened room, however, it was by means of many red light bulbs at any rate light enough – at least for my vision – to distinguish objects and people.'[52] Similarly, the biologist and vitalist philosopher Hans Driesch noted that 'all light except for a red electric lamp was extinguished; one still saw the outline of all participants.'[53] The emphasis placed in such protocols on the manner in which the laboratory was lit and on how well participants could see in these conditions was deliberate. The use of red light, to illuminate proceedings and to allow the cameras' shutters to remain open throughout experiments, was a distinguishing feature of this environment.[54] While by no means bright, as Professor Ernst Aster's use of the term 'ein sehr abgedämpftes rotes Licht' ['very muted red light'] suggests,[55] this form of illumination helped distinguish the experiments of parapsychologists from those routinely conducted in the dark by spiritualists. [56]

The number of participants who attended the Baron's experiments also tended to differentiate parapsychology from experimentation in other fields. In experimental psychology, for example, it was often necessary for the experimenter and subject to occupy separate rooms, in order to ensure that the subject was not influenced by those observing him or her.[57] Indeed, this separation between experimenter and subject, along with the subject's ignorance of the purpose of the experiment, was one of Wundt's rules of experimentation.[58] In contrast, experiments conducted in the Baron's laboratory involved large groups, who actively engaged with and attempted to influence the experimental subject, who was well aware and continually reminded of the purpose of the experiment. Driesch, for example, noted the presence of eleven people, besides the medium and his attendant, at a sitting held on 20 February 1920.[59] He mentioned also the manner in which participants asked the medium's trance personality to remove a towel from the lamp it was covering.[60] Mann's protocols also pointed to the attendance of large numbers of people at the Baron's experimental evenings. He wrote, for example, of the necessity of forming a row behind the séance circle to accommodate all those present.[61] Despite the admonitions of men like Grunewald to strictly limit the number of participants during mediumistic sittings in order to minimise interference and suggestion, Schrenck-Notzing, whose aims were polemical as well as scientific, encouraged large numbers of people to attend his experiments.[62] Since critics had argued that his early experiments with mediums such as Eva C. had lacked a sufficient number of witnesses, the Baron dedicated himself to getting as many scientifically educated people as possible to bear witness to the phenomena produced in his laboratory.[63] If Oesterreich's estimate was correct and over two dozen scholars had authenticated the phenomena they had observed in the presence of Willy Schneider, these promotional efforts met with some success.[64]

Like a spiritualist séance, an evening in the Baron's laboratory could be understood not only as an opportunity for experimentation, but given the combination of scientific precaution, idle banter and sensation that marked these occasions, as a social or theatrical event. That the Baron was aware that his experiments were viewed as a form of entertainment by some participants was evident in a letter he wrote to a Dr Edith Ebees, an attendee who had been deeply impressed by what she experienced in the Karolinenplatz laboratory.

> For those with a scientific interest with the necessary literary knowledge, in particular those from the official circles of the alma mater, I am always happy to be at their disposal, but not people who come to the sittings out of curiosity and desire for sensation, as if to a theatrical performance.[65]

The idea that scientific experimentation with mediums was a form of entertainment, a variety show combining conjuring and cabaret, was compounded by the sense of anticipation fostered by the dim red lights and the darkness of the medium cabinet and by the musical performances that tended to accompany mediumistic sittings. Mann wrote in this regard:

> [T]he sporting zoology professor... armed himself with an accordion. It appeared that he was a skilled performer on this instrument, in demand for excursions and summer evening garden-parties, and particularly welcome in such gatherings as the present one, for a medium needs music, almost continuous music, for his demonstrations – a temperamental requirement which it would be foolish not to gratify.[66]

The combination of these elements, the comfortable furnishings, the cameras, stethoscopes and balances, the muted red light, and the whine of the accordion, all conspired to lend these occasions a chaotic feel and to strengthen the impression that this environment was indeed some strange hybrid between a spiritualist séance, a theatrical performance and a scientific experiment. As Mann noted of one of the sittings he attended, it was 'a masculine lying-in, in a reddish darkness, amid chatter and shouting and jazz. It was like nothing in the world.'[67]

Mediums in the laboratory

While the physical environment provided by the parapsychological laboratory played a significant role in Germans' engagement with and experience of the paranormal, the principal precondition for this interaction was the participation of a medium, a person whom, according to Grunewald, should be understood as a type of human conductor capable of transferring and reorganising energy in unusual ways.[68] As the only known means of producing phenomena such as materialisation and telekinesis, these paraphysically endowed individuals stood at the centre of parapsychological research, at once privileged vessels graced with natural or spiritual power, and interesting, possibly pathological, specimens demanding study, but worthy of suspicion. This dependence on mediums for the production of paranormal phenomena forced on parapsychologists a compromise, embodied in the parapsychological laboratory, between the experimental approach they wished to take and the spiritualist rituals to which mediums were deeply attached. The power differential between mediums and parapsychologists, their education within the spiritualist paradigm and the lack of knowledge surrounding the psychic and moral conditions of mediumship ensured that interactions between these two groups were and would remain problematic.

Despite their elevated psychical and physical abilities, these human conduits, often adolescents, tended to be poorly educated and to issue from the lower echelons of society. The Polish medium Stanislava P., for example, with whom the Baron experimented between September 1912 and February 1913, had been brought up by a gardener after the death of her parents and had remained illiterate up until her tenth year, still exhibiting difficulty with reading and writing when she first took part in a mediumistic sitting at the age of eighteen.[69] Mann also took an interest in, and noted the background of, the physical medium Willy Schneider, citing the Austrian dialect spoken by the young man as evidence of his humble origins.[70] It was typical also for these individuals, whose contact with and understanding of the scientific world was minimal, to have first discovered their mediumistic talent within a spiritualist setting, often in the family home or in the abode of close friends.[71] The medium Rudi Schneider, for example, began at twelve years of age to produce weak physical phenomena after watching the mediumistic performances of his older brother Willy in his home in Braunau am Inn.[72] While Willy was occupied in Munich, experimenting with Schrenck-Notzing, the boys' father dedicated himself to the mediumistic apprenticeship of his younger son, inculcating in Rudi an adherence to spiritualist rituals, including that of the trance personality.[73]

Bourgeois scientists' examinations of lower-class mediums, whose abilities had been discovered and fostered in domestic circles, ensured that the parapsychological laboratory became the site of a complex interaction between the classes and tension over mediums' reliance on spiritualist ritual.[74] Eager to transform the study of the paranormal from a religious enterprise into an experimental science, parapsychologists became increasingly aware of the necessity of ridding mediums of their spiritualist preconceptions and educating them in the scientific method. The Baron, for example, was convinced that while the physical aids used in the laboratory, including thermometers, cameras and balances, were of great importance in parapsychologists' struggle to gain scientific recognition, the correct training of mediums for scientific investigation would ultimately prove of much more significance in this endeavour. Such training was essential, Schrenck-Notzing stressed, because:

[W]e may be sure that absence of criticism, credulity, and the fanaticism of spiritists, have greatly hindered the education of mediums for scientifically useful objects…. The whole method of the spiritistic education of mediums, with their ballast of unnecessary conceptions, gives indeed encouragement to fraud.[75]

The spectre of fraud in the parapsychological laboratory was, as many researchers noted, highly problematic, an issue that had its roots in the spiritualist education of mediums and in the as yet opaque relationship between mediumship and hysteria, a well-known symptom of which was simulation. The medium, an instrument peculiarly sensitive to both the physical and psychical environment, required an atmosphere free of scepticism or suspicion in order to function optimally. Grunewald stressed that:

The behaviour of the experimenter towards the medium and the external intelligences manifested through them is a point, the importance of which can not be stressed enough. If one does not know from the beginning how to win the trust of the medium, success is already doubtful. Mediums are psychically mostly extremely sensitive people. Mistrustful scepticism or complete disbelief, open or concealed from view, will be felt by most mediums as extremely disturbing, so that in many cases in the presence of particularly mistrustful persons the phenomena will partially or totally fail to appear.[76]

In a similar fashion, T.K. Oesterreich suggested that mediums might be subject to *inhibition sociale*, which he described as an extreme sensitivity to mistrust. Under no circumstances, he declared, should the possibility of fraud be discussed in the medium's presence, he or she should be convinced of the participants' absolute belief in the phenomena.[77] This precaution might prove insufficient, he warned, in cases where the medium possessed telepathic abilities and was able to sense scepticism even when it was not articulated. In these circumstances, Oesterreich concluded, it was unsurprising that the best phenomena were frequently restricted to spiritualist séances where mediums felt most at ease.[78]

Those dedicated to the application of the scientific method to the paranormal soon became aware of the difficulties implicit in such an approach. The sceptical stance adopted by those involved in such experimentation and made explicit in the checks and controls to which the medium was subject appeared to drastically inhibit the ability of these individuals to produce paranormal phenomena. The very conditions required to satisfy standards of scientific proof, it seemed, were inimical to the phenomena they attempted to verify. There existed a conviction among

148

parapsychologists, for example, that their ignorance of the psychic and moral conditions required for mediumship was responsible in large part for the fraudulent production of paranormal phenomena by mediums. The restrictions and controls demanded by the scientific method, they believed, prohibited mediumship in much the same manner as a room devoid of oxygen would prohibit fire. In such circumstances the lability of mediums, – subject, as they were thought to be, to the hystero-hypnotic complex – was believed to contribute to conscious or unconscious fraud. Schrenck-Notzing wrote:

> [I]ndeed, it almost seems as if the tendency towards deception and to the mechanical production of mediumistic occurrences is a frequent quality of mediumship, just as simulation appears as a symptom of hysteria, or as *pseudologia phantastica* is inseparable from certain degenerative conditions of the brain.[79]

But while it was crucial to reassure the medium of the open-mindedness of the experimenter, it was equally important, given the propensity of such paraphysically endowed individuals to both consciously and unconsciously aid in the production of their phenomena, and parapsychologists' investment in moulding the study of the paranormal into a science, to ensure that precautions were taken to prevent fraud.

The sense of *Gemütlichkeit* fostered by the laboratory's domestic furnishings and the congenial banter of the experimenters was juxtaposed with the series of invasive checks and controls to which the medium was subject in order to vouchsafe their phenomena. While precautionary measures were also taken in the spiritualist context, the procedures carried out in the laboratory tended to be of a much more intrusive and clinical nature. Mediums were routinely asked, for example, to remove their clothes, in the presence of several people, in order to undergo a series of thorough oral, gynaecological and anal examinations.[80] According to one participant, who attended a mediumistic sitting during November 1917, even the space under the medium's fingernails was checked for hidden devices by means of a manicuring device.[81] Mediums were usually dressed in a simple one-piece outfit, often a type of body stocking, which was sewn up the back and supervised as they took their place in the medium cabinet. These measures were intended to exclude the possibility of the medium smuggling material into the laboratory.[82] It was also typical for the medium to be restrained in some manner, either by participants who held their wrists and feet, or by some form of device, an electrical medium control, for example, which would register movement through a flickering light, or a gauze-covered cage in which they would be locked. Mann, like many other participants in

Schrenck-Notzing's experimental evenings, took an active part in the examination and restraint of the medium particularly at the first sitting he attended. As a precautionary measure he was instructed to watch the medium, Willy Schneider, dress and to inspect his mouth for hidden devices. He was also asked to act as a control, that is, to sit facing the medium, to clasp the young man's hands and to secure his knees between his own.[83] Driesch noted similar checks and controls in a protocol dated 20 February 1922, describing his perusal of the cabinet and the medium's clothing prior to the séance and detailing the manner in which Willy's hands, legs and feet were restrained by other participants during the proceedings.[84] Despite the invasive and restrictive measures to which the medium was subject in the laboratory, the sitting remained a forum in which he or she exhibited impressive control and was given sanction, by virtue of their mediumship, to subvert both social and moral norms.

The coquettish behaviour of Mina, the female trance personality of the medium Willy Schneider, and the sexually suggestive sounds and motions that accompanied the production of his phenomena, combined not only to give sittings, such as that attended by Mann, a sensational character, but an overtly sexual tone.[85] The retiring working-class adolescent that had been introduced to guests before the experiment was replaced in the laboratory by an assertive medium who demanded that the participants talk, reminded the Baron of precautions that had been overlooked, and called for intermissions when he felt fatigued. The participants, as Mann noted, encouraged the medium, asking his trance personality what they might do to speed up the phenomena, they cajoled him and stroked his hands in the hope of persuading him to perform, they entered into the delusion of his trance personality, entreating Mina to show them some phenomena. The medium, however, persisted in making them wait nearly two hours before he manifested his power. The medium's moans and the writhing of his or her body was likened by many participants to the act of childbirth, an impression that was strengthened by the emission of phenomena from the breasts and genitals of female mediums.[86] Willy Schneider's trance behaviour was of an even more overtly sexual and startling nature. Mann wrote to the Baron in December 1922, for example, that he was not surprised to hear that Willy's phenomena were on occasion accompanied by erections and ejaculations, often actively induced.[87] The nature of Willy Schneider's behaviour, the transformation he made during the séance from a deferential youth to a self-assured conduit of unknown biological and psychological power, was understood by the Baron and the participants to be a concomitant of mediumship. Behaviour that would have been considered socially and morally subversive in another context was accepted in the laboratory as an integral part of these ill-understood phenomena.

The mediumistic manifestations witnessed by séance participants such as Mann and Oesterreich were of a physical rather than a psychical nature, consisting almost exclusively of the movement of objects at a distance. The telekinetic phenomena exhibited by Willy Schneider included the levitation of a handkerchief, which appeared to be lifted from within by a claw-like limb, the ringing of a small table bell by some unseen force, and the tap-tap-tap of an invisible hand on a typewriter. Oesterreich, who was witness to such phenomena, wrote:

> A bell (made visible through fluorescent paint) placed on the floor by Schrenck-Notzing lifted itself and swayed backwards and forwards in space in front of the participants. The music box began to play, sounded again anew from the beginning and as many times as the participants wished.[88]

Elsewhere he noted the brief appearance of an ectoplasmic limb, which although he never saw it clearly, resembled the end of a large finger.[89]

Other mediums with whom Schrenck-Notzing experimented, including the talented French medium Eva C., more routinely produced ectoplasmic forms rather than telekinetic movements. These protrusions might be amorphous, issuing from the nose, mouth or genitals, or resemble body parts, such as limbs and heads. Eva C's materialisations tended to be two dimensional images of heads, which bore a strong resemblance to pictures that had appeared in the French newspaper *Le Miroir* and even reproduced, as some participants noted, the creases and tears one might expect to see on a piece of paper that had been folded and secreted away (see Image 3.2 overleaf).[90] This medium also, on occasion, produced large quantities of pale muslin-like ectoplasm, some of which spewed forth onto her dress and some of which swathed the ideoplastic heads that she produced, quickly reabsorbing into her body as the phenomena dematerialised or if the medium was touched or threatened in some manner. These phenomena, many of which were captured by the stereoscopic cameras which dominated Schrenck-Notzing's laboratory, were the central ingredients of the parapsychological experience and received extensive coverage in the protocols provided by those that participated in experiments at the Karolinenplatz laboratory.

Photography in the laboratory

The camera, ostensibly immune to the weaknesses characteristic of the senses, was understood by parapsychologists to offer an objective and unmediated form of testimony. Schrenck-Notzing, like Enrico Imoda in Italy and Harry Price (1881–1948) in England, used this technology to capture the fleeting phenomena of mediumship, granting its emissions

Image 3.2

Eva C. with materialised head, 1913.
Reproduced with permission from the Institut für Grenzgebiete der Psychologie
und Psychohygiene e. V., Freiburg im Breisgau (IGPP collection).

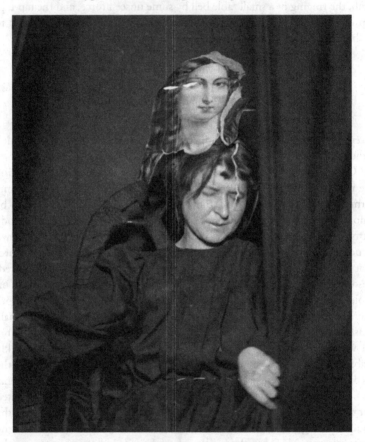

evidentiary status. The Baron, who took hundreds of photographs of the materialisations produced by the physical mediums Eva C., Willy Schneider and Stanislava P., published these pictures alongside experimental protocols as tangible evidence of some as yet unknown natural force. This peculiar use of photography, referred to in some instances as the 'Fotographie des Unsichtbaren' [photography of the invisible], purported to be an accurate and uncompromised record of the mediumistic phenomena produced in the course of parapsychological experiments; images differentiated from those taken in the spiritualist context by strict control of the medium's body and constant illumination of the experimental space.[91]

Spirit photography had emerged during the 1860s offering what many believed was convincing evidence of spiritualist contentions about the afterlife and fostering a lucrative business in images of the dead, which fed off both sensation and grief.[92] Such photographs, taken in a studio, tended to consist of a subject – not usually a medium – who sat or stood unaffected by and unaware of the spectre in the background. In nineteenth-century spirit photographs it was not normally necessary for a medium to be present, the camera acted as the mediator for the supernatural, materialising what was invisible to the naked eye.[93] Early on in the history of spirit photography, however, it became apparent that such otherworldly portraits could be and were being faked – photographers developing ever more ingenious techniques in order to keep up not only with advances in the technology but the public's knowledge and understanding of it.[94] Despite multiple exposures for fraud, spirit photography proved resilient, surviving well into the twentieth century where it experienced a revival following the First World War.[95] For some observers, most particularly spiritualists, the reproduction of ghostly images on photographic plates provided compelling evidence for the immortality of the soul, for others, however, including critics of both spiritualism and psychical research, such photographs served only to foster debate over the nature of objective knowledge.[96]

The photographic images produced in the course of parapsychological experiments, although superficially similar to spirit photographs, differed from them in at least one significant way. This was the centrality of the human medium in these images and the demotion of the camera from its role as the mediator of the supernatural to dispassionate observer and recording device. Parapsychologists used photography to capture the dynamic and often violent production of ectoplasm from mediums' bodies, which in stark contrast to the calm, composed bodies of those who sat for spirit photographs were often seen contorted in pain or in furious motion.[97] These images were understood by parapsychologists to exist less in the tradition of the spirit photograph, with its chequered history of both commercialism and fraud, and more in the tradition of scientific or medical photography. During the nineteenth century a number of new scientific fields, including meteorology and bacteriology, used photography as part of their bid for epistemic authority and professional status. For these emergent sciences, as with parapsychology, the camera seemed to offer a means of capturing elusive or invisible phenomena and eliminating human prejudice and error from observations.[98] This belief in a kind of unmediated seeing was also apparent in the photographic work undertaken by Jean-Martin Charcot with Parisian hysterics.[99] Charcot, who made use of historical paintings of witches and demoniacs as well as photographs in his attempt to establish the immutability of his hysteric nosography, believed that visual inscription allowed the truest account of clinical practice, transforming the bodies of hysterics into psychic canvases and rendering symptoms self-evident to the observer.[100] Similarly, parapsychologists maintained that the photographs they took of materialised heads and amorphous strands of ectoplasm were unmediated images of self-evident biological and psychological realities. Although historian Jennifer Tucker has shown that during the mid-nineteenth century peak of fascination with, and height of faith in, photography, there was concern and debate about its value as scientific evidence, it is apparent that the trope of photography as an objective and unmediated portrait of nature continued to be used by parapsychologists and others to support claims to scientific legitimacy long after this naïve notion had been debunked.[101]

The photographs of materialised forms published by the Baron were perhaps the most evocative of the proofs he produced in order to verify the objective existence of the physical phenomena of mediumship. These images conveyed, in a way in which written protocols could not, the sensory experiences of those who visited Schrenck-Notzing's laboratory. They also demonstrated the manner in which the Baron believed he had transformed the study of mediumship into a truly scientific endeavour. While Schrenck-Notzing advocated the importance of those instruments imported from the physical and psychological sciences, he was convinced that the introduction of the camera to the parapsychological laboratory was of even greater significance. In his book *Materialisations-Phänomene* [*The Phenomena of Materialisation*], in which he made extensive use of photography, he argued, 'better even than dynamometers, balances and metronomes is the photographic camera, since it gives positive proofs in the real sense of the word.'[102]

Schrenck-Notzing's introduction of photographic equipment to his laboratory and to his mediums was a gradual process. In his initial experiments with the medium Eva C., with whom most of his materialisation photographs were taken, the Baron used only a single camera. Nearing the end of his four-year investigation with this medium, however, he routinely used up to nine photographic devices, including several stereoscopic cameras, at the same time.[103] With the Polish medium Stanislava P., he also had some success in producing cinematographic images, which demonstrated vividly the manner in which ectoplasm, issuing from the medium's mouth, expanded and contracted.[104] For Schrenck-Notzing, the evidentiary power of these photographic and cinematographic images was such that he believed himself justified in declaring the birth of a new scientific discipline.[105]

The Baron's use of photography impressed many of those who attended his sittings or read his books. The correspondence he received on this matter reveals a shared conviction of photography's importance to the field and a concern with perfecting the conditions under which such pictures were taken. The cinematographer Ernst Haberkorn, for example, wrote to the Baron in order to tell him that he found his photographic technique extraordinary and to offer his services should Schrenck-Notzing ever require them.[106] E. Westlake of the Society for Psychical Research also wrote, making a few suggestions on how the Baron could improve his photographic method. The future of mediumistic research, it seemed to Westlake, depended on a better means of illumination than the flashbulb. This device had the double disadvantage of allowing only one photo to be taken at a time and of distressing the medium to the extent that the phenomena usually terminated.[107] He suggested the use of tanks, attached to the ceiling and filled with a solution of ammonia-copper-sulphate, which would cut off all rays except ultraviolet light.[108] If it were possible to obtain cinematographic pictures in this light, he maintained, the field would undergo an enormous advance. He wrote, 'The new era in astronomy began with Galileo's glasses. Similarly, I conceive the discovery of light in which mediums could be properly observed would initiate a new era in psychology.'[109] While such suggestions helped refine the use of photography in the Karolinenplatz laboratory they did little to clarify the meaning of those phenomena captured by the Baron's cameras.

Interpretations and theories

The materialisation and dematerialisation in Schrenck-Notzing's laboratory of teleplastic limbs and heads, and the movement of objects at a distance by the invisible ectoplasmic protrusions that issued from mediums' bodies were understood by some observers not only as strange or entertaining experiences, but as phenomena revealing of Germany's prevailing social, moral and epistemological situation. Mann's essay 'Okkulte Erlebnisse' ['An Experience in the Occult'] analysed the emergence of experimental parapsychology in this manner, pointing to the social and moral void that parapsychology helped fill in the wake of the First World War and to the contemporary epistemological changes to which the scientific study of the paranormal was linked. The lust for the occult exhibited in the Baron's laboratory was symptomatic, according to Mann, of the *weltanschauliche* changes brought about by the war.[110] The social and moral uncertainties of the Weimar period were apparent in Germans' loss of faith in institutions, such as the Church and the Government, and in their attempts to locate alternatives to them. The surge of occultism that followed the war, for instance, of which experimental parapsychology was an example, was one such attempt to supplement or by-pass traditional means of social and moral support and to regain the sense of equilibrium in German life that had been disrupted by the hostilities. The attempt in Germany to create an experimental parapsychology was also regarded by Mann as a response to the series of epistemological changes that had occurred around the turn of the century in sciences such as physics, biology and psychology. He noted, for instance, the manner in which he believed Einstein's doctrine of relativity had made fluid the border between mathematical physics and metaphysics, and the way in which the influence of vitalism in biology had allowed materialisation and telekinesis to be theorised as forms of supernormal biology.[111] Mann's musings reflected contemporary social, moral and epistemological tendencies and the radically different ways in which spiritualists and parapsychologists interpreted the phenomena of mediumship.

The experiential fissure between what transpired in the laboratory and what occurred in the domestic séance room, a gap that parapsychologists were naturally eager to widen, was less to do with the nature of the phenomena produced in these venues, or the differences between these venues themselves, and more to do with the different epistemological lenses through which parapsychologists and spiritualists chose to view these manifestations. While spiritualists understood and theorised these phenomena in terms of an afterlife or some other less tangible form of survival (the spiritist paradigm), parapsychologists, many of whom were also doctors, psychologists or biologists, tended to favour a natural, albeit pathological, explanation (animist paradigm) for the materialised forms and telekinetic movements they witnessed in the laboratory. The adoption of this epistemological approach saw the disembodied heads and limbs produced by mediums such as Eva C. interpreted not as spiritual messengers, but as materialised thoughts, memories or ideas.[112] These ideoplastic protrusions, as Schrenck-Notzing dubbed them, were mental images that had, in some as yet unexplained way, been made material and projected outside, but in connection with, the medium's body. Telekinesis, similarly, was believed to be achieved by invisible ideoplastic or ectoplasmic threads that grew out of the medium's body, wrapping themselves around distant objects in order to effect movement. The ectoplasmic material that on occasion issued from medium's orifices and reproductive organs also lent itself to a natural or super-normal explanation.[113] As previously mentioned, Schrenck-Notzing managed to obtain pieces of ectoplasm and sent samples to laboratories in Munich for microscopic analysis.[114] This approach to mediumistic phenomena was based on the conviction that these manifestations were of psycho-biological origin, a hypothesis that came to dominate parapsychologists' theoretical engagement with the paranormal during the 1920s and 1930s.

The clash of these two paradigms occurred in the transference of mediums from the spiritualist context, where they tended to receive their initial training, to that of parapsychology, where there existed a strong desire to achieve differentiation from spiritualism and recognition from the scientific community. Parapsychologists' reliance on mediums for the production of the phenomena they wished to study created a series of problems between these two groups, who found themselves in a struggle over the manner in which mediumistic experiments should be conducted and over the meaning – spiritual, biological or psychological – that was to be attributed to these phenomena. The power play that occurred between mediums and parapsychologists in the laboratory around the categories of gender, class and knowledge played a significant role in parapsychologists' attempts to win acceptance for their nascent experimental science.

Gender, class and power in the laboratory

The parapsychologist's circumscription of meaning within the laboratory, as a consequence of their analysis of paranormal phenomena within the biomedical and psychological paradigms in which they received their formal training, constrained the flexibility of gender and class relations that has been noted as a characteristic of the domestic séance.[115] In this context, the medium was less the empowered conduit to the other world found in the spiritualist séance, than an experimental subject whose agency was restricted by a lack of control over the circumstances under which he or she performed and of the meaning given to that performance. The medium as a privileged or superior being is absent from experimental protocols and works of parapsychological theory, replaced by the immature young adult of somewhat suspect character, hysteric constitution, and limited social graces. The medicalisation and psychologisation of mediumship, which took place in the laboratory, produced a meaning entirely different from that generated within the spiritualist context, altering the manner in which mediums were able to exert power and control in the production of their phenomena.[116] Contrasting the gender and class relations typical of spiritualism with those of experimental parapsychology in the German context, this section explores the struggle over meaning and power that took place in the parapsychological laboratory.

Mediums were understood by spiritualists to be people who, as a result of either spiritual superiority or psychic talent, were capable of acting as intermediaries between this world and the next.[117] In their capacity as messengers for the departed, mediums helped transmit information or images through automatic writing, direct speech and materialisation.[118] A medium might, for example, establish contact with spirits and then submit them to written or oral interrogation, they might become possessed by a spirit who sought to communicate with the séance participants or act as a source of matter and energy for a spirit who wished to take on physical form. By mediating the discourse between this and the other world and by transforming the immaterial into the material these individuals provided evidence for the immortality of the soul and sustenance for flagging religious convictions.[119] Understood as conduits to the spirit realm, privileged vessels, spiritualist mediums could, to a large extent, dictate the conditions under which they performed and the meaning of the phenomena they produced.

The domestic nature of spiritualism, as we have seen above, distinguished it from parapsychology and lent séances an atmosphere of trust and intimacy that could not be replicated in the laboratory. While checks and controls were practised in some domestic séances and in those sittings conducted for profit, for many spiritualists it seemed unnecessary, if not insulting, to frisk one's friends, family or servants. The use of domestic space for spiritualist séances also saw large numbers of women take on the role of medium, a part that proved liberating for those whose opinions on religious, social and political matters were not normally given an airing.[120] Mediumship also allowed both men and women to play with or distort concepts of gender and thereby subvert societal norms.[121] A female medium, for example, might adopt a male spirit guide or trance personality whose behaviour was lewd and uncouth, or perform in an unbecoming manner, sitting on men's laps and kissing them, as did the English medium Florence Cook.[122] In a similar manner, male mediums like Willy Schneider often employed female trance personalities, many of whom were outrageous flirts. A spiritualist séance might also provide opportunities for advancement or the transgression of class boundaries in cases where domestic servants became mediums in the homes in which they worked. Spiritualist mediumship, thus, was a phenomenon that not only offered participants a reward, that is, contact with their dead relatives or confirmation of their religious beliefs, but also benefited mediums who might derive from their role power and freedom, if only temporarily, from restrictive gender roles and societal norms. This was particularly liberating for female mediums who in this forum could throw off the shackles of gender without fundamentally questioning accepted ideas about women's nature.[123]

The power derived from female mediumship, however, was of a peculiarly limited nature, feeding off socially constructed ideas about women's innate passivity and receptivity.[124] Contemporary stereotypes of femininity bore a striking resemblance to the ideal medium, who was unsophisticated, innocent, passive, young, tender, feeling and intuitive.[125] While mediumship allowed unheard of freedom of expression, its foundation in an essentialist theory of womanhood restricted the performance of these freedoms to the séance room and the trance state. Spiritualists commonly believed that spirits could only enter the bodies of those, like women, whose wills were weak or easily supplanted. In this understanding of mediumship, the act of spirit communication or possession operated as a type of spiritual penetration to which women were naturally susceptible given their presumed passive role in the sexual act and their subservience under God's law to the will of men. This theory was also responsible for the homosexual taint that attached itself to male mediums. In his book on sexual inversion (homosexuality), Albert Moll noted that, '[Eduard von] Hartmann has observed that among spiritualists and mediums in particular, are a great many sexual inverts.'[126] Homosexuality was seen by many observers as a requisite of male mediumship, which, understood as sexual inversion, that is a desire to take on the passive role in the sexual act, explained the mediumistic power of certain men.[127] The spiritualist belief in this theory ensured that the power and freedom that both female and male mediums derived from mediumship did not pose a serious threat to normative gender or class roles because mediums' subversive performances were understood only to be possible because of their innate inferiority.

The limited powers and freedoms that accompanied the role of medium underwent further circumscription in the parapsychological laboratory where the phenomena of mediumship were interpreted within psychological and biological paradigms. In this context, mediums' powers were understood as the result of both their innate passivity and receptivity, and as a signifier of their abnormality or pathology; a link made explicit in parapsychologists' emphasis on the relationship between mediumship and hysteria.[128] The psychologist and parapsychologist Richard Baerwald (1867–1929), for example, argued that hysteria and a mediumistic predisposition were so intimately linked that they were almost identical.[129] This relationship, he argued, helped explain the tendency of mediums towards fraud. Baerwald wrote in this regard that in the dissociative state many mediums committed fraud, unaware of what they were doing.[130] The perceived connection between hysteria and mediumship was also apparent in those theories that regarded materialisation and telekinesis as physical manifestations of the mental distress and unchannelled sexual energy of hysterical women.[131] The sexual nature of much of the phenomena encouraged such interpretations. The opposite sex trance personalities exhibited by mediums like Willy Schneider, for example, were understood as the result of frustrated sexual desires. The parapsychologist and psychoanalyst Richard Winterstein assigned such spirit personifications an erotic meaning, writing:

In the majority of cases the controlling spirit belongs to another sex than the medium ('Nell' of Frau Silbert, 'John' of Eusapia Palladino) and personifies then either a love object or the strongly pronounced sympathies of the medium with the opposite sex.[132]

The sexual behaviour of mediums and their trance personalities, many of whom were adolescents, also led a number of parapsychologists to make a connection between sexual development and mediumship.[133]

The agency and dignity that mediums enjoyed in the spiritualist context was largely absent from parapsychological sittings. In the laboratory, experimenters conducted invasive searches of the medium's person and belongings, intimated, through the use of physical restraint and medical discourse, that the medium was a pathological fraud and interpreted what the medium understood to be their spirit guide or trance personality as a spiritualist crutch or symptom of nervous or sexual disorder.[134] The spiritual significance that mediums and spiritualists gave paranormal phenomena was, in the laboratories of parapsychologists such as Schrenck-Notzing, disregarded as childish fantasy.[135] In this context, the medium lost both their role as a mediator and their right to interpret or decide the meaning of their phenomena. Like the magnetic somnambulists of the early nineteenth century, the hypnotised medium might be able to dictate some conditions in the laboratory, but ultimately the interpretation of any phenomena would be decided by the magnetiser or, in this case, the parapsychologist.[136]

The medium's subjectification within the laboratory took a number of forms. By accepting an engagement with a parapsychologist the medium tacitly agreed to undergo a series of examinations, often of an uncomfortable and humiliating nature. It was standard procedure, as we have seen, to be asked to remove all of one's clothes prior to and following a séance and not uncommon to be required to submit to anal, oral and vaginal searches in order to establish that the phenomena produced during the sitting were not the result of props hidden on or in the body.[137] These precautions were necessary, according to parapsychologists, because mediums, despite or perhaps because of their psychic and physical abilities, were consummate frauds. The ability of mediums to produce ectoplasmic substances from their mouths, for example, was considered suspicious by sceptics who hypothesised that mediums might be individuals who possessed the ability to regurgitate objects they had swallowed at will.[138] In order to insure against this possibility mediums were fed liquids or foods, such as berries, which would dye their stomach contents. Other mediums were fed purgatives to ascertain whether they had 'dematerialised' any of their phenomena by swallowing them or were examined by x-ray to ensure that they did not hide props in their stomachs. X-ray technology was also used to discover whether mediums were subject to any physiological abnormality, such as two stomachs, which they could exploit to produce fraudulent phenomena. The medium Eva C. underwent just such an examination in Paris in May 1921. Louis Beaupres and Emile Vallet, both physicians, wrote:

We now let her have milk and sponge to drink and noticed that the passage of the sponge through the oesophagus was carried out in an absolutely normal manner and that the oesophagus showed no peculiarities whatever, like, for example, narrowing, widening or other abnormalities. The stomach appears to be a hollow pouch of normal volume and fills itself in a normal manner…. One observed neither gastric hyperkinesis nor autoperistaltic movements or regurgitation.[139]

Within the sitting itself, mediums also found themselves disempowered by the physical restraints and mechanical devices used to restrict and monitor their movements.

The measure of agency that mediums did manage to maintain in the laboratory frequently came at the price of their waking personalities. Mediums' trance personalities were shown a level of respect that mediums themselves could not expect in their waking state. While the medium was subject to examinations and suspicion, trance personalities or spirit guides, while not taken seriously by parapsychologists, were often the recipients of praise and flattery. 'Mina', the trance personality of the medium Willy Schneider, for example, was cosseted by admirers, demanded subtle changes to her environment, and made her audience wait up to two hours before she revealed any phenomena.[140] But while participants were respectful of these spirit guides or trance personalities, parapsychologists tended to view them as a nuisance, another spiritualist ritual, that might eventually be discarded once the medium understood the principles of scientific experimentation and had undergone a process of re-education.

The experimental protocols produced in the Baron's home illustrate the transformation that the meaning of mediumship and the balance of power underwent in its transition from the séance room to the laboratory. In his book *Materialisations-Phänomene*, published in 1913, Schrenck-Notzing prefaced his reports on the phenomena of the medium Eva C. with a description of his laboratory, a discussion of theoretical and methodological considerations, and with details of how he had successfully re-educated her for laboratory experiments. All of this gave the impression of mastery over the circumstances under which such experimentation took place and of the medium. Analysis of his correspondence, however, reveals more than the image that Schrenck-Notzing – focused on achieving differentiation from spiritualism and recognition from the scientific community – hoped to project. Indeed, they expose the complex set of class, gender and power relationships operating within the parapsychological laboratory. While these relationships may at first glance appear straightforward – a wealthy medically trained aristocrat exploiting lower middle- or working-class female or adolescent male mediums – the reality was often more complex. The medium's control of the 'means of production', that is, their status as the only known means of producing paranormal phenomena, gave them a measure of power over the parapsychologist that could be and in some cases was used to their advantage.

Willy versus the Baron

Schrenck-Notzing's near monopoly of German parapsychology during the 1920s was in part due to his use of medium contracts. These agreements allowed the Baron to re-train those mediums who clung stubbornly to spiritualist traditions and to conduct a volume of sittings, which was not possible with freelance mediums. In return, the contracted medium received board and remuneration. In the case of Willy Schneider, an Austrian boy from a printer's family, Schrenck-Notzing not only provided a small allowance and private board with a Frau Prestele, but a dental technician's apprenticeship under the tutelage of the dentist Herr Delmuth.[141] This arrangement was intended to provide security for both parties, protecting Willy from the police prosecution he would have faced as a freelance medium under Bavarian law and enabling the Baron to conduct a series of experiments with a talented physical medium without fear of competition. A contract of this nature should have ensured the parapsychologist's dominance in his relationship with his medium, but Schrenck-Notzing's dependency on the mediumistic powers of his disobedient charge made the dynamic between them more complex. In spite of the Baron's warnings that Willy would be subject to prosecution should he breach his contract, the medium threatened on multiple occasions to withdraw his services if his demands were not met.[142] Willy accused Schrenck-Notzing of exploiting him, claiming that he withheld the money generated through his performances. The argument that followed in a series of letters exchanged between Schrenck-Notzing and Herr Schneider, the medium's father, revealed a conflict in which the balance of power between medium and parapsychologist exhibited an unexpected plasticity.

In October 1922, Herr Schneider wrote to Schrenck-Notzing accusing him of using his son in order to bolster his academic reputation, a charge that the outraged Baron fervently denied. He wrote:

> It is a complete mistake, if you believe that Willy is for me a means of gaining prestige in the intellectual world. My scientific position is completely

162

Image 3.3

Willy Schneider gives a séance in Braunau am Inn.
Reproduced with permission from the Institut für Grenzgebiete der Psychologie
und Psychohygiene e. V., Freiburg im Breisgau (IGPP collection).

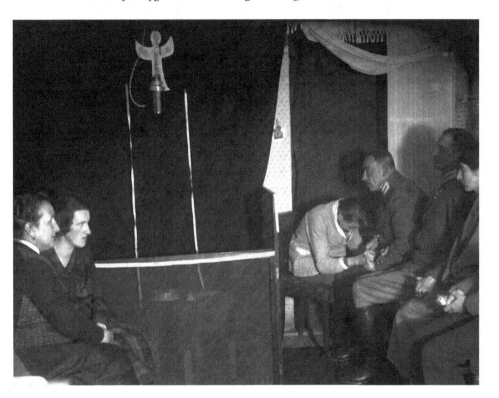

ensured through decades of work done. On the other hand, however, I must
claim credit, if it succeeds in making Willy a world-famous medium....[143]

According to the Baron, Willy was lazy, unreliable and tardy. In his work
as a dental technician he was clumsy, taking inadequate care with the
application of gold, and frequently arrived at work late. The boy's lack of
money was not due to the inadequacy of his allowance, Schrenck-Notzing
claimed, but was a result of his indiscriminate spending on items such as
cigarettes. This same lack of discipline was apparent in his performance as a
medium, his failure to concentrate on the task at hand inhibiting his
production of phenomena.[144] Willy, the Baron maintained, was a liar,
although this, he conceded, might be an attribute of his mediumship.[145]

Early the next year began another barrage of letters in which Herr Schneider made it clear that he no longer wanted Willy to work with Schrenck-Notzing, hinting that his son aspired to be a professional medium.[146] It also became apparent at this time that other researchers, including J. Hewat McKenzie of the British College of Psychic Science, were attempting to lure Willy away, offering the boy a far more substantial salary than he was receiving from Schrenck-Notzing.[147] The Baron's retort stressed that he had done everything in his power to comply with Schneider's wish that Willy be provided with an education and that he should not become a professional medium. He reminded Schneider that:

> You must also reckon with the possibility that one day the mediumistic power expires. Then, if he is not in the position to be gainfully employed as a dental technician, he will be a loafer and black marketeer on the street.[148]

In answer to Schneider's accusation that he deprived Willy of money that was rightfully his, Schrenck-Notzing explained, that he asked participants only for a small contribution towards the cost of the experiments and that he made no profit from these donations.[149] Sadly, the Baron wrote, Schneider's threat to withdraw his son's services came at a most inopportune moment for both parties because the press and the public were only just becoming interested in Willy and his phenomena.[150]

Two years later, during which time Willy's younger brother Rudi had developed as a powerful physical medium, the recalcitrant medium returned to the Baron's employ.[151] Relations between the two, however, remained strained with Willy ignoring the Baron's repeated invitations to give sittings in Munich and allowing other researchers, in deliberate breach of his contract, to experiment with him.[152] In spite of the dire consequences threatened by Schrenck-Notzing, who stressed that under both German and Austrian law Willy was bound to him by a one-year contract, the medium continued to push the boundaries. The final act of this drama was played out in 1927 when Willy allowed an English researcher to investigate his phenomena. This man accused Willy of fraud and circulated his report in the press. The Baron wrote angrily to Schneider, whom he held responsible for this mess, 'now you, as a perpetual know-it-all, have clumsily destroyed the work that I have for years laboriously built up and have shamefully destroyed the good reputation of your two sons'.[153] The medium's command of the power relations within the laboratory, while never particularly great, was most apparent, as in Willy's case, when they threatened to withdraw their services. As the conduits of paranormal power the medium's psychical or physical talents were their most important bargaining chips in their interactions with parapsychologists.

The grand seignior

Schrenck-Notzing's dominance within the German parapsychological community began to generate discontent during the mid-1920s among those who sought a more democratic approach to the study of the paranormal. These critics, the majority of whom were of a younger generation than the Baron, resented the power that his money gave him to shape and direct parapsychological research in the German context. The Baron's monopolistic grasp on the *Psychische Studien* and later the *Zeitschrift für Parapsychologie*, allowed him, they maintained, to dictate the content of these journals, to hire and fire editorial staff at will, and to set the agenda for parapsychological research in Germany, deciding, for example, which researchers would represent German interests at international congresses.[154] These complaints were not without foundation. Schrenck-Notzing's aggressive promotion of parapsychology as a nascent science and his large financial contributions to the field led him to demand deference and gratitude from his colleagues. Fashioning himself as the 'Grand Seignior' of German parapsychology, his paternalistic and adversarial attitude towards other members of the parapsychological community provoked a series of bitter conflicts during the mid- to late 1920s.[155]

Schrenck-Notzing's heavy-handed directorship of the journal *Psychische Studien* during the early 1920s led a number of researchers, in particular those with an interest in the psychical phenomena of mediumship, to found a new periodical under the leadership of Richard Baerwald in 1925. This periodical entitled, *Zeitschrift für kritischen Okkultismus* [*Journal for Critical Occultism*], was supported by researchers including Albert Hellwig, Graf Carl Klinckowstroem (1884–1969) and Rudolf Tischner (1879–1961), and took a far more critical approach to parapsychology than that sanctioned in the *Psychische Studien*.[156] The Baron's initial reaction to the foundation of this new journal was to attempt to become a member of its editorial board, a move that would have negated its purpose as an organ immune to his influence. When this strategy proved unsuccessful, Schrenck-Notzing undertook the transformation of the *Psychische Studien* into a scientific format, a process that resulted in the birth of the *Zeitschrift für Parapsychologie*. The Baron's immense financial contribution to this conversion ensured his control of the new periodical's content and editorial procedure.[157] While this new journal was intended to project a scientific image and to provide a forum for research from every part of the spectrum, many researchers remained concerned by its polemic tone and its exclusionary editorial practices. Hans Thirring, for example, whom Schrenck-Notzing offered an editorial position at the *Zeitschrift für*

Parapsychologie, asked that the argumentative mode of writing that had characterised the *Psychische Studien* be abandoned in this new periodical.

> Exactly at this point when parapsychology feels safer, it is no longer necessary for [the journal] to serve as a polemical organ, rather a sober objective periodical requires that it publishes objective and critical works relevant to the field…. We hope therefore that the *Zeitschrift für Parapsychologie* under the skilful leadership of Dr Sünner will be a worthy organ for this new branch of research.[158]

In his reply, the Baron acknowledged Thirring's concern but argued that a polemical tone was still required in order to combat the attacks of critics.[159] Tensions over Schrenck-Notzing's role within the parapsychological community came to a head in 1927 in a confrontation with Rudolf Tischner and Rudolf Lambert (1866–1964).

Early in September of 1927, Tischner and Lambert wrote to Schrenck-Notzing complaining that the Baron's dismissal of a number of workers from the *Zeitschrift für Parapsychologie*, including Walther Kröner, Edgard Dreher, Carl Bruck and Eberhard Bruchner, had caused a state of crisis within the German parapsychological community, which could only be resolved by his resignation as the unofficial director of the journal.[160] They maintained that the current situation, in which the field was dominated by one man of great financial means, was disastrous. No one, Tischner and Lambert argued, could challenge Schrenck-Notzing because his fortune gave him the power to do whatever he wanted.[161] They wrote, 'the more profound reason is above all that you attempt dictatorially to lead occultism and in particular the *Zeitschrift für Parapsychologie* in your way and to practise an overriding control, that in a community of scholars is inappropriate.'[162] Claiming concern for the future of parapsychological research in Germany, they wrote:

> We must, because of the serious reasons cited, demand that you step down from your position as unofficial leader of the *Zeitschrift für Parapsychologie*…. Should you reject our suggestions or want to make difficulties after your passing of the *Zeitschrift für Parapsychologie*, we will have to announce this communication to all those working on the *Zeitschrift für Parapsychologie*, in particular Driesch and Oesterreich, whose judgement will not allow any doubt, we will also in the interest of the cause necessarily turn to the broader public.[163]

Schrenck-Notzing disputed these claims arguing that the chief editor of every journal had the right to overall control and that this did not constitute a dictatorship. Having dedicated both his time and money to the promotion of parapsychology as a legitimate field of scientific inquiry, he felt that such a leadership role was his due.

Schrenck-Notzing put this vicious attack on his person down to a number of factors. The first was Tischner's desire to replace Dr Paul Sünner as editor of the *Zeitschrift für Parapsychologie*. While the Baron conceded that Sünner's work was flawed and that Tischner might be a popular choice for the editorship, he was constrained, he contended, by the fact that the publisher Ostwald Mutze was against such an appointment. In subsequent correspondence, however, it became apparent that Schrenck-Notzing was equally opposed to Tischner gaining editorial control. While Tischner's work on telepathy and clairvoyance belonged to some of the best scholarship in the field, the Baron argued, it remained unclear, due to his vacillating nature, with which party he was affiliated. Tischner's editorial experience was also a cause for concern according to Schrenck-Notzing. During his brief time as the editor of the periodical *Der Okkultismus*, subscriptions, which had been at four thousand, fell dramatically. It was also noteworthy, he argued, that Tischner had been a member of the editorial board of the opposing journal the *Zeitschrift für kritischen Okkultismus*. But the most compelling reason against Tischner's editorship, Schrenck-Notzing maintained, was his involvement with the spiritualist group Eclaros. Tischner's talks on parapsychological topics to this group of amateurs, the Baron believed, compromised the nascent science of parapsychology. He wrote to Lambert, 'I now ask: can you still really give your trust to a man, who in a public manner supports occult quackery.'[164] Ironically, this was a similar argument to that made by Moll during Schrenck-Notzing's association with the *Traumtänzerin* Magdeleine G.

The second factor was less tangible. Stunned by the ungratefulness of a man he had helped educate as a parapsychologist, Schrenck-Notzing could only conclude that Lambert's behaviour was a result of an unresolved father complex.[165] He reminded his younger colleague of the contribution he had made to the field and the reasons why he was entitled to demand respect. He wrote:

> You forget completely, that it was not you who interested a large number of university lecturers in parapsychology and arranged the gentlemen who took over the protectorate of our journal; that it was not you who moulded mediums for scientific experiments; that it was not you who undertook the extraordinarily difficult transformation of *Psychische Studien* into a scientifically acceptable periodical – *rather all these achievements are thanks to me*. I would like you apart from that to remember, that during the inflation I supported the *Psychische Studien* financially and thereby protected it against folding, that I never took a fee for the printing of my work, that I made a

large series of royalty free contributions accessible to the journal, that I gave up the greater part of the dividends I was entitled to from the publishing house to propaganda purposes....[166]

This exchange between Schrenck-Notzing and his provocateurs was, as the Baron's instincts told him, to a large extent a generational conflict. Tischner and Lambert desired a greater role in the leadership and administration of parapsychology in Germany, but were prevented from doing so by Schrenck-Notzing, whose money allowed him to control the means of both production and publication.

The crucial role played by money in the development of parapsychology in the German context was also evident in several other attempts to release German parapsychology from the yoke of Schrenck-Notzing's dictatorship. In December 1925, Tischner established the Okkultische Gesellschaft [Occult Society] in Munich, the purpose of which was to conduct research across the entire field on a scientific basis. By January 1930, however, the group had collapsed. 'In the club register was today entered: Occult Society, Munich: Through complete loss of members the club is dissolved.'[167] There were efforts also to establish a Deutsche Gesellschaft für Parapsychologie [German Society for Parapsychology] along the lines of the London-based Society for Psychical Research and a Deutschen Zentralinstituts für parapsychologische Forschung [German Central Institute for Parapsychological Research]. Both ventures, however, required substantial financial backing, support that their advocates found difficult to locate. Oesterreich acknowledged this problem when he attempted to solicit donations in a pamphlet, which prefaced the third edition of his book *Der Okkultismus in modernen Weltbild* [*The Occult in the Modern World*]:

> The further development of parapsychology is in a not insignificant part a question of material means.... Who will give the first million as a foundation grant? His name will remain unforgettable. And the call also goes out to Germans abroad: Give money! German parapsychology cannot win and maintain the necessary contacts with foreign parapsychology, if the foreign literature remains inaccessible.[168]

Tischner and Oesterreich negotiated with sponsors, continuing their efforts even after Schrenck-Notzing's death in February 1929. A few months later, however, the project had to be abandoned, because of the stock market crash.[169]

Schrenck-Notzing's attempt to nurture and promote experimental parapsychology in the German context was obviously not appreciated by everyone. It is clear that those with an interest in the psychical phenomena of mediumship felt excluded by the emphasis the Baron placed on the physical phenomena and that younger parapsychologists resented his domination of the field. It was money that allowed him to play this role and a lack of funds that prevented others from moulding the study of the paranormal in a way they might have preferred. For these reasons the *Geisterbaron*, while Germany's most prominent propagandist for parapsychology, became a controversial figure among his peers. Schrenck-Notzing's critics, of course, did not all derive from within the parapsychological community, his most ferocious opponents hailed from other fields.

Scientific knowledge, authority and experimental parapsychology

In the preface to his 1914 book, *Materialisations-Phänomene*, Schrenck-Notzing wrote of his hesitation in publishing the results of his four-year long study of the physical medium Eva C. and his six-month observation of Stanislava P., the Polish medium. The Baron's misgivings, based on the treatment of men such as Charles Richet, William Crookes and Johann Karl Friederich Zöllner, who had been subject to public ridicule and reproach in the wake of their forays into the occult, were tempered by the belief that his experiments with mediums, as far as was feasible with such labile subjects, had met rigorous standards of scientific inquiry.[170] The method of experimentation utilised, apparent in the meticulous protocols produced in the Karolinenplatz laboratory and in the prolific use made of photography in this forum, signified, according to Schrenck-Notzing, a significant advance in this field.[171] While he declined to attempt any thoroughgoing explanation of the ectoplasmic protrusions and telekinetic movements produced by his mediums, claiming that such hypotheses were premature, the Baron contended that the publication of these results would help focus both the public's and the scientific community's attention on the dark, unexplored realms of the psyche, fostering further research of the problematic relationship between body and mind.[172]

In spite of the refinement of methodology and adherence to scientific method that Schrenck-Notzing claimed this work represented, the reception of *Materialisations-Phänomene* during 1913 mimicked closely that of Richet's, Crookes' and Zöllner's occult works; the author, his work and his methodology became the target of public ridicule. The Baron's claim, for instance, that the photographic images reproduced in his book provided indisputable evidence for the existence of paraphysical powers was discredited by a host of newspapers and journals.[173] In spite of his insistence on elaborate precautionary measures, the press were also able to demonstrate Schrenck-Notzing's credulity by revealing that Eva C. was identical to the fraudulent medium Marthe Béraud, who had been exposed during a series of experiments with Richet in Algiers in 1909.[174] The lambasting of this work and its author was not, however, limited to the scathing satirical reviews that appeared in the popular press, but included a number of more thoroughgoing critiques, which hypothesised the ability of mediums to regurgitate the contents of their stomachs at will and sought to quash the Baron's claims that his experiments, which he maintained rigorously applied the scientific method to the phenomena of mediumship, signified the emergence of parapsychology as an experimental science.[175]

Similar critiques emerged during the 1920s in response to Schrenck-Notzing's continued publication of his findings in the field of physical mediumship and to the collections of experimental protocols, provided by respected figures in areas such as physics, psychology and biology, that he argued offered overwhelming evidence of the reality of the physical phenomena. While in *Experimente der Fernbewegung* [*Telekinetic Experiments*] (1924) he recommended direct experience of the phenomena of mediumship, he assured his readers that the protocols that appeared here, contributed by men whose social, cultural and scientific authority was beyond reproach, negated the need to make one's own observations.[176] Critics conceded the impressive persuasive power that the large number of positive reports received by Schrenck-Notzing from well-respected scientists, doctors and authors wielded, it proving difficult to dismiss these accounts without impugning the honour, sanity and expertise of such witnesses. They argued, however, that the Baron's fetishism of authority served only to emphasise parapsychology's innate distance and difference from science, deriding also his claim to have excluded the possibility of fraud from his experiments. Schrenck-Notzing's contention that he had met rigorous standards of scientific inquiry through the constant refinement of his methodology and precautionary measures and that he had provided hard evidence of the physical phenomena of mediumship through the publication of large numbers of experimental protocols and photographs, was rejected by critics who argued that his concessions to mediums' eccentricities fundamentally flawed his methodology and rendered the exclusion of mechanical causes, specifically fraud, difficult if not impossible.[177] These responses to the Baron's work and his replies to such critiques represented an ongoing debate between parapsychologists and sceptics over the nature of scientific knowledge and authority, which did not differ substantially from that which had taken place between Wundt and Zöllner half a century earlier. This seemingly interminable argument illustrated the irresolvable paradox at the heart of parapsychology, embodied in the parapsychological laboratory's fusion of spiritualist and scientific space, which saw the application of a methodology that was apparently unfavourable to the phenomena it was intended to verify.

In the introductory passages of *Materialisations-Phänomene*, Schrenck-Notzing insisted that the scientific study of mediumship be conducted under circumstances in which the possibility of a mechanical explanation was definitively excluded. Yet, according to his critics, the approach that he had utilised in his experiments with the two mediums Eva C. and Stanislava P. stood in stark contrast to this precautionary method. Mathilde von Kemnitz, later Mathilde von Ludendorff, (1877–1966), for example, whose book *Moderne Mediumforschung* [*Modern Medium Research*] (1914) the Baron felt compelled to respond to at length, argued that had the author provided evidence of just one materialisation under strict experimental conditions, rather than the numerous accounts of sittings, one hundred and fifty illustrations and thirty tables of which his work consisted, his case for the existence of materialisation would have been immeasurably strengthened.[178] The possibility of actually conducting such an experiment, however, was minimal, according to Kemnitz, given the control that mediums, whose powers she understood to be mixed with both conscious and unconscious fraud, exercised over experimental conditions in this field.[179] A 1925 critique of Schrenck-Notzing's work written by Walter Gulat-Wellenburg (b.1877), Carl von Klinckowstroem and Hans Rosenbusch (b.1888), and known as the *Dreimännerbuch* [*Three-Man Book*] made a similar point, arguing that in scientific experiments, as opposed to parapsychological examinations, the investigator exercised strict control of the circumstances under which they conducted their observations, dictating the place, time, apparatus and number of repetitions of the phenomena required.[180] In contrast, the parapsychologist, constrained by a lack of knowledge about the conditions under which paranormal phenomena manifested themselves and reliant on the goodwill of a medium, exhibited a distinct lack of power to mould the experimental conditions under which they observed their subject matter. Hellwig, another critic of the Baron's advocacy of parapsychology as an experimental science, argued that the term experiment should refer exclusively to research conducted under conditions over which the experimenter had control and that the accommodation of spiritualist ritual and mediumistic whim that typified experimentation in the Karolinenplatz laboratory made explicit Schrenck-Notzing's lack of mastery in his interactions with mediums.[181]

The use of private mediums in parapsychological research was, according to Kemnitz, responsible for the considerable power that mediums exhibited in the laboratory. While it might be supposed, she argued, that prolonged experimentation by scientists with mediums would ensure the swift exposure of frauds, the use of private rather than professional mediums, who offered their services without the expectation of financial gain, made the adherence to strict scientific conditions difficult.[182] While the exposure of professional mediums proved straightforward because of the tacit authority, derived from the commercial transaction between the medium and the researcher, to apply thoroughgoing experimental conditions to mediumistic phenomena, private mediums, by virtue of their refusal to accept money for their manifestations, were more difficult to examine. The private medium, whose goodwill the parapsychologist needed to maintain in order to study their phenomena, was in a position to demand the alteration or refinement of experimental conditions in a manner in which the professional medium could not. Kemnitz noted on this point the way in which private mediums' demands – requests ostensibly made due to the labile nature of the phenomena and the sensitivity of mediumistic constitutions – coincidentally tended to negate the ability of the parapsychologist to definitively exclude the possibility of fraud from their experiments.[183]

The problematic status of fraud and simulation in this field was, according to Gulat-Wellenburg, Klinckowstroem and Rosenbusch, a peculiarity of experimental parapsychology.[184] In the physical and chemical sciences, they contended, the possibility of deception was almost non-existent, but in the human sciences also, psychiatry in particular, the potential for fraud could be kept to a minimum through the repetition of experiments and through the use of observational techniques of an objective physical (reflex phenomena) and psychological (variations methods) variety.[185] In the field of experimental parapsychology, however, fraud and simulation were understood to be concomitant with mediumistic ability, an innate attribute of those who derived their psychic or physical abilities from the hystero-hypnotic complex, and thus an integral component of this nascent science.[186] In order to meet the rigorous standards of inquiry typical of established sciences, parapsychology required a methodology capable, not only of guarding against deception and distinguishing between real phenomena and fraud but of coping with mediums' sensitivity to disbelief and scepticism, a requirement which Schrenck-Notzing's critics, including Kemnitz, Hellwig, Gulat-Wellenburg, Klinckowstroem and Rosenbusch, had demonstrated, through their critiques of parapsychological methodology, had not been and perhaps could not be fulfilled.

Schrenck-Notzing's attempt to combat the implications of fraud and the accusations of sensory deception levelled at him by his critics consisted of both angry retorts in books and journals and the collection and collation of large numbers of positive reports from participants with expertise in a vast range of disciplines.[187] The evidentiary weight of these protocols and the social, cultural and scientific authority of their authors were intended to override concerns about methodology or individual bias. In his book, entitled *Experimente der Fernbewegung*, largely composed of the positive experimental protocols of luminaries from both the arts and sciences,

Schrenck-Notzing's stress on methodological precision and precaution gave way to an emphasis on authority and its evidentiary status. His reliance on authority was such that he contended that the quality and authority of the remarks of these witnesses, who were members of the most varied vocations, was, despite their lack of experience or expertise in this field, beyond all doubt.[188] On the issue of bias as it concerned this collection of reports, the Baron noted that, of the fifty-six people invited to take part in experiments with the physical medium Willy Schneider during 1922, only seven had prior experience of paraphysical phenomena, the remaining forty-nine approaching these sittings with a healthy scientific scepticism.[189] Despite the Baron's conviction that the evidence he had compiled was indisputable, his critics were once again swift to dispute his claims.

The possible sources of error in the observations and conclusions of those unaccustomed to the eccentricities of mediumistic phenomena, regardless of their expertise in other fields, were multiple, according to the authors of the *Dreimännerbuch*.[190] The possibility of accurate observation, they contended, was to a high degree contingent upon the functionality of the senses or, where these were not precise enough, on the use of instruments and apparatus intended to supplement or replace the sense organs.[191] In parapsychological research, however, the obstruction of the senses as a result of the experimental conditions, for example, the dim lighting, the use of a cabinet, and the medium's abhorrence to their phenomena being touched, made accurate observation difficult, although some attempt was made to remedy this problem through the construction of instruments such as the electrical medium control.[192] In their defence, parapsychologists pointed to their ceaseless efforts to improve experimental conditions, an attempt that Kemnitz understood not as an elimination of fraud, but as a hindrance that simply encouraged mediums to improve their technical dexterity.[193] Even those participants skilled in scientific observation in another field, according to the critics, might prove incapable of judging the veracity of mediumistic phenomena because of their inexperience with simulation and fraud, which remained unlikely to be exposed by those without an intimate knowledge of trickery and conjuring. Critics were also concerned with the manner in which observer–participants, such as those who had taken part in Schrenck-Notzing's experiments, might feel themselves constrained by politeness and social convention when asked by their host to pass comment on the phenomena they had witnessed.[194]

Perhaps the most pressing concern of those who critiqued Schrenck-Notzing's work, however, was the manner in which he had elevated the concept of authority, be it social, cultural or scientific, to the status of irrefutable evidence. Indeed, as the authors of the *Dreimännerbuch* noted, the mere authority of names played a substantial role as a means of evidence in experimental protocols, their incantation assuming an almost magical power.[195] While scientific authority was understood to be based on training, experience and observational skill and was not awarded evidentiary status above personal observation and experiment, Schrenck-Notzing, transferring the authority and prestige that participants enjoyed in other fields to the realm of parapsychology, asked his readers to grant these protocols the status of evidence, arguing that they negated the need for personal investigation of the phenomena in question.[196] In this manner, that is, through the force of authority, he hoped to establish for a wider circle of people than could actually experience these elusive phenomena the objective reality of physical mediumship.[197] Hellwig argued on this point that although in certain circumstances the reports of researchers who are known to be reliable and expert can convince us, we cannot then say, however, that we possess a well-founded scientific knowledge of paranormal facts, rather we only have good grounds to believe.[198] This was a distinction, he claimed, that was not appreciated by parapsychologists.

The debate surrounding the attempt of Schrenck-Notzing and others to claim scientific status for experimental parapsychology was primarily a dispute about the nature of scientific knowledge. The evidence for physical mediumship, according to critics, offered no irrefutable certainty and could therefore not form the basis of a science; a claim that parapsychologists disputed, arguing not only that devices such as the electrical medium control excluded the possibility of fraud, but that the photographic images taken during parapsychological experiments constituted hard evidence of the physical phenomena of mediumship. The critics argued furthermore that those competent to make a decision about the reality of physical mediumship derived not from parapsychology – a new science of doubtful legitimacy – but rather, given the centrality of issues such as observational skill and difficulty to this field, from observational psychology.[199] This argument perhaps referred to attempts on the part of psychologists and critical occultists to create a psychology of occult belief, an endeavour to which we will return in a later chapter.

Conclusion

In the opening pages of his 1924 book on telekinesis, Schrenck-Notzing noted the repeated requests of those intellectuals who had attended sittings with Willy Schneider in the Karolinenplatz laboratory that further experiments be conducted with this medium in a neutral environment.[200] Concerned, as were other participants, that the medium's power might in some way be dependent on this space or that the Baron's laboratory might contain hidden devices, Dr Erich Becher (1882–1929) provided a room at the Psychologisches Instiut [Psychological Institute] at the University of

Munich for the months of September and October 1922. While some equipment, including stools, tables, waste paper baskets and lighting, was provided by the Psychological Institute, more specialised utensils such as the medium's costume, luminous ribbons and a gauze-covered cage were taken from the Karolinenplatz laboratory. In total, fifteen sittings took place in this context, the conduct and results of which were similar to those experiments conducted in the Baron's laboratory. These experiments bore a striking similarity to a series of sittings that had been carried out two years earlier with the medium Eva C., in the Faculté des sciences [Faculty of Science] at the Sorbonne.[201] In an auditorium, four scientists, Henri Piéron (1881–1964), George Dumas, Louis Lapicque (1866–1952) and Henri Laugier (1888–1973), all of whom were professors of psychology or physiology, waited for the medium, who was seated in her cabinet, to produce phenomena. Their protocols, although devoid of phenomena, did supply detailed measurements of the level of light, the length of the curtain, and the size of the cabinet.[202]

The transfer of these telekinetic experiments to the Psychological Institute at the University of Munich and the Faculty of Science at the Sorbonne, illustrates quite explicitly the complex and not entirely successful manner in which parapsychologists attempted to differentiate themselves from spiritualists. While these experiments might have represented another step away from the domestic séance and a further refinement of methodology and controls through the application of techniques and instruments designed specifically to examine human behaviour, they also served to highlight parapsychology's distance from established sciences. Despite the fact that these sittings had been carried out in spaces specifically designed for scientific observation and by people trained in psychological and physiological method, both sets of experiments differed little from spiritualist séances because of the mediums' insistence on conditions mimicking those of the séance room. Indeed, these experiments demonstrated, in their continued use of the props of spiritualism, and in their failure to adapt their methodology or evidentiary standards, the inability of parapsychology to shake off its spiritualist past, and to rid itself of its dependence on authority. The use of mediums, with their sensitivity to certain stimuli, including bright light and touch, rendered them problematic objects of scientific experimentation; this was the biggest stumbling block for those attempting to employ strict scientific controls in parapsychological research, a situation that remained unchanged on the unexpected death of Schrenck-Notzing from appendicitis in 1929.

During the 1930s, a young doctoral student at the University of Bonn carried out a series of experiments on automatic spelling and automatic writing in which he became convinced that he had detected the operation of telepathy. This preliminary research led to a dissertation entitled *Psychologische Automatismen* [*Psychological Automatisms*], in which the student Hans Bender (1907–1991) linked subconscious productions to extrasensory perception.[203] While Bender's thesis met with resistance from the academic community it became the first dissertation submitted at a German university on a parapsychological theme that had yielded positive results.[204] Supported by researchers including Driesch, E.R. Jaensch (1883–1940), the psychiatrist Gruhle, and the Gestalt psychologist Gottschaldt, and encouraged by the publication of J.B. Rhine's (1895–1980) *Extrasensory Perception* (1934), Bender continued his work in this field, completing his postdoctoral thesis (*Habilitation*) on crystal vision in 1941.[205] Determined to integrate parapsychology into an academic framework, Bender introduced the topic of parapsychology into his lectures in psychology and psychopathology at the University of Freiburg, following the Second World War. In 1950, he set up the Institüt für Grenzgebiete der Psychologie und Psychohygiene [Institute for the Border Areas of Psychology and Psycho-Hygiene], the dual focus of which was scientific research into the reality of the paranormal and the changing attitudes of the general public towards these phenomena.[206] The result of these endeavours was the establishment of a chair of psychology and the border areas of psychology in 1954.[207]

Significantly, it was the psychical rather than the physical phenomena that found their way into German universities and became the focus of experimental parapsychology in the years following Schrenck-Notzing's death. This was the case not only in Germany but also in the United States, where Rhine experimented with so-called extra-sensory perception, i.e. telepathy and clairvoyance, rather than materialisation and telekinesis.[208] Not only were the physical phenomena of mediumship burdened with the stigma of fraud and spiritualism, from which experimental parapsychologists never seemed fully to rid themselves, but they ultimately bore little relationship to, and thus exhibited little relevance for, experimental sciences such as physics, biology and psychology. In contrast, by the mid-twentieth century the psychical phenomena appeared more conducive to thoroughgoing control than that achievable with the manifestations of physical mediumship. This was the case because ordinary subjects rather than mediums could be tested, making it possible to implement the kind of scientific checks and controls at which mediums would have balked. Experiments with telepathy and clairvoyance also bore a closer relationship to mainstream work being carried out in the field of psychology than the physical phenomena. Bender's experiments with automatic writing and extrasensory perception, for example, bore a strong relationship to Pierre Janet's (1859–1947) work on automatism and personality disorders. It was with research of this nature, conducted within psychological laboratories in universities, that an experimental parapsychology, although of a different kind to that envisioned by Schrenck-Notzing, can be said finally to have emerged in the German context.

Notes

1. 'Sanitisation' is the term Roy Wallis has coined to describe the process by which a pseudo-science distances itself from the theory and practice of its more notorious proponents or predecessors, using professional associations, memberships, and the incorporation of methodologies utilised by accepted scientific disciplines to differentiate itself. See R. Wallis, 'Science and Pseudo-Science', *Social Science Information,* 24, 3 (1985), 585–601; Wolf Lepenies uses the term 'purification' in a similar sense to describe the process by which the nascent field of sociology tried both to adopt scientific methods and distance itself from literature. Lepenies argues that this process stranded sociology between science and literature, making it what he calls a 'third culture'. My argument about the hybrid nature of parapsychology, stranded between spiritualism and science, is similar. See W. Lepenies, *Between Literature and Science: The Rise of Sociology,* R.J. Hollingdale (trans.) (Cambridge: Cambridge University Press, 1988), 7.

2. Schrenck-Notzing complained that savants were forced to recreate the physical environment typical of spiritualist séances in order to experiment with mediums. See A. von Schrenck-Notzing, *Phenomena of Materialisation: A Contribution to the Investigation of Mediumistic Teleplastics,* E.E. Fournier d' Albe (trans.), (London: Kegan Paul, Trench, Trubner & Co., 1920), 11. Originally published as A. von Schrenck-Notzing, *Materialisations-Phänomene: Ein Beitrag zur Erforschung der mediumistischen Teleplastie* (Munich: Verlag von Ernst Reinhardt, 1914).

3. *Ibid.,* 12.

4. *Ibid.,* 12.

5. *Ibid.,* 21.

6. 'Aus dem Laboratorium des Geisterbarons', *Welt am Sonntag,* (3 March 1929), in: ZA, Personen Schrenck-Notzing, StArMü. On Schrenck-Notzing's domination of the field as a result of his wealth, see E. Bauer, 'Periods of Historical Development of Parapsychology in Germany - An Overview', in *Proceedings of the Parapsychological Association 34th Annual Convention* (Petaluma: Parapsychological Association, 1991), 11.

7. R. Tischner, *Geschichte der Parapsychologie: Von der Mitte des 19. Jahrhunderts bis zum ersten Drittel des 20. Jahrhunderts* (Tittmoning/Obb: Walter Pustet, 1960), 214–16.

8. A significant number of these participants seem to have been members of Berlin and Munich's artistic or literary communities. The link between

occultism and the avant-garde has been explored at great length in V. Loers (ed.), *Okkultismus und Avantgarde: Von Munch bis Mondrian, 1900–1915* (Frankfurt: Schirn Kunsthalle, 1995). The symbiotic relationship between spiritualism and literary modernism has also been the topic of a recent symposium, *Spiritismus und ästhetische Moderne: Berlin und München als Zentren,* 29 July to 1 August 2004, at the Fürstenzimmer of Schloss Hohentübingen, University of Tübingen.

9. The experimental protocol, the written record of events that occur in the course of a mediumistic sitting, represents an important source for a history of parapsychology. Intended to provide an account of the paranormal phenomena experienced by its author and to authenticate those phenomena by describing the controls and conditions under which they manifested themselves, the protocol offers the historian access to the experiential heart of parapsychology.

10. T.K. Oesterreich, *Der Okkultismus im modernen Weltbild,* 3rd edn (Dresden: Sibyllen-Verlag, 1923), 21.

11. A. von Schrenck-Notzing, 'Die Entwicklung des Okkultismus zur Parapsychologie in Deutschland', *Zeitschrift für Parapsycholgie,* 7, 1 (1932), 28–42; 7, 3 (1932), 115–25; 7, 5 (1932), 211–23; 7, 6 (1932), 265–76; 7, 7 (1932), 307–16; 7, 8 (1932), 347–57; 7, 9 (1932), 398–406; 7, 10 (1932), 456–69; 7, 11 (1932), 504–9.

12. L.A. Shepard (ed.), *Encyclopedia of Occultism and Parapsychology,* 3rd edn. (Detroit: Gale Research, 1991), 485.

13. *Ibid.,* 1167.

14. M.B. Brower, 'The Fantasms of Science: Psychical Research in the French Third Republic, 1880–1935.' (unpublished PhD dissertation: Rutgers University, 2005), 280.

15. *Ibid.,* 307.

16. F. Grunewald, *Physikalisch-mediumistische Untersuchungen* (Pfullingen i. Wurtt.: Johannes Baum Verlag, 1920), 13.

17. O. Lodge, 'Address by the President', *Proceedings of the Society for Psychical Research,* 17 (1902), 47; Grunewald, *ibid.,* 13–14.

18. Schrenck-Notzing, *Phenomena of Materialisation, op. cit.* (note 2), 21.

19. On Krall's laboratory, see K. Amereller, 'Das Krall'sche Institut für Tierpsychologie und parapsychologische Forschung, München', *Zeitschrift für Parapsychologie,* 3 (1929), 165.

20. A. Schrenck-Notzing, 'Ein elektrischer Apparat für Medienkontrolle', *Zeitschrift für Parapsychologie,* 9 (1926), 513–14.

21. 'Das Material wurde zunächst in Wasser und Glycerin beobachtet; ferner nach Behandlung mit Jogjodkali und Anilinfarbstoff-Lösungen in Glycerin-Gelantine. Die Präparate zeigen grössere Epithelgruppen und einzeln gelagerte Epithelien, deren Kerne vielfach deutlich erkennbar sind. Als

Verunreinigungen finden sich Baumwollfäden, Stärkekörner und Pilzsporen. Bacterien (Stäbchen-Formen) wurden in geringer Menge beobachtet.' Letter from Dr A. Schwalm (Öffentliches Laboratorium für chemische, mikroskopische und bakteriologische Untersuchungen zu medizinisch-diagnostichen und technischen Zwecken) to Albert von Schrenck-Notzing, 18 February 1916, Korrespondenz 1, Nachlaß Albert von Schrenck-Notzing, IGPP.

22. K.B. Staubermann, 'Tying the Knot: Skill, Judgment and Authority in the 1870s Leipzig Spiritistic Experiments', *British Journal for the History of Science,* 34 (2001), 78.

23. *Ibid.*

24. *Ibid.*

25. D. Cahan, 'The Institutional Revolution in German Physics', *Historical Studies in the Physical Sciences,* 15, 2 (1985), 4, 12.

26. *Ibid.,* 6–12.

27. M.G. Ash, 'Academic Politics in the History of Science: Experimental Psychology in Germany, 1879–1941', *Central European History,* 13, 3 (1980), 257: 260–1.

28. S. Nicolas and L. Ferrand, 'Wundt's Laboratory at Leipzig in 1891', *History of Psychology,* 2, 3 (1999), 198–9.

29. Grunewald, *op. cit.* (note 16), 34.

30. Cahan, *op. cit.* (note 25), 32.

31. Grunewald, *op. cit.* (note 16), 34.

32. Nicolas and Ferrand, *op. cit.* (note 28), 198–9.

33. Grunewald, *op. cit.* (note 16), 35–7.

34. A. von Schrenck-Notzing, 'Über die Anwendung automatischer Registriermethoden bei paraphysischen Untersuchungen', in Gerda Walther (ed.), *Grundfragen der Parapsychologie* (Stuttgart: W. Kohlhammer, 1962), 156.

35. A. von Schrenck-Notzing, *Die Phänomene des Mediums Rudi Schneider* (Berlin: Walter de Gruyter & Co., 1933), 95–6; For a description of the Zeigeapparat, see A. von Schrenck-Notzing, *Experimente der Fernbewegung* (Stuttgart: Union Deutsche Verlagsgesellschaft, 1924), 11–12.

36. Schrenck-Notzing, *op. cit.* (note 34), 157.

37. Grunewald, *op. cit.* (note 16), 14.

38. 'Mir war es vielmehr von Beginn meiner laboratoriumsmässigen Untersuchung an lediglich darum zu tun, in das Wesen der eigenartigen Erscheinungen immer tiefer einzudringen. Ich sah denn auch sehr bald ein, dass hierzu ein umfangreicher physikalischer Apparat notwendig wäre, in Form eines aufs beste eingerichteten Laboratoriums. Das Ideal, das mir bereits in den Jahren 1908 und 1909 vorschwebte, ist vorläufig allerdings

nochlange nicht erreicht. Dazu waren die begleitenden Umstände zu
schwierig und die Mittel zu unzureichend'. Grunewald, *op. cit.* (note 16), 14

39. Following Grunewald's death in 1925, Schrenck-Notzing attempted to have
the engineer's laboratory transported to Munich. Grunewald's family,
however, was determined that it remain in Berlin. See letters from Dr W.
Kröner to Albert von Schrenck-Notzing, 27 July 1925 and 29 July 1925,
Korrespondenz Berlin, Nachlaß Albert von Schrenck-Notzing, IGPP.

40. On the significance of these epistemological revolutions for the study of the
paranormal, see Oesterreich, *op. cit.* (note 10), 11–27.

41. Schrenck-Notzing, *op. cit.* (note 2), 7.

42. See J. Winter, *Sites of Memory, Sites of Mourning: The Great War in European
Cultural History* (Cambridge: Cambridge University Press, 1995), 54–77.

43. T. Mann, 'An Experience in the Occult', in *Three Essays,* H.T. Lowe-Porter
(trans.), (London: Adelphi, 1932), 219–61. This chapter makes use of
Mann's essay, which represented a reworking of three experimental protocols
that Mann wrote in response to sittings with the medium Willy Schneider
during December 1922 and January 1923. These protocols, which are also
used here, were published in Schrenck-Notzing, *Experimente der
Fernbewegung, op. cit.* (note 35). While 'An Experience in the Occult' has
traditionally been regarded as a satirical essay, Mann's personal
correspondence reveals a more complex attitude to the occult. More
importantly, however, Schrenck-Notzing considers Mann the best observer
he had ever encountered, see letter from Albert von Schrenck-Notzing to
T.K. Oesterreich, 11 July 1928, Nachlaß T. K. Oesterreich, 399/12, UAT.
For a more detailed analysis of Thomas Mann and the occult, see A. Rausch,
Okkultes in Thomas Manns Roman Der Zauberberg (Frankfurt am Main: Peter
Lang, 2000).

44. E. Buchner, 'Der Mollprozeß in zweiter Auflage', *Zeitschrift für
Parapsychologie,* 1, 3 (1926), 156.

45. T.K. Oesterreich, 'Mediumismus und Wissenschaft. Ein Medium in der
Münchener Universität', in: Nachlaß T.K. Oesterreich, 399/15, UAT.

46. Schrenck-Notzing, *Experimente der Fernbewegung, op. cit.* (note 35), 68.

47. See for example, Schrenck-Notzing, *ibid.;* Schrenck-Notzing, *Phänomene des
Mediums Rudi Schneider, op. cit.* (note 35).

48. Mann, *op. cit.* (note 43), 231, 233, 235.

49. 'In ersten Teil der Sitzung befand sich in der Mitte des Teilnehmerhalbkreises
der Gazekäfig, der mit Ausnahme des Schlitzes geschlossen war. In ihm stand
ein Tisch, auf demselben eine Spieldose, die mit einem doppelt gesiegelten
Bindfaden umwunden war.' T.K. Oesterreich, 'Bericht über die Sitzung am
24 Juni 1922', in: Nachlaß T.K. Oesterreich, 399/15, UAT.

50. 'Die Beleuchtung was wesentlich heller als Anfang April'. *Ibid.*

51. Schrenck-Notzing, *Experimente der Fernbewegung, op. cit.* (note 35), 254.

52. 'Die Sitzung fand in einem verdunkelten Zimmer statt, jedoch war es durch mehrere rote Glühlampen immerhin hell genug - wenigstens für meine Sehkraft -, Gegenstände und Personen zu unterscheiden.' Schrenck-Notzing, *ibid.*, 252.

53. 'Alles Licht wird bis auf eine rote elektrische Lampe ausgelöscht; man sieht noch die Umrisse aller Teilnehmer.' Schrenck-Notzing, *ibid.*, 70.

54. R.H. Kraus, *Beyond Light and Shadow: The Role of Photography in Certain Paranormal Phenomena: An Historical Survey* (Munich: Nazraeli Press, 1995), 166. Andreas Fischer has argued that the use of photography as a control altered the conditions of the séance room, bringing light into the darkness. See A. Fischer, 'Ein Nachtgebiet der Fotographie', in Loers (ed.), *op. cit.* (note 8), 510.

55. Schrenck-Notzing, *Experimente der Fernbewegung, op. cit.* (note 35), 76.

56. Kraus, *op. cit.* (note 54), 166.

57. Nicolas and Ferrand, *op. cit.* (note 28), 198.

58. Staubermann, *op. cit.* (note 22).

59. Schrenck-Notzing, *Experimente der Fernbewegung, op. cit.* (note 35), 69.

60. *Ibid.*, 71.

61. *Ibid.*, 253; Mann, *op. cit.* (note 43), 234.

62. Grunewald, *op. cit.* (note 16), 34.

63. Schrenck-Notzing, *op. cit.* (note 11) 7, 5 (1932), 218.

64. T.K. Oesterreich, 'Der Nachweis der Echtheit von Telekinesie und Materialisation am Willy S. Bericht über drei Sitzungen.', in: Nachlaß T.K. Oesterreich, 399/15, UAT.

65. Für wissenschaftliche Interessenten mit den nötigen litterarischen Erkenntnissen namentlich aus den officiellen Kreisen der alma Mater stehe ich immer gern zur Verfügung, nicht aber Leute, die zu den Sitzungen aus Neugierde und Sensationslust, wie zu einer Theatervorstellung kommen. Letter from Albert von Schrenck-Notzing to Dr Edith Ebees, 19 October 1924, Sammlung Albert Freiherr von Schrenck-Notzing, Monacensia Literaturarchiv, Stadtbiblothek München.

66. Mann, *op. cit.* (note 43), 234.

67. *Ibid.*, 239.

68. Grunewald, *op. cit.* (note 16),16.

69. Schrenck-Notzing, *Phenomena of Materialisation, op. cit.* (note 2), 251.

70. Schrenck-Notzing, *Experimente der Fernbewegung, op. cit.* (note 35), 253.

71. Schrenck-Notzing, for example, notes the inability of Stanislava P. to fully comprehend the necessary conditions for experiments because of her low level of education. See Schrenck-Notzing, *Phenomena of Materialisation, op. cit.* (note 2), 251.

72. Schrenck-Notzing, *Phänomene des Mediums Rudi Schneider, op. cit.* (note 35), 1–2.

73. *Ibid.*, 2.
74. Mediumship, in this context, might be considered a specialised form of domestic service.
75. Schrenck-Notzing, *Phenomena of Materialisation, op. cit.* (note 2), 20–1.
76. Das Verhalten des Experimentators gegenüber dem Medium und den sich durch dasselbe äussernden Intelligenzen ist überhaupt ein Punkt, dessen Wichtigkeit nicht genug betont werden kann. Versteht man es nicht von Anfang an, das Vertrauen des Medium zu gewinnen, so ist der Erfolg schon zweifelhaft. Die Medien sind psychisch meist äusserst empfindliche Personen. Misstrauischer Skeptizismus oder gar vollkommen unbekehrbarer, offen oder versteckt zur Schau getragen, wird von den meisten Medien als äusserst störend empfunden, so das vielfach in Gegenwart besonders misstrauischer Personen die Phänomene teilweise oder ganz ausbleiben. Grunewald, *op. cit.* (note 16), 19.
77. Oesterreich, *op. cit.* (note 64).
78. *Ibid.*
79. Schrenck-Notzing, *Phenomena of Materialisation, op. cit.* (note 2), 20.
80. Schrenck-Notzing, *op. cit.* (note 11), 7, 1 (1932), 39.
81. Letter from R. Schott to A. von Schrenck-Notzing, November 1917, in: Korrespondenz 5, Nachlaß Albert von Schrenck-Notzing, IGPP.
82. Schrenck-Notzing, *Phenomena of Materialisation, op. cit.* (note 2), 39.
83. Schrenck-Notzing, *Experimente der Fernbewegung, op. cit.* (note 35), 253–4.
84. *Ibid.*, 69.
85. *Ibid.*, 255.
86. Schrenck-Notzing, *Phenomena of Materialisation, op. cit.* (note 2), 15; Schrenck-Notzing, *op. cit.* (note 11), 7, 1 (1932), 40.
87. Schrenck-Notzing, *Experimente der Fernbewegung, op. cit.* (note 35), 255.
88. 'Eine von Schr. N., auf den Boden gestellte Glocke (durch Leuchtfarbe sichtbar gemacht) erhob sich und schwebte im Raum vor den Teilnehmern hin und her. Die Spieldose begann zu spielen, hörte wieder auf begann von neuem und so mehrmals je nach Wunsch der Teilnehmer.' Oesterreich, *op. cit.* (note 45).
89. *Ibid.*.
90. 'Stellungnahme von M. K. Fragment', 4, in: L4401, Sammlung Max Kemmerich, Monacensia Literaturarchiv Stadtsbibliothek München.
91. On photography as a way in which to make the invisible visible, see Fischer, *op. cit.* (note 54), 503–45; A. Fischer, *Im Reich der Phantome: Fotografie des Unsichtbaren* (Ostfildern-Ruit: Cantz, 1997).
92. Kraus, *op. cit.* (note 54), 99–107; Winter, *op. cit.* (note 42), 54–77.
93. K. Schoonover, 'Ectoplasms, Evanescence, and Photography' *Art Journal,* 62, 3 (2003), 33
94. *Ibid.*, 35.

95. Winter, *op. cit.* (note 42), 54–77

96. J. Tucker, 'Photography as Witness, Detective, and Impostor: Visual Representation in Victorian Science' in B. Lightman (ed.) *Victorian Science in Context* (Chicago: University of Chicago Press, 1997), 378–408.

97. Schoonover, *op. cit.* (note 93), 33, 39.

98. Tucker, *op. cit.* (note 96), 380.

99. Schrenck-Notzing had attended a number of lectures given by Charcot at the Salpêtrière and had made a study of the photographs that formed Charcot's iconography of hysteria. See A. von Schrenck-Notzing, 'Albert von Keller als Malerpsychologe und Metaphysiker', *Psychische Studien,* 48 (April-Mai 1921), 194. For the connection between the photography of hysterics and mediums, see also M. Roth, 'Hysterical Remembering' *Modernism/Modernity,* 3, 2 (1996), 1–30.

100. Brower, *op. cit.* (note 14), 226–7; See U. Baer, 'Photography and Hysteria: Towards a Poetics of the Flash', *Yale Journal of Criticism,* 7, 1 (1994), 41–78.

101. Tucker, *op. cit.* (note 96), 380

102. *Ibid.,* 12.

103. *Ibid.,* 22.

104. Kraus, *op. cit.* (note 54), 169.

105. Schrenck-Notzing, *op. cit.* (note 11), 7, 1 (1932), 40.

106. Letter from E. Haberkorn to A. von Schrenck-Notzing, 22 October 1924, in Korrespondenz München, Nachlaß Albert von Schrenck-Notzing, IGPP.

107. Letter from E. Westlake to A. von Schrenck-Notzing, 29 July 1922, in Korrepondenz 1, Nachlaß Albert von Schrenck-Notzing, IGPP.

108. *Ibid.*

109. *Ibid.*

110. Mann, *op. cit.* (note 43), 225.

111. *Ibid.,* 223–4: 257–8.

112. Schrenck-Notzing, *op. cit.* (note 11), 7, 1 (1932), 41.

113. *Ibid.,* 40–2.

114. A. Schwalm to A. von Schrenck-Notzing, *op. cit.* (note 21).

115. On parapsychologists' socialisation within the biomedical and psychological paradigms, see B. Wolf-Braun, 'Zur Geschichte der Parapsychologie in der Weimarer Republik: Deutungen des Mediumismus', (Report for the Institut für Grenzgebiete der Psychologie und Psychohygiene, University of Bonn, 2002), 14; On spiritualism and freedom from gender roles, see A. Owen, *The Darkened Room: Women, Power, and Spiritualism in Late Victorian England* (London: Virago Press, 1989), 202.

116. For the interpretation of mediumship within the psychiatric paradigm in Germany, see Wolf-Braun, *ibid.,* 1–17.

117. J. Oppenheim, *The Other World: Spiritualism and Psychical Research in England, 1850–1914* (Cambridge: Cambridge University Press, 1988), 7.

118. R.L. Moore, *In Search of White Crows: Spiritualism, Parapsychology, and American Culture* (Oxford: Oxford University Press, 1977), 15.

119. Oppenheim, *op. cit.* (note 117), 63.

120. Owen, *op. cit.* (note 115), 1–6.

121. J. Walkowitz, 'Science and Séance: Transgressions of Gender and Genre in Late Victorian London', *Representations* 22, 2 (1988), 9.

122. Oppenheim, *op. cit.* (note 117), 21.

123. A. Braude, *Radical Spirits: Spiritualism and Women's Rights in Nineteenth-Century America* (Boston: Beacon Press, 1989), 82.

124. Owen, *op. cit.* (note 115), 6–12.

125. V. Skultans, 'Mediums, Controls and Eminent Men', in Pat Holden (ed.), *Women's Religious Experience* (London: Croom Helm, 1983), 23.

126. A. Moll, *Perversions of the Sex Instinct: A Study of Sexual Inversion*, Maurice Popkin (trans.), (Newark: Julian Press, 1931), 62.

127. On the tension between sexologists' and occultists' understandings of homosexuality, see J. Dixon, 'Sexology and the Occult: Sexuality and Subjectivity in Theosophy's New Age', *Journal of the History of Sexuality* 7, 3 (1997), 409–33.

128. Wolf-Braun, *op. cit.* (note 115), 13.

129. R. Baerwald, *Okkultismus und Spiritismus und Ihre weltanschaulichen Folgerungen* (Berlin: Deutsche Buch Gemeinschaft, 1926), 136.

130. *Ibid.*, 147.

131. See, for example, P. Sünner, 'Ein Beitrag zur Frage des Zusammenhanges zwischen Hysterie und Mediumismus', *Zeitschrift für Parapsychologie,* 5 (1931), 265–77.

132. 'Der Kontrollgeist gehört ja in der Mehrzahl der Fälle einem anderen Geschlecht an als das Medium ('Nell' der Frau Silbert, 'John' der Eusapia Palladino) und personifiziert dann entweder ein Liebesobjekt oder die stark ausgeprägten gegengeschlechtlichen Anteile des Mediums.' A. Winterstein, 'Die Bedeutung der Psychoanalyse für die Parapsychologie', *Zeitschrift für Parapsychologie* 7 (1930), 428.

133. Wolf-Braun, *op. cit.* (note 115), 14. Chapter 4 looks at this connection in greater detail.

134. While Schrenck-Notzing dismissed his mediums' trance personalities as a concomitant of either hysteria or psychological disturbance, he was loath to submit them to analysis. As Gerda Walther noted in the case of Rudi Schneider, he rejected psychoanalytic treatment of this medium for fear that Rudi might lose the ability to produce paranormal phenomena. See G. Walther, *Zum anderen Ufer: Vom Marxismus und Atheismus zum Christentum* (Remagen: Otto Reichl, 1960), 451.

135. Mann, *op. cit.* (note 43), 237.

136. D. Sawicki, *Leben mit den Toten: Geisterglauben und die Enstehung des Spiritismus in Deutschland, 1770–1900* (Munich: Schöningh, 2002), 175–6.

137. It is perhaps worth noting here the remarkable parallels between the treatment of mediums and that of early modern witches and demoniacs whose bodies were also subjected to humiliating searches and tests. The temporary freedom from gender roles enjoyed by mediums was also evident among demoniacs, whose relationships with their exorcists exhibited similar power dynamics to those between mediums and parapsychologists. See, for example, M. De Certeau, *The Possession at Loudun,* M.B. Smith (trans.), (Chicago: University of Chicago Press, 1990).

138. On the regurgitation theory, see Gulat-Wellenburg's contribution in, M. von Kemnitz, *Moderne Mediumforschung: Kritische Betrachtungen zu Dr von Schrenck-Notzing's 'Materialisationsphaenomene'* (Munich: J.F. Lehmann, 1914).

139. Wir liessen sie nun Milch und Bisquit trinken und konstatierten, dass der Durchgang des Bisquits durch den Oesophagus sich durchaus normaler Weise vollzog und dass der Oesphagus keinerlei Besonderheit zeigt wie z. B. Verengerung, Erweiterung oder sonstige Abnormalitäten. Der Magen stellt eine hohle Tasche von normalem Volumen dar und füllt sich in normaler Weise.... Man beobachtet weder gastrische Hyperkinese noch autoperistaltische Bewegungen oder Regurgitation. 'Gutachten', in Nachlaß T.K. Oesterreich, 399/15, UAT.

140. Mann, *op. cit.* (note 43), 242–3.

141. Letter from A. von Schrenck-Notzing to Herr Schneider, 26 February 1923, in: Korrespondenz 1, Nachlaß Albert von Schrenck-Notzing, IGPP.

142. Letter from A. von Schrenck-Notzing to Herr Schneider, 24 October 1925, in: Korrespondenz 1, Nachlaß Albert von Schrenck-Notzing, IGPP.

143. 'Es ist ein vollkommener Irrtum, wenn Sie glauben, dass Willy für mich ein Werkzeug sei für Lorbeeren in der Gelehrtenwelt. Da meine wissenschaftliche Stellung durch Jahrzehnte hindurch geleistete Arbeiten vollkommen gesichert ist. Auf der anderen Seite muss ich es als mein Verdienst in Anspruch nehmen, wenn es gelingt, aus Willy ein weltberühmtes Medium zu machen....' Letter from A. von Schrenck-Notzing to Herr Schneider, 11 October 1922, in: Korrespondenz 1, Nachlaß Albert von Schrenck-Notzing, IGPP.

144. *Ibid.*

145. *Ibid.*

146. Letter from A. von Schrenck-Notzing to Herr Schneider, 13 March 1923, in: Korrespondenz 1, Nachlaß Albert von Schrenck-Notzing, IGPP.

147. Letter from J. Hewat McKenzie to A. von Schrenck-Notzing, 23 March 1923, in: Korrespondenz 3, Nachlaß Albert von Schrenck-Notzing, IGPP.

148. 'Sie müssen auch mit der Möglichkeit rechnen, dass die mediumistische Kraft eines Tages erlischt. Dann sitzt er, wenn er nicht in der Lage ist, sich genügend als Zahntechniker zu erwerben, als Bummler und Schieber auf der Strasse.' Letter from A. von Schrenck-Notzing to Herr Schneider, 18 February 1923, in: Korrespondenz 1, Nachlaß Albert von Schrenck-Notzing, IGPP.

149. Schrenck-Notzing, *op. cit.* (note 146).

150. Letter from A. von Schrenck-Notzing to Herr Schneider, 21 March 1923, in: Korrespondenz 1, Nachlaß Albert von Schrenck-Notzing, IGPP.

151. In 1925 Schrenck-Notzing organised an apprenticeship for Rudi with the Stockdorfer Motor Factory near Pasing-Munich and began to conduct experiments with him. Letter from A. von Schrenck-Notzing to Herr Schneider, 16 September 1925, in: Korrespondenz 1, Nachlaß Albert von Schrenck-Notzing, IGPP.

152. Letter from A. von Schrenck-Notzing to Herr Schneider, 18 September 1925, in: Korrespondenz 1, Nachlaß Albert von Schrenck-Notzing, IGPP. Letter from A. von Schrenck-Notzing to Herr Schneider, 24 October, 1925, in: Korrespondenz 1, Nachlaß Albert von Schrenck-Notzing, IGPP.

153. 'Sie haben nun mit täppischer Hand als ewiger Besserwisser das Werk zerstört, das ich seit Jahren mühevoll aufgebaut und den guten Ruf Ihrer beiden Söhne in schändlicher Weise preisgegeben.' Letter from A. von Schrenck-Notzing to Herr Schneider, 17 September 1927, in: Korrespondenz 1, Nachlaß Albert von Schrenck-Notzing, IGPP.

154. Letter from R. Tischner and R. Lambert to A. von Schrenck-Notzing, 5 September 1927, in: Korrespondenz 3, Nachlaß Albert von Schrenck-Notzing, IGPP.

155. M. Kemmerich, 'Die Wissenschaft des Humbugs: Eine Abrechnung m. Dr med. Albert Frhrn. von Schrenck-Notzing' (typescript), 7, in: L 4400 (Kemmerich, Max), Monacensia Literaturarchiv, Stadtbibliothek, München,.

156. Tischner, *op. cit.* (note 7), 215.

157. *Ibid.,* 216.

158. 'Gerade, wenn die Parapsychologie sich nunmehr sicherer fühlt, hat sie es nicht mehr notwendig, sich eines Kampforganes zu bedienen, sondern bedarf eines nüchtern sachlichen Fachblattes, das objective und kritische Arbeiten des einschlägigen Gebietes bringt.... Hoffen wir also, daß die Zeitschrift für Parapsychologie unter der geschickten Leitung Dr Sünners ein würdiges Fachorgan des neuen Forschungszweiges werde.' Letter from Professor H. Thirring to Albert von Schrenck-Notzing, 18 October 1925, in: Korrespondenz 1, Nachlaß Albert von Schrenck-Notzing, IGPP.

159. Letter from A. von Schrenck-Notzing to Professor H. Thirring, 20 October 1925, in: Korrespondenz 1, Nachlaß Albert von Schrenck-Notzing, IGPP.

160. Tischner and Lambert, *op. cit.* (note 154).

161. Letter from R. Tischner to A. von Schrenck-Notzing, 2 November 1927, in: Korrespondenz 3, Nachlaß Albert von Schrenck-Notzing, IGPP.

162. 'Der tiefere Grund ist von all dem der, dass Sie versuchen den Okkultismus und im besonderen die ZfP diktatorisch in Ihrem Sinne zu leiten und eine Oberkontrolle auszuüben, die in einer Gelehrtenrepublik unangebracht ist'. Tischner and Lambert, *op. cit.* (note 154).

163. 'Wir müssen deshalb aus den angegebenen schwerwiegenden Gründen fordern, dass Sie von Ihrer Stellung als unoffizieller Leiter der ZfP zurücktreten.... Sollten Sie unsere Vorschläge ablehnen oder nach deren Annahme der ZfP Schwerigkeiten machen wollen, so müssten wir dieses Schreiben allen Mitarbeiten der ZfP inbesondere den Herrn Driesch und Oesterreich mitteilen, deren Urteil nicht zweifelhaft sein dürfte, auch wären wir im Interessen der Sache genötigt uns an die breitere Oeffentlichkeit zu wenden.' *Ibid.*

164. 'Ich frage nun: können Sie einem Manne, der in so offenbarer Weise das okkultistische Kurpfuschertum unterstützt, wirklich noch Ihr Vertrauen schenken.' A. von Schrenck-Notzing to R. Lambert, 15 September, 1927, in: Korrespondenz 3, Nachlaß Albert von Schrenck-Notzing, IGPP.

165. Letter from A. von Schrenck-Notzing to R. Lambert, 12 September 1927, in: Korrespondenz 3, Nachlaß Albert von Schrenck-Notzing, IGPP.

166. 'Sie vergessen ganz, dass nicht Sie es waren, der die grosse Zahl Hochschullehrer für die Parapsychologie zu interessieren wusste und die Herrn veranlasste, das Protektorat über unsere Zeitschrift zu übernehmen; dass nicht Sie es waren, der die Medien zum wissenschaftlichen Experiment erzogen hat; dass nicht Sie es waren, der die ausserordentlich schwierige Umwandlung der *Psychischen Studien* in ein wissenschaftlich anehmbares Fachblatt vernahm – *sondern das alle diese Leistungen mein Verdienst sind.* Ich möchte Sie ausserdem daran erinnern, das während der Inflationzeit ich die *Psychischen Studien* pekuniär gestützt habe und sie dadurch vor dem Eingehen bewahrte, dass ich niemals für den Abdruck meiner Arbeiten ein Honorar nahm, dass ich eine grosse Reihe honorarfreier Beiträge der Zeitschrift zugänglich machte, dass ich den grössern Teil der mir zustehenden Dividende dem Verlag für Propagandazwecke überliess....' *Ibid.*

167. 'Im Vereinsregister wurde heute eingetragen: Okkultische Gesellschaft e. V. München: Durch Wegfall sämtlicher Mitglieder ist der Verein aufgelöst', in: StArMü , Polizedirekton 5610.

168. 'Die weitere Entwicklung der Parapsychologie ist zu einem nicht unerheblichen Teile eine Frage der materiellen Mittel.... Wer gibt die erste Million als Gründungsstifung? Sein Name wird unvergessen bleiben. Und auch an die Deutschen des Auslandes ergeht der Ruf: Gebt Geld! Die deutsche Parapsychologie kann sich nicht entwickeln und kann nicht den

notwendigen Kontakt mit der Parapsychologie des Auslandes gewinnen und aufrechterhalten, wenn uns die fremde Literatur unzugänglich bleibt.' Oesterreich, *op. cit.* (note 10).

169. Tischner, *op. cit.* (note 7), 216.
170. Schrenck-Notzing, *Phenomena of Materialisation, op. cit.* (note 2), v.
171. *Ibid.*, vi.
172. *Ibid.*,
173. On the public response to *Materialisations-Phänomene*, see Mann, *op. cit.* (note 43) , 224–5.
174. Kraus, *op. cit.* (note 54), 162.
175. See Kemnitz, *op. cit.* (note 138).
176. Schrenck-Notzing, *Experimente der Fernbewegung, op. cit.* (note 35), xii.
177. A. Hellwig, *Okkultismus und Wissenschaft unter besonderer Berücksichtigung der Telekinese und der Materialisationen* (Stuttgart: Ferdinand Enke, 1926), 10–1.
178. Kemnitz, *op. cit.* (note 138), 6.
179. *Ibid.*, 6–7.
180. W. von Gulat-Wellenburg, C. von Klinckowstroem and H. Rosenbusch, *Der Physikalische Mediumismus* (Berlin: Ullstein, 1925), 15.
181. Hellwig, *op. cit.* (note 177), 10.
182. Kemnitz, *op. cit.* (note138), 7.
183. *Ibid.*, 7.
184. Gulat-Wellenburg, *et al., op. cit.* (note 180),16.
185. *Ibid.*,16.
186. Kemnitz, *op. cit.* (note 138), 6.
187. Schrenck-Notzing, *Experimente der Fernbewegung, op. cit.* (note 35), xi.
188. *Ibid.*, xii.
189. *Ibid.*, xii.
190. Gulat-Wellenburg, *et al., op. cit.* (note 180), 16.
191. *Ibid.*, 16.
192. Schrenck-Notzing, *op. cit.* (note 20), 513–19.
193. Kemnitz, *op. cit.* (note 137), 9.
194. Gulat-Wellenburg, *et al., op. cit.* (note 180), 17.
195. *Ibid.*, 488.
196. Schrenck-Notzing, *Experimente der Fernbewegun, op. cit.* (note 35), xii.
197. Brower has pointed to this same difficulty in the French context. While there was popular interest in physical mediumship in France during the 1920s, the rarity of the physical phenomena meant that the public had to rely on the good faith of those who witnessed materialisations and ectoplasm. For French critics, like their Germany contemporaries, this was a major weakness in parapsychology's bid to contribute to the scientific construction of public knowledge. See Brower *op. cit.* (note 14), 320.

198. Hellwig, *op. cit.* (note 177), 9.
199. Gulat-Wellenburg, *et al., op. cit.* (note 180), 489.
200. Schrenck-Notzing, *Experimente der Fernbewegung, op. cit.* (note 35), 1.
201. F. Parot, 'Psychology Experiments: Spiritism at the Sorbonne', *Journal of the History of the Behavioral Sciences* 29 (1993), 22.
202. *Ibid.*, 23.
203. H. Bender, 'A Positive Critic of Superstition', in R. Pilkington (ed.), *Men and Women of Parapsychology: Personal Reflections*, (Jefferson: McFarland & Company, 1987), 114.
204. E. Bauer, 'Hans Bender und die Gründung des "Instituts für Grenzgebiete der Psychologie und Psychohygiene"', in J. Jahnke, *et al.* (eds), *Psychologiegeschichte: Beziehungen zu Philosophie und Grenzgebieten* (Passauer Schriften zur Psychologiegeschichte; Vol. 12) (Munich: Profil, 1998), 461.
205. 'Hans Bender im Gespräch mit Johannes Mischo (1983)', *Zeitschrift für Parapsychologie und Grenzgebiete der Psychologie* 33 (1991), 7.
206. Bauer, *op. cit.* (note 6) , 15; Bauer, *op. cit.* (note 204), 466–7.
207. Bender, *op. cit.* (note 203), 115.
208. See S.H. Mauskopf and M.R. McVaugh, *The Elusive Science: Origins of Experimental Psychical Research* (Baltimore: Johns Hopkins University Press, 1980).

4

An Holistic Science:
Philosophical Renewal and Official Response

Introduction

At the International Congress for Parapsychology held in Athens in 1930, a significant shift in focus was apparent among the German representatives. The death of Schrenck-Notzing, whose virtual monopoly of the German parapsychological scene had ensured an emphasis on experimentation, allowed those with an interest in the analysis and interpretation of paranormal phenomena to come to the fore. On the opening day of proceedings, three of the German participants gave papers on philosophical and theoretical themes. The biologist and philosopher Hans Driesch, for example, spoke about the person and supraperson from both a spiritualist and biological perspective, the philosopher T.K. Oesterreich considered the psycho-physical problem in terms of mediumistic phenomena while K.C. Schneider looked at the relationship between physics, empiricism and Gestalt psychology on the one hand, and parapsychology on the other.[1] This retreat from experimentalism – a result of the methodological and financial difficulties posed by research with mediums – saw a concentration on the aetiology and mechanism of physical mediumship and an attempt to reconcile these phenomena with new developments in fields such as biology, physics and psychology.[2] Speculation as to the meaning of materialisation and telekinesis also led these researchers to contemplate parapsychology's potential as the basis for both scientific advance and philosophical renewal.

The Athens congress was a watershed for German parapsychology from another perspective also, as it was the last that German parapsychologists were permitted to attend. In 1935, the National Socialist government denied German parapsychologists permission to travel, preventing them from participating in the International Congress for Parapsychology held in Oslo.[3] In 1938, as preparations were being made for the sixth International Congress for Parapsychology in Budapest, the Auswärtiges Amt [Foreign Office] informed the Unterrichtsministerium [Ministry for Education] that the possibility of Germans attending this gathering was ruled out until normal circumstances once again prevailed in Europe.[4] While these

191

restrictions suggested that the Nazis harboured a negative or at least suspicious attitude towards parapsychology, a number of other initiatives, including the attempt of an official within the Propaganda-Ministerium [Propaganda Ministry] to establish a parapsychological research group, indicated a more complex relationship between National Socialism and parapsychology.[5]

Shifting the focus away from the laboratory, where the emphasis remained almost exclusively on the observation and verification of the physical phenomena during this period, this chapter considers contemporary attempts to explain and theorise the phenomena of mediumship. The first section briefly describes the manner in which a number of German researchers who were deeply affected by the social, political and economic crises wrought by the First World War, most notably the philosopher and psychologist T.K. Oesterreich, used epistemological tensions within biology, physics and psychology to portray their discipline as a complete science, capable of expanding scientific and philosophical horizons. This attempt to create an holistic science, a project similar to that advocated by du Prel and his followers, and to use it as the basis for scientific reform and social and spiritual renewal, was nowhere more evident than in the work of Hans Driesch; a man who, along with Oesterreich, was regarded as one of the leaders of German parapsychology following the death of Schrenck-Notzing in 1929. The second section is thus an exploration of Driesch's contribution to parapsychology in the German and international contexts, tracing his development from biologist to philosopher and outlining his problematic relationship with the National Socialists. Using the Nazis' ambivalence towards Hans Driesch as a starting point, the third section attempts to cast light on their attitude towards parapsychology. It asks how the Nazi stance on this nascent science coincided with or differed from their stance on occultism; and to what extent their position was a continuation of the policies of Weimar governments, whose legislation reflected the concerns of interest groups, including the medical community and the churches?

Materialism, parapsychology and philosophical renewal

The sense of existential crisis that had characterised the writings of men like Carl du Prel and Wilhelm Hübbe-Schleiden during the late nineteenth century was renewed by the events of 1914 to 1918. While most representatives of psychical research had abandoned their pursuit of a transcendental psychology during the late 1880s in favour of an experimental psychology based on mediumistic research, the First World War saw a revival among German parapsychologists of passionate anti-materialism and the renewal of that stream of thought that regarded research with mediums as an antidote to the philosophical problems posed by modernity. This school of thought was most prominently represented by T.K. Oesterreich, whose philosophical and psychological interest in split consciousness had led him to parapsychology.[6] According to Oesterreich, the Great War was the logical conclusion of the mechanistic worldview that had dominated nineteenth-century thought and bore the responsibility for the revolutionary events in Russia, from whence civil war and mass terror threatened to spill out to engulf the continent.[7] The atavistic and destructive tendencies that dominated the social and cultural life of Europe were, Oesterreich argued, also evident within the sciences. Convinced that the scientific project inaugurated by Copernicus, Kepler, Galilei and Newton, was one sided and incomplete due to its exclusive focus on matter and motion, Oesterreich and a number of like-minded colleagues looked to contemporary developments in biology, physics and psychology both to explain the phenomena of mediumship and to overthrow materialism.[8]

Following the First World War in Germany, a period characterised by civil unrest and political uncertainty, large numbers of Germans found solace and security in occult practice and belief. Contemporaries who noted this surge of interest in the occult labelled this phenomenon an 'okkulte Welle' ['occult wave'], blaming the war and revolution for the revival of belief in astrology, mysticism and fortune telling. Attempts to quantify this development, like that undertaken by the Protestant church, estimated the number of fortune-tellers active in Berlin at around three thousand, and the number advertising their services in Leipzig at two hundred and fifty.[9] Such reports also noted the manner in which these savvy occultists loitered outside department stores and factories at closing time touting for subscriptions among the women and girls who worked there.[10] Contemporary analyses made clear that the market for such services was also experiencing rapid expansion, observers calculating both the large numbers of Germans with an interest in the occult, several million by one count, and the demographic make-up of this group. According to such reports, the occult epidemic had spread quadratically, permeating every level of society, high and low, rich and poor, belying claims that this contagion was restricted to those of limited education or means.[11] Commentators agreed that this astounding growth in occultism was a result of a well-known historical law, according to which intellectual developments occurred in a wave- or pendulum-like pattern, rising up or swinging in an opposing arch in response to earlier ideologies.[12] According to this theory, the mechanisation and rationalisation of life that had reached its peak in the war, set in motion an intense reaction that was apparent not only in the drive towards occultism but in the revival of mysticism and Catholicism.[13]

While many observers located the cause of the 'occult wave' in the war and the economic crisis that followed it, others, including Oesterreich, provided a more nuanced analysis. Oesterreich, in an effort to explain what he saw as the arrested development of parapsychology in the German context, was careful to stress that while the war had provided the immediate impetus for this upsurge in occult activity, the underlying cause should be located in a series of philosophical developments that had occurred during the nineteenth century.[14] Occultism, he maintained, had emerged in Germany, as elsewhere, in response to the materialistic philosophy that had dominated scientific discourse from the 1850s onwards. This mechanistic worldview, Oesterreich argued, had demoted the mind to a function of the brain, impoverishing philosophy and relegating psychology to a branch of physiology.[15] While in France and Anglo-Saxon countries philosophy and psychology had managed to free themselves from materialism by the end of the nineteenth century, in Germany materialism remained a prominent feature of the philosophical landscape up until the First World War.[16]

That parapsychologists like Oesterreich viewed materialism as a peculiarly German malaise was evident in their complaints that Germany lagged behind other countries in the acceptance of the paranormal as a legitimate field of study.[17] The reason for materialism's stranglehold in the German context, they argued, was the emergence during the early nineteenth century of a uniquely German form of Romanticism.[18] This philosophy, as it became manifest in Germany, celebrated non-rational aspects of human thought and action, placing emphasis on feeling and intuition rather than reason and research. The development of German philosophy along materialistic lines during the mid-nineteenth century was thus a knee-jerk reaction to the idealistic excesses of German Romanticism.[19] Materialism, these researchers maintained, remained entrenched in Germany because the rabid anti-Idealism inspired by the Romantics had an insulating effect, shutting German philosophy and psychology off from developments in other countries where a more balanced approach to mind and matter evolved during the *fin de siècle*.[20]

At the same moment at which experimental psychology in the German context confined itself to the study of objective phenomena, France and the Anglo-Saxon nations expanded their experimental method to investigate the entire spectrum of mental events, including those occult phenomena exhibited in unconscious and somnambulistic states.[21] Viewing these putative paranormal powers as a product of abnormal psychology, these researchers attempted to separate reality from superstition. While this research, situated alongside normal psychology on the one hand and psychopathology on the other, was conducted by such intellectual luminaries as William James (1842–1910), it received minimal attention in Germany where a materialistic worldview largely militated against similar investigations.[22] The estrangement of German psychology from that practised in both the Anglo-Saxon world and in France also saw the neglect of subconscious phenomena. Pierre Janet's and Alfred Binet's (1859–1911) pioneering studies of the subconscious were all but ignored in Germany due to a focus on the psychology of conscious events in healthy individuals.[23] For these reasons, Oesterreich maintained, Germany had produced few significant philosophical or psychological advances during the late nineteenth and early twentieth centuries. Once a nation of philosophers, Germany's philosophy and psychology had become stunted and deformed by its servitude to materialism, the consequence of which, Oesterreich argued, was the failure of parapsychology in Germany to develop with the same vigour that it had in other countries.[24]

Oesterreich contended that while the mechanistic worldview that dominated German philosophy after the collapse of Idealism had acted as a barrier against the recognition and advance of parapsychology in Germany, its disintegration in the early twentieth century, under pressure from modern physics and biology, finally enabled Germans to equal their English, American, French and Italian counterparts.[25] Responsible for this change were the revolutionary theories and research of scientists like Einstein, whose theory of relativity radically altered the manner in which science conceived of matter and energy, and Driesch, whose neo-vitalism suggested that there existed teleology in biological development.[26] In psychology also there was recognition that while the mind could not be explained simply as a function of the brain, it was intimately connected to the body.[27] The result of this realisation was the creation of a new sub-discipline known as psychobiology.[28] These epistemological changes negated materialism and helped construct a *Weltanschauung* into which seemingly occult phenomena could be more easily fitted. In this new intellectual climate, telekinesis and materialisation no longer seemed to circumvent the laws of nature, but to reinforce them.

The engineer and parapsychologist Fritz Grunewald, who constructed a laboratory for parapsychological research in Berlin prior to the First World War, employed modern physics to explain the phenomena of mediumship. He argued that the materialisation process offered concrete proof that energy could be changed into matter and matter into energy.[29] If one took the point of view, he maintained, that the matter out of which materialisations took shape was simply a reorganisation of the material that constituted the medium's body, one need look no further for an explanation.[30] Even in those cases where no visible link between the medium's body and the materialisation could be seen, Grunewald contended, the two were connected by either a field or band of energy. A parallel for this exchange between matter and energy existed, he argued, in modern physics in the phenomenon of radioactivity. With radioactive atom disintegration, he wrote, there occurs a separation of energy in the form of radiation, allied with a simultaneous transformation of the atom.[31] The atom, however, is not completely converted into radiating energy, rather only a part of it, a material component being retained.[32] Grunewald maintained not only that physics provided parapsychology with theoretical and methodological succour, but that the experimental study of mediumship would prove important for the development of physics in the future.[33]

While Grunewald looked to modern physics to help explain materialisation, men like Richet and Schrenck-Notzing consulted the new biology as a means of accounting for the sexually suggestive phenomena associated with physical mediumship.[34] The conviction that the physical phenomena of mediumship bore some as yet ill-defined connection to normal reproductive energies or processes was widespread during this period. In a letter to the Austrian physicist, Professor Hans Thirring, for example, Schrenck-Notzing thought it relevant to note that a fifteen-year-old 'Spuk' [poltergeist] medium he had recently discovered had not yet begun to menstruate. He also mentioned the correspondence he saw between Willy Schneider's maturation and the steady decline of his mediumistic powers. He declared:

> In correspondence with your views I am of the opinion that sexual factors play a decisive role in these manifestations. Hence the occurrence of these phenomena between the thirteenth and twenty-third years of life. It is possible that these powers will completely disappear on the maturation of the youth into a man.[35]

The sexual nature of the physical phenomena was also highlighted by its connection with the reproductive organs. Ectoplasm was often seen to issue from the breasts and vagina of the medium Eva C., and the writhing and moaning of the medium as phenomena were produced was reminiscent of both sexual intercourse and childbirth. Hypotheses regarding these phenomena, which argued that materialisation and telekinesis were some kind of exteriorisation of reproductive or biological processes, fitted nicely with the vitalistic theories postulated by Henri Bergson (1859–1941) and Hans Driesch.

Driesch's work in particular proved useful in linking biology and parapsychology, suggesting that the construction of the organism was due to some kind of vital energy or unconscious function.[36] If reproduction, as Driesch maintained, was an example of this vitalistic force at work, it seemed possible that in certain individuals these powers might be harnessed, given direction and form in the mind, and projected outside the body as so-called pseudopodia or materialisations. While critics such as Richard Baerwald argued that should the materialisation of organic forms from mediums' bodies prove a reality, this would be of physiological significance but would have no bearing on philosophical problems, parapsychologists maintained that proof of a vitalistic force would be of enormous philosophical importance.[37] For Oesterreich, the knowledge, provided by mediumistic research, that the world was infused with meaning, would enable Europe to turn back from the brink of destruction. Echoing du Prel, he wrote:

> The future, the question of the decline or further development of European and American culture depends on whether man learns to see the structure of the world and his place in it with other eyes. And I do not know what kind of facts there should be more readily suitable for leading to this than mediumistic phenomena. They will, if they are capable of philosophical conviction, exert a profound influence on the life of man and the entire structure of culture, providing the basis for a reorganisation and intellectual rebirth of the world.[38]

Driesch wrote similarly:

> We say openly: paraphysics (*Paraphysik*) is our hope in matters of biology, just as parapsychics (*Parapsychik*) is our hope in matters of psychology. Both however, are our hope in the matter of a well-founded metaphysics and worldview.[39]

For Driesch like Oesterreich, then, parapsychology was the basis not only for scientific reform, but also for philosophical renewal.

Supernormal biology

In 1923, a mere three years before he became the president of the Society for Psychical Research, the German biologist and philosopher Hans Driesch made explicit for the first time, in an article entitled 'Der Okkultismus als neue Wissenschaft' ['Occultism as a New Science'], the links he perceived between his vitalistic theory of entelechy, new directions within biology and psychology, and occult phenomena.[40] With reference to his own experiments in the field of embryology, Driesch argued that modern academic biology had definitively proven the inability of the mechanistic model of life to account for the purposive nature of biological development.[41] He postulated instead a teleological vital force, entelechy, which guided the construction and regeneration of organic matter.[42] Mechanism, Driesch noted here, had been rejected not only by biologists, but also by the proponents of the 'new' psychology, who regarded the machine model of mind as inadequate to explain psychical factors.[43] Significantly, Driesch argued, the decision to abandon a rigidly materialistic view of life and mind allowed phenomena traditionally ignored by science, for instance, telekinesis, materialisation, telepathy and clairvoyance, to be investigated and explained in scientific terms.[44] The mediumistic materialisation of limbs, heads and amorphous forms, for example, could be understood in terms of a vitalistic biology. In this view, certain people possessed the ability not only to harness the vitalistic force, but also to reorganise it outside their bodies in the shape of both conscious and unconscious ideas – a process which might be called 'supernormal biology'.[45] The elucidation of these links in 'Occultism as a New Science', signified Driesch's retreat from experimental work and his immersion in questions of the 'soul-life', a focus that would allow him not only to voice epistemological concerns about science, but social, cultural and political concerns about modernity in the German context.[46]

During the 1890s, unease with some of the more bewildering aspects of modernity, including rapid industrialisation, urbanisation, and economic instability, saw significant numbers of Germans experience what has been termed a crisis of modernity. Germans, like many other Europeans, were concerned that the forces of modernisation would undermine traditional values and leave them adrift without moral or social anchors. While some Germans undoubtedly indulged in cultural despair and rabid anti-modernism in response to this crisis others, as we have seen, channelled their discontent into reformist projects, which aimed at improving health care, housing and workers' rights, and which utilised both economics and biology as the impetus for social, cultural and political change.[47] Within the life and mind sciences, discomfort with modernity was focused on positivism, which in the eyes of critics reduced life to a base mechanistic process and the mind to predictable and quantifiable mechanical and chemical changes in the brain. For opponents of these mechanistic and atomistic tendencies within biology and psychology, a reassessment of scientific epistemology, one that would enable life and mind to be understood holistically, seemed imperative.[48] Embryology's transformation during the early 1890s from a purely morphological and descriptive discipline to an analytical science concerned with the mechanism of organic development, promised to provide an empirical basis for such epistemological reform.[49]

The ostensibly purposive nature of life, that is the capacity of organisms to develop, change and heal themselves, had precluded, for many German scientists, the extension of the principles of physics and chemistry to biology.[50] Seeking instead a theory that would explain the dynamic nature of life, these scientists looked to the field of embryology where, to some observers at least, a mechanical view of organic development was becoming increasingly untenable.[51] With the aim not only of describing changes in the form and structure of embryos, but also of explaining them, Wilhelm Roux (1850–1924) had introduced an analytical approach to embryology during the early 1890s.[52] This new focus, known as 'Entwicklungsmechanik' [developmental mechanics], encouraged biologists to study and contemplate the apparently purposive nature of growth and development. During 1891, as part of this shift in disciplinary focus, Hans Driesch, Roux's former student, conducted a series of experiments designed to test and develop the model of inheritance posited by August Weismann (1834–1914). Driesch's manipulation of sea urchin eggs elicited surprising results, results that in Driesch's view not only offered definitive proof that life was not a mechanical process, but which hinted at some as yet undiscovered life force.

Driesch had travelled to Naples in 1891 in the hope of repeating a series of experiments on heredity initiated by Roux. Roux had attempted to test Weismann's hypothesis that a complicated structure exists which promotes ontogeny by its disintegration during cell division, by destroying one of the first two blastometres of a frog's egg following its first cleavage.[53] These experiments, as Roux had expected and as Weismann's theory had predicted, resulted in the formation of half embryos indicating the operation of mechanical laws of development during embryogenesis. Driesch, keen to recreate these results, repeated Roux's experiments substituting the eggs of frogs for those of the more resilient sea urchin. Separating the cells of a number of sea urchin eggs at the two-cell stage by violent shaking, Driesch observed the development of one of the severed cells:

> It went through cleavage just as it would have done in contact with its sister-cell and there occurred cleavage stages which are just half the normal ones.... I now expected that the next morning would reveal to me the half organisation of my subject once more.... But things turned out as they were bound to do and not as I had expected; there was a typically whole gastrula on my dish the next morning, differing only by its small size from a normal one; and this *small but whole* gastrula was followed by a whole and typical small pluteus-larva.[54]

The results were similar when two eggs were forced to join, they did not create conjoined organisms, as Weismann's theory might suggest, but one giant one. Driesch wrote:

> I have succeeded in raising *one giant* organism from *two* sea-urchin eggs, fused in the blastula stage.... This, of course is the real counterpart of my first experiments: in these I got *many* (two or four) complete organisms from a material that normally should have given *one*; now there is *one* instead of many.[55]

This was the opposite result to that of Roux whose experiments had suggested that embryonic development proceeded according to a mosaic-like blueprint, the proof of which was evident in the half or mutilated organisms produced by the disruption of this process.[56] Driesch's small, but whole, sea urchin larvae contradicted both Weismann's hypothesis and Roux's experimental results, demonstrating for him not only the limitations of mechanism, but also the possibility that a purposive force existed within nature.

By the late 1890s, Driesch had deduced a theory from his findings in the field of embryology. On the basis of his results with sea urchin eggs he postulated a non-material teleological principle called entelechy, which he argued guided the development and regeneration of organic life. This vitalistic interpretation of embryogenesis had, however, taken a number of years to evolve. Following his experiments in 1891, Driesch had attempted to understand his findings in purely mechanistic terms. Settling briefly, around 1894, on a mechanical theory of ontogeny, which became known as Driesch's 'machine theory of life', he soon became dissatisfied with the inability of this theory to explain the harmonious nature of development.[57] The extremely fragmentary view of ontogeny that such mechanical hypotheses provided led Driesch to the conclusion that a teleological approach was necessary to explain the apparent harmony of embryonic development.[58] By 1896, he had declared all organisms subject to teleological laws, dividing them into 'determined equipotential systems', such as frogs' eggs, where developmental potential is divided among the parts of the system, and 'harmonious equipotential systems', such as sea urchins' eggs, where it is not.[59] The reality of these harmonious equipotential systems, as demonstrated by his sea urchin egg experiments, proved for Driesch the existence of a vitalistic force within nature. He wrote in this regard:

> The forces of matter are at work in the organism; there is no doubt about this. But something else is at work in it also, directing the material forces without changing the amount of energy, to put it shortly. And to this unifying, non-material, mind-like something I have given the Aristotelian name of *entelechy*....[60]

The development and publication of this theory around 1899 marked Driesch's movement away from biology and towards philosophy and parapsychology. Unable to reproduce the results of his sea urchin experiments with other species, and thereby increase the empirical basis for his theory of entelechy, Driesch sought other fields where his hypothesis might be applied and developed. With this in mind, he began to acquaint himself during the last years of the decade with the literature of both philosophy and parapsychology.

When Driesch attempted to expand his empirical base, from sea urchin eggs to those of other organisms, in the early 1890s, he had discovered that they did not reveal the same plasticity, that is, they consistently produced, in accordance with the findings of Weismann and Roux, half or mutilated organisms. Turning instead to the philosophy of Kant, Schopenhauer, Eduard von Hartmann, Locke and Alois Riehl, Driesch expanded his teleological principle beyond biology and into philosophy, where it contributed to the movement among a diverse group of Germans for holism, and psychology, where it acted as critique of contemporary mechanistic theories of mind.[61] In the period prior to the First World War, Driesch also began to take an interest in the work of the Society for Psychical Research, slowly becoming convinced that parapsychology could provide the empirical proof required to validate his theory of entelechy.[62] By the mid-1920s, he had persuaded himself that the physical phenomena of parapsychology, if they were in fact real, could provide definitive proof of vitalism. In this regard, Driesch informed an audience at Clark University in 1927 that:

> [I]t is here [with the physical phenomena] that Parapsychology is in closer connection with well-established and well-known facts of science than anywhere else. I may even go as far as to say: modern biology is already 'psychical research', along the physical side... the action I have called Entelechy in the field of biology proper does not 'create' matter but is only ordering pre-existing matter. And it is only this action of ordering, of directing which we have to assume in parapsychology, matter being everywhere.[63]

Driesch argued that his vitalism had 'bridged' the gap between the world of matter and the world of parapsychology, allowing occult phenomena to be understood as extensions or exaggerations of normal biological and psychological processes. To Driesch's mind, parapsychology not only disproved the mechanistic models of life and mind, but also provided the basis for an holistic *Weltanschauung*, the implications of which would extend beyond biology and psychology into the realm of culture and politics.[64]

Driesch's interest in parapsychology had begun prior to the First World War, as a result of his reading in this area.[65] His familiarity with scholarship in this field was evident as early as 1908 when he mentioned, as part of his Gifford Lectures, his conviction that telepathy existed and his knowledge of a popular contemporary theory which likened telepathy to the wireless telegraph.[66] In this forum, he also considered the spiritualist hypothesis suggesting that the vitalistic force might survive death in a personal form. The advantage of this theory, Driesch argued, was that it explained, in an uncomplicated manner, the strong resemblance that some mediums' trance personalities bore to those of deceased persons.[67] In the course of another lecturing engagement in England, during 1913, Driesch met Mrs Eleanor Sidgwick (1886–1919), widow of the philosopher Henry Sidgwick and an active member of the Society for Psychical Research, who since the 1880s had utilised her formidable skills as a mathematician and physicist in the field of psychical research.[68] He wrote of his encounter:

> The acquaintance with Mrs Sidgwick, a clever, intellectual woman, was significant for me in that she brought me nearer that subject, that in England has been called Psychical Research, by us *Parapsychologie*… and of which I hitherto knew little, but which had, mind you, influenced me strongly.[69]

It was during 1913 also that Henri Bergson, whose vitalist philosophy was influential on Driesch's theory of entelechy, had taken up the presidency of the Society for Psychical Research.[70] In his inaugural address to the society, Bergson used his conviction that the mind and brain did not exist in strict parallelism as a means of explaining both telepathy and 'phantasms of the living'.[71] Conversation with Mrs Sidgwick and the explicit mixing of vitalism and psychical research in Bergson's speech fostered Driesch's burgeoning interest in the study of the paranormal encouraging him to become a member of the Society for Psychical Research and to incorporate the facts of parapsychology, as he saw them, into his scientific and philosophical worldview. It was not until after the Great War however, which impacted on the pacifistic and cosmopolitan Driesch profoundly, that he began in earnest to develop and to publicise his interest in parapsychology.

Perusal of the Society for Psychical Research's results had rapidly convinced Driesch of the reality of the so-called psychical phenomena of mediumship, including, telepathy, clairvoyance and psychometry.[72] He believed that these psychical phenomena could be understood in scientific terms with reference to the new psychology's concept of 'Gestalt' and theories of sub- and co-consciousness.[73] Driesch was more reluctant, however, to admit the reality of physical phenomena, such as materialisation, levitation and telekinesis, which although impressive were frequently performed under conditions unsuitable for scientific observation. He noted:

> With the physical para-phenomena I remained more sceptical, even though in 1922 I attended with Schrenck-Notzing a sitting with Willy Schneider that was very influential. I found no possibility of deception… but the experimental conditions were just not completely satisfactory in a scientific sense.[74]

In 1928, however, after attending another séance with Schrenck-Notzing, Driesch informed his host that, 'the sitting with Rudi convinced me more than everything that I have seen up until now, of the reality of the physical phenomena. I have repeatedly thought about the phenomena: there really is no loophole.'[75] While Driesch's scepticism appears to have dissipated somewhat as a result of further observation, he was never entirely convinced that the conditions under which physical mediumship was performed were sufficient to prevent fraud. Driesch's cautious stance on the physical phenomena did not, however, prevent him from hypothesising a link between vitalistic biology, materialisation, levitation and telekinesis. This enthusiasm for the paranormal, its theorisation in vitalistic terms, and the widespread influence of neo-vitalism in the fields of biology, psychology and philosophy, saw Driesch, who had made no parapsychological experiments of his own, become an important figure within the international parapsychological community.

In 1926, Driesch, a man with negligible experience in the field of experimental parapsychology, became the first German to be appointed president of the Society for Psychical Research. In his presidential address he confessed:

> To tell the truth at the very beginning: I have never made a successful psychical experiment myself, though I have tried to do so. I have seen some phenomena, but only as a spectator. Thus the only possible thing that I may claim to have done for the elucidation of our great object is this, that I have prepared its road in a certain way.[76]

Even before he had made his interest in the paranormal explicit, Driesch's ideas had been popular within the parapsychological community in Europe. Driesch's vitalism had challenged the epistemological assumptions of a number of sciences, including biology and psychology, and had presented the parapsychological community with an ostensibly scientific basis for their rejection of both mechanism and materialism. Driesch, cognisant of his influence in this field, stated, in the course of his presidential address, that his work in biology and psychology had led him to certain theoretical ideas according to which the phenomena of mediumship existed in connection with established facts of modern science. He designated his contribution to parapsychology, therefore, as that of a bridge builder, his vitalistic theory forming the bridge between the biological and psychological sciences, and paranormal phenomena, such as telepathy and materialisation.[77] This approach allowed Driesch not only to explain telepathy by analogy with cases of dissociation but to argue also that materialisation might be understood as the externalisation, through some unknown mechanism, of the body's vitalistic forces in the form of memories and ideas.

Despite Driesch's reluctance to commit to the reality of the physical phenomena of mediumship it was, arguably, in this branch of parapsychological endeavour that his theories had the most impact. Supernormal biology or super-vitalism, as Driesch sometimes called it, appealed to large numbers of those with an interest in the physical phenomena, including materialisation, levitation and telekinesis. For example, Driesch's vitalistic hypothesis provided an elegant explanatory model for those ectoplasmic forms which issued from the orifices and reproductive organs of both male and female mediums and which had long been thought to be of organic origin. Driesch used his theory of entelechy to explain the process of materialisation as a form of super-normal biology, hypothesising that materialisation was simply an externalisation of vitalistic processes in connection with the body of a medium. He stressed that there was little that separated normal vitalistic processes within the organism from super-normal or parapsychological projections outside the body. He argued:

> The only difference between ordinary vitalistic and parapsychological control relates to the range or area of controlling; this area being of far greater extent in the second case than in the first. But in a sense embryology is already 'materialisation' from the vitalist's point of view. Think of the little material body, called an egg, and think of the enormous and very complex material body, say, an elephant, that may come out of it: here you have a permanent stream of materialisations before your eyes, all of them occurring in the way of assimilation, ie. of a spreading entelechial control.[78]

One needed only to assume, according to Driesch, that some people possessed the ability, consciously or unconsciously, to harness the vitalistic force and to externalise their ideas and memories in material form. Connected to the medium by an ectoplasmic umbilicus this material could quickly be re-absorbed back into the medium's body leaving no trace. In this regard he wrote:

> Thus, whenever there is a physical phenomenon occurring in connection with the body of a particular paraphysically endowed individual... we should assume that the unconscious mental part of that individual has the capacity in his purposive action on matter to extend this action beyond its normal range to the extent of as much as several yards, but always in connection with the body. Materialisation would then be organised assimilation in an extended field. In fact, normal organisatory and constructive assimilation as it appears, for instance, in regeneration, would have to be amplified only in regard to its effects.... Materialisation would at the same time be a supernormal embryology.[79]

For those who had rejected the spiritualist hypothesis, which interpreted materialisations as the spirits of the dead, Driesch's theory was attractive. While the sudden appearance and disappearance of ectoplasmic protrusions might seem fantastic, those with an interest in the physical phenomena of mediumship were quick to note that they had analogies in a range of well-established biological events.

In a series of posthumously published articles entitled 'Die Entwicklung des Okkultismus zur Parapsychologie in Deutschland' ['The Development of Occultism into Parapsychology in Germany'] (1932), Schrenck-Notzing indicated the widespread acceptance that the vitalistic philosophy of Driesch had achieved within the German parapsychological community by the mid-1920s, particularly as it pertained to the question of physical mediumship.[80] The Munich-based zoologist Karl Gruber (1881–1927), for instance, had attempted during the twenties to prove that a relationship existed between occult phenomena and certain natural but purposive events within the realm of biology.[81] Schrenck-Notzing's work at this time also demonstrated a familiarity with Driesch's vitalistic theories and a strong conviction that the phenomena of materialisation were of psycho-biological origin. He wrote in this regard, 'it seems certain primitive processes from the field of biology provide important contributions to the explanation of mediumistic materialisation problems.'[82] Utilising Driesch's entelechy and the 'supra-normal physiology' of the French biologist Gustave Geley (1868–1924), whose ideas were similar to those of Driesch,[83] Gruber, Schrenck-Notzing and others argued that the mediumistic materialisation of limbs, heads and amorphous forms was analogous to well-established biological phenomena, including the regeneration of limbs in certain organisms and the projection and retraction of pseudopodium from the cells of protozoa.

The dominance of biological theories and the influence of Driesch's vitalism within the parapsychological community were also evident to the casual observer. Annie Francé-Harrar (b.1886) noted in her autobiography that her experiences with the medium Eva C. had convinced her that occult phenomena belonged to the field of biology.[84] This belief was confirmed for her not only by reading Rhine, Jung and Driesch, but also by the microscopic analysis of a piece of ectoplasm obtained by her husband during a séance. This porous, dry substance, the cells of which were larger than those usually produced by humans, was, in Francé-Harrar's opinion, undoubtedly from a living body.[85] Thomas Mann was also of the opinion that the occult phenomena he had witnessed in Schrenck-Notzing's laboratory were of organic origin. He informed his host:

> There can be no question of a swindle in any mechanical sense. Here we are dealing with the occult jugglery of organic life, with processes whose

abnormal reality strikes me as unquestionable, with intricate constellations deep down in man.... Today when matter has been understood to be a form or, one might say, another aggregate state of energy, there would seem to be nothing very fantastic about an ephemeral materialisation of energy outside the medium's organism, about psycho-physical telepathy.[86]

The link established not only within the parapsychological community, but also within the public mind between parapsychology and biology, the discourse of which had by the early twentieth century permeated German social, cultural and political life, ensured that parapsychology, like biology, would be of import beyond the laboratory.

The use both of Driesch's vitalism, which had helped foster epistemological change within the life and mind sciences, and of analogy between supernatural and natural events, allowed those within the parapsychological community to understand their work on a continuum with established sciences such as biology and psychology, and to imagine their enterprise as the establishment of a new holistic science with implications for all realms of human endeavour. During the 1930s, as Germany's political climate became increasingly nationalistic and anti-Semitic, Driesch himself came to understand his super-normal biology as scientific proof that the aggressive and racist policies of the National Socialists should be abandoned and pacifism and cosmopolitanism embraced. Driesch, whose political convictions led to his dismissal from the University of Leipzig in 1933, had long been dedicated to both pacifism and cosmopolitanism. In his autobiography he noted, 'From my youth I had been a cosmopolitan and a pacifist. War in general seemed to me to be humanity's greatest disaster, but this war [the First World War] seemed absolute craziness'.[87] Following the First World War, Driesch travelled throughout China and Japan in the hope of re-establishing relations between German and Asian intellectuals.[88] Convinced that all races were related, Driesch argued that the study of other cultures would reveal universal laws and promote both understanding and peace.[89] In order to validate these convictions scientifically, however, Driesch needed to extend the findings of his 1891 sea urchin egg experiments to both metaphysics and international relations.

Driesch had succeeded in the course of his brief career in embryology in creating many organisms from material that under normal circumstances should have provided one – i.e., he produced clones – and one organism from material which normally should have provided two – i.e., he enabled one organism to absorb and subsume another. This demonstrated, in Driesch's mind at least, not only the simultaneous individuality and multiplicity of organic life, but that the *One* was the basis of all life. He wrote:

> It is a well founded metaphysical hypothesis that all Egos and minds and entelechies are ultimately *one*... though this One may under certain circumstances appear as *the many*. Let me only mention some of the results of my own former embryological work: One egg may give two or four organisms a*nd souls*, if only you separate the blastomeres; and two eggs may give one organism and *one soul.* Can souls divide and unite? Would it not be more adequate to say that Oneness and Manyness in these cases depend on material conditions and have both their last root in The One?[90]

Driesch used this argument as the basis of his theory of telepathy, hypothesising each individual's connection to a non-spatial framework of souls, and as the foundation of his belief that the state, as conceived of by the National Socialists, possessed no super-personal entelechy and therefore was not an organism.[91] He argued:

> The fact that mankind can create states qualifies it to be in a certain sense a *single* 'organism'; however the empirical *individual* states are, in their logical essence, much more like [inorganic] rocks than like some special construction in the context of the organic world.[92]

This was an explicit rejection of the Nazi holists' contention that each racial group constituted a *Volk*, which was not only biologically distinctive from all others, but also antagonistic to them.[93] According to Driesch, the only biological whole to which one could belong was humanity.[94]

Driesch's transference of his scientific and political convictions into the realm of parapsychology provided him with the opportunity to speak publicly about his disenchantment with the dominance of a mechanistic and positivistic epistemology within the natural sciences and the ascendancy of fascism in public life. Driesch's use of parapsychology as a form of critique and as a basis for scientific progress and philosophical renewal was not however unique, a number of well-known and respected European scholars also conceived of parapsychology as a form of oppositional or reformist politics. The Nobel Prize-winning physiologist Charles Richet, for example, also touted parapsychology as a basis for pacifism. Driesch noted in his autobiography that Richet had given a talk at the Paris International Congress for Parapsychology in 1928:

> [I]n which he pointed to the *weltanschauliche* significance of psychical research, and expressed his great trust in its future; he then turned to general questions, professed himself a committed pacifist, and attributed a great role specifically to Parapsychology in maintaining peace between nations. Each

time he closed with the words 'the future is in our hands'. After consulting with my German colleagues, I took it upon myself to reply; I professed my complete accord with everything that Richet had said, and closed with the same confident words that he had used.[95]

In his report on this Congress, which appeared in the journal *Unterhaltung und Wissen* [*Conversation and Knowledge*], Driesch echoed Richet. The article concluded by describing a dinner held at a Parisian hotel during which it became apparent to him that parapsychology was not just of theoretical significance, but meaningful also in terms of worldview and ethics. The power of the greatest science to bind peoples together and to reconcile them, Driesch wrote, was apparent on this evening more than any other.[96]

Driesch's efforts at promoting parapsychology, particularly after 1933 when he lost his position at the University of Leipzig because of his pacifism, were not a retreat from scientific or political life, but an engagement with them in a language that allowed him to be publicly, if somewhat covertly, critical of the Nazi regime.[97] This freedom did not last long, however. In 1935, the National Socialist government forbade Driesch and his wife from travelling and from giving public talks both within and outside Germany.[98] Despite this, Driesch remained a focus for parapsychological research in Germany and, as the letters that fill his *Nachlaß* demonstrate, a mentor to younger researchers. It is here also among these letters that one finds an indication of the Nazi attitude towards parapsychology.

Responses to parapsychology

In a letter to Driesch, dated 4 April 1938, Walther Kröner, a homeopath and parapsychologist, informed his addressee that he had been in discussions with a member of the Propaganda Ministry about the possibility of a state-sanctioned parapsychological research group.[99] Kröner stressed that this group would enjoy official protection as well as freedom in both scientific research and publication, but was to remain secret until the public could be presented with convincing results.[100] He encouraged Driesch to add his name to this project, warning that if parapsychologists did not take this opportunity to show what they were capable of, the border sciences might find themselves subject to a general ban.[101] This letter reflected not only Kröner's fear that parapsychology, like occultism, might be outlawed but the ambivalence of the Nazis towards parapsychology, which some regarded as useful but others found ideologically suspect. The ambivalent response of the National Socialists to parapsychology needs to be understood both in the context of their attitude to occultism and as a continuation of previous governments' policies. For this reason it is necessary to explore the stance of successive Weimar governments on occultism and to discuss the attitudes towards both occultism and parapsychology harboured by the medical and religious groups that informed their policy-making decisions before considering the Nazi response to these cultural phenomena.

The emergence in Germany during the late nineteenth century of modern occultism, a movement with scientific and philosophical ambitions as well as practical potential in fields such as medicine and law enforcement, quickly attracted the attention of both the local and national authorities. While the philosophising of men like du Prel, the quasi-religious rituals of spiritualists, and the tinctures, tonics and magnetic passes of occult healers may have seemed benign to many Germans, the authorities, including regional police commissioners and the Reich ministers for health and social welfare, quickly became convinced of occultism's dangers. It became apparent during the 1870s, for example, that the darkened séances attended by spiritualists acted as forums not only between the living and the dead but between the sexes and those with socialist tendencies, constituting a social, moral and political threat. Occult practitioners' claims to heal without recourse to invasive surgical procedures or expensive pharmaceuticals also caused official concern, the authorities perceiving a threat to both the public's health and its purse from lay healers. Police and legislators, prompted by concerned individuals and interest groups, were swift to appreciate both occultism's potential for social, political and financial disruption and the need for its containment. Their responses, although constantly evolving in order to deal with new species of occult practice and the ideological stances of successive governments on occultism, typically took the form of bans and prohibitions, most commonly those against public performances and the promotion and remuneration of occult services.

During the Weimar Republic, modern occultism elicited responses not only from the local authorities and the state but also from those groups that represented the interests of the medical profession and the churches. Occultism's infiltration of both the medical marketplace in the form of faith healing and magnetism, and the religious sphere in the guise of spiritualism and theosophy, created tension between occultists, who offered an alternative to established means of physic and salvation, and those groups, including doctors and ministers, who wished to maintain their monopoly in these areas. These two groups were instrumental in helping shape the state's and public's responses to occultism. The medical community, for example, focused its efforts throughout the Weimar period on those lay practitioners who purported to heal by occult means or who utilised techniques, including hypnosis and suggestion, that doctors were eager to appropriate for themselves. The medical community's campaign against occultists and lay hypnotists was conducted in books, pamphlets, newspapers and petitions, which argued the danger to public health and liquidity posed by occult medicine and the necessity of legislation against it. Protestant and Catholic responses to occultism, in contrast, placed less emphasis on legal measures, preferring to remind their parishioners of the mortal danger in which spirit conjuring and magic placed their souls. Occult practices with religious pretensions, such as spiritualism, were combated by both denominations in books, pamphlets and church newspapers as errors, temptations and sins, which the Protestant and Catholic faithful must resist at all costs. Just as physical health and financial solvency were at stake in the practice of occult medicine, according to vocal opponents of occultism within the medical community, so was spiritual and moral health at risk in the séance room, in the view of the Protestant and Catholic churches.

While the medical profession and the churches maintained a consistently hostile stance towards those forms of lay occultism that were conducted for financial gain or that in some way threatened the monopoly they enjoyed over the body or the soul, their attitude towards the scientific study or use of occultism remained open, as did that of the state. Differentiating between vulgar occultism, that species of occult practice conducted for profit by uneducated people, and parapsychology, the purview of an educated élite experimenting as a means of intellectual or philosophical fulfilment, the state, medical profession and the churches allowed parapsychologists, by means of exceptions within the relevant legislation, to work largely unmolested by the police. The justification for this stance was the belief that such experiments were of both scientific value and practical potential. This approach ensured a share in the spoils should the phenomena of mediumship prove of practical or theoretical significance. It acknowledged also that occultism had been the source of important discoveries, such as hypnosis and suggestion, in the past and might prove useful to medicine, religion and the state in the future. If, for example, clairvoyant powers could be harnessed to detect criminals and locate missing persons, or divining used to accurately predict the presence of water, metals and minerals, the benefit to law enforcement, mining and town planning would be enormous. The tolerance exhibited by the medical community, the churches and the government towards parapsychology, apparent in those pieces of legislation that allowed for occult demonstrations as long as they were of scientific merit, not only contrasted with, but undermined their efforts to control lay occultism. Lay occultists took advantage of the ambiguity surrounding concepts such as scientific merit and educational value, advertising their performances as scientific demonstrations and relocating them to private venues, strategies that made it difficult, if not impossible, for the authorities to root out occultism in its popular form.

The medical community's response

During the Weimar Republic, a concerted effort was made on the part of the German state to control the practice of lay occultism. While these measures pertained chiefly to that species of occultism carried out for profit or in public, attempts were also made to outlaw occult practices in private and domestic spaces. The growing number of occult practitioners touting their services in the wake of the war and the expansion of the market for these alternatives to healthcare and spiritual solace, were viewed by the medical profession and the churches as problems in dire need of solution.

During the 1920s, the German government made repeated attempts, often under intense pressure from medical interest groups, to restrict the practice and performance of hypnotism and occultism in both public and private, a goal that had proved elusive during the 1880s and 1890s, at which time medical hypnotists had campaigned vigorously to gain a medical monopoly over hypnosis and suggestion. In 1925, the Preußische Ministerium für Volkswohlfahrt [Prussian Minister for Social Welfare] proposed the reconstitution of a bill prohibiting the application of hypnosis by 'nicht approbierte Personen' [persons without medical qualifications], in order to stamp out those instances of public hypnosis that masqueraded either as 'talks' or private performances.[102] The restrictions on such events suggested by the minister were greeted with enthusiasm by government and medical advisors at the local level, who demanded that:

> All public or professional and all private exhibitions of hypnosis, suggestion, magnetism, occultism, muscle reading and similar themes [should be] forbidden, so long as they are not of scientific worth and are not approved of by the local police authorities.[103]

The rationale behind such demands was the threat posed by hypnotism and occultism to the public's physical and psychological well-being, a threat considered so serious that the government attempted to ban even the cinematic representation of hypnosis, the fear being that audiences might succumb to an irresistible hypnotic influence.[104] This concern for public health was reiterated by a number of medical pressure groups, including the Deutsche Gesellschaft zur Bekämpfung des Kurpfuschertums [German Society for the Combatting of Quackery] and the Deutscher Ärztevereinsbund [German Doctors' Organisation], both of which campaigned vigorously throughout the 1920s and 1930s for more comprehensive legal measures against occult practitioners, particularly those who infringed in some way on the medical profession's monopoly on health care.[105]

In April 1922, the German Doctors' Organisation informed the Prussian Minister for Social Welfare of their concern that as yet there existed no law or ministerial decree in Germany or Prussia prohibiting the application of hypnosis by those without medical qualifications.[106] Arguing that the therapeutic application of hypnosis required both an accurate diagnosis of the patient's condition and a careful assessment of the appropriateness of hypnotic treatment in their case, they pronounced as ridiculous the contention that hypnosis could be safely and beneficially utilised by amateurs. Any such equality between doctors and lay people in this area, they argued, would undermine the professional and social standing of doctors.[107] In a similar manner, the German Society for the Combatting of Quackery expressed their concern about the threat that hypnotists and occultists posed for a medical monopoly on healthcare. In a letter to the Innenminister [Minister for the Interior], dated November 1924, this group pressed for legislation in which the advertisement of so-called miracle pills, balms and treatments would become illegal.[108] The campaigns of both organisations against occult practitioners betrayed a deep-seated anxiety on the part of the medical community about the integrity of their jurisdictional claim over medicine, an anxiety that manifested itself in rhetoric about occultism's physical, mental and social dangers.

Most medical commentators identified the contemporary interest in occultism with a tendency towards mysticism that, they believed, had reached epidemic proportions at all levels of society since the war. Worryingly, they argued, occult phenomena such as spiritualism were all too often a front for other forms of quackery, including abortion and lay healing.[109] The danger that hypnosis represented for the community – as a form of both lay therapeutics and occult entertainment – was portrayed by medical practitioners largely in psychological and social terms. It was believed, for example, that in those with a predisposition, particularly women, the application of hypnosis might not only adversely affect the nervous system, but also encourage in the patient a dangerous mental and sexual uninhibitedness, with dire social consequences.[110] A fear existed also that the unrestrained and unmonitored use of hypnosis by lay people would lead to an occult crime wave in which large numbers of Caligari-like figures would compel their unwitting somnambulists to commit offences of every kind. An official in Breslau, for example, cited a case in which a twenty-year-old man charged with breaking and entering claimed to have been hypnotised by an unknown assailant who, by means of post-hypnotic suggestion, had persuaded him to commit the crime.[111] The criminal misuse of hypnosis was considered a danger in another area also, that of sexual assault. This had been a concern since the turn of the century and was one of the most compelling reasons for legislation against the use of hypnosis by people without medical qualifications. The trope of crime and suggestion, which had developed within medico-legal discourse, on the basis of a series of hypnotic crimes simulated by members of the Nancy school, and which had been appropriated by popular culture, featured in a series of Weimar films including Robert Wiene's *Das Cabinet des Dr Caligari* [*The Cabinet of Dr. Caligari*] (1919), Arthur Robinson's *Schatten: Eine nachtliche Halluzination* [*Shadows: A Nocturnal Hallucination*, also known in English as *Warning Shadows*] (1922) and Fritz Lang's *Dr Mabuse, der Spieler* [*Dr Mabuse, the Gambler*] (1922).[112] The association these films fostered in the public mind between hypnosis and crime helped reinforce doctors' claims that they were the only group capable of safely applying this technique, and provided criminals, such as the aforementioned Breslau burglar, with an excuse for their societal trespasses.

While that species of lay occultism with pretensions to healing power was rejected by physicians, some medical practitioners showed themselves willing to investigate paranormal phenomena scientifically. The audience for Schrenck-Notzing's experiments had always contained a high percentage of doctors and the Berliner Gesellschaft für Experimental-Psychologie also attracted its fair share of physicians during the late nineteenth century. There were a number of societies founded during the inter-war period, however, that made the interest of the medical community in parapsychology explicit. During the early 1920s, the Ärztliche Verein München [Munich Medical Club], for example, formed an Ärztekommission für Okkultismus [Medical Commission for Occultism], which held seminars on the physical phenomena of mediumship and discussions of parapsychological literature.[113] In 1922, an Ärztliche Gesellschaft für parapsychologische Forschung [Medical Society for Parapsychological Research] was founded in Berlin by the psychiatrist Paul Sünner, who at that time also edited the *Psychische Studien*. With around one hundred members, many of whom were psychiatrists and neurologists, this society dedicated itself to telepathic experiments as well as explorations of telekinesis and materialisation. This demonstrated doctors' differing attitudes to occultism on the one hand and parapsychology on the other, an ambivalence that was reflected in those pieces of legislation that allowed for so-called scientific demonstrations of occultism.

The response of the churches

The official response to occultism was shaped not only by the medical profession, but also by representatives of Germany's Protestant and Catholic communities, who recognised in the spiritualist séances of the late nineteenth century and in the occult wave that followed the war, a challenge to their monopoly on both spiritual solace and pastoral care. Spiritualism claimed to offer believers experimental proof of an afterlife and to reunite them with departed friends and relatives, providing great reassurance to those Germans suffering personal loss in the wake of the war. Like other forms of occultism with religious pretensions, spiritualism's promotion of an unmediated knowledge of the spiritual realm and its organisational structure, often a rejection of the hierarchies found in Protestant and Catholic churches, offered an implicit criticism of organised religion's ability to meet people's spiritual and pastoral needs. In this context, occultists and, in particular, spiritualists were viewed as competitors by the representatives of organised religion, who could ill afford to lose parishioners given the ever increasing numbers of Germans abandoning their churches and their faith.[114] The response of both denominations to occultism was overwhelmingly negative, their understanding of spiritualism, fortune telling and card reading derived from a paradigm in which conjuring and magic, in which categories these phenomena were placed, were regarded as sins or satanic temptations.

Within the Protestant community the occult threat was monitored by a group known as the Apologetische Centrale [Centre for Apologetics] (1921–37), which collected information on sects and occult groups in Germany and publicised the Church's stance on modern occultism.[115] This group argued, in a large number of articles and pamphlets, that those forms of occultism with religious pretensions, including spiritualism with its attempts to contact the dead in order to establish the immortality of the soul, posed a spiritual, physical and mental threat to Christians.[116] Eager not only to establish the reason for the German public's interest in the occult, but also to suggest solutions to this problem, the Apologetische Centrale argued that superstitions, beliefs ranging from spiritualism to astrology, were the result of materialism, curiosity, fear, and ignorance.[117] In the thousands of Germans who flocked to consult fortune tellers, card readers and spiritual healers, the Apologetische Centrale recognised a desire to secure personal health and fortune, a morbid curiosity about the future, a fear of death and a profound ignorance of both the causes and consequences of superstition. Protestant commentators argued that manifestations of the occult wave, including astrology, amulets, fortune telling, theosophy, spiritualism and psychography, were atavistic cultural tendencies, which had their roots in the social, financial and spiritual uncertainty brought about by the war. Those wishing to free themselves from the power of such superstitions, they argued, must acknowledge them as a sin, that is, as nothing less than an insult to the majesty of God.[118]

While many spiritualists believed their faith to be compatible with, if not complementary to, Christianity, Protestant thinkers made it clear that this belief was erroneous in the eyes of the Church. Asking what it was that spiritualism wished to achieve, Friedrich Walcher answered that it sought to mediate congress with the spirits of the dead, providing proof by means of this interaction of the immortality of the soul, and functioning as a support for disintegrating belief in both the Bible and Church doctrine.[119] The Protestant Church, however, believed the spiritualist project, which attempted to provide the living with definitive proof about the fate of their departed friends and relatives, to be implicated in this process of disintegration. Not only, they argued, had Jesus made clear that discourse with the dead was impossible, but that it was unnecessary given his sacrifice, a sacrifice that vouchsafed immortality for believers. Christianity, predicated on this belief, required a leap of faith not scientific proof. Participation in spiritualist gatherings indicated a lack of faith and a desire, despite God's prohibitions, to tear down the veil he had erected to obscure the nature of the after-life.[120] The church's exhortation to leave the mysteries surrounding death intact was an attack on a competitor and on the scientific impulse, that helped inform spiritualism, an impulse that it saw as steadily undermining Germans' faith in religion and the answers it offered.

The social consequences of the public's fascination with occultism were also of particular concern to Protestant writers who claimed that the incidence of 'Sittlichkeitsverbrechen' [crimes against morality] including murder, suicide and the disintegration of family groups, were demonstrably related to the contemporary mania for magic and superstition.[121] These social calamities, according to one author, had their origin in the physical changes brought about by the practice of spiritualism, hypnosis and fortune telling, that is, paralysis of the inner and outer organs leading to pressure around the heart, blurred eyes, loss of peace, suicidal thoughts and neuroses.[122] Neglect of these symptoms and the continued reliance of Germans on magicians and occultists rather than on God would, he argued, lead to social and cultural catastrophe.[123] In order to protect the public from this threat, groups within the Church, including the Women's Association of the Berlin Women's Conference [Die Frauenverbände der Berliner Frauenkonferenz], petitioned the government to include within existing legislation on fortune-telling – §263 Strafgesetzbuch or StGB [criminal code] – a clause, that would ensure the punishment of those occultists who accepted payment for their prognostications.[124] Conscious of the spiritual crisis experienced by Germans in the wake of the war and the public's desire for some contact with or confirmation from those family members who had perished in the fighting, the Protestant authorities claimed both to comprehend and sympathise with their parishioners' interest in occultism, but felt compelled to remind them that true solace could only be found in the teachings of the Church.

The Catholic authorities, like their Protestant counterparts, denounced both occultism and spiritualism as false religions, forbidding their

215

parishioners, by means of a holy ordinance dated 24 April 1917, from participating in spiritualist séances.[125] Spiritualism, they claimed, strove to be a religion based on a set of new revelations, derived from dialogue with the spirits of the dead, that were antithetical to those of the Catholic faith.[126] These teachings posed a danger to the spiritual well being of Catholics, not least because, according to many commentators, they were of diabolical origin. In harmony with those folk beliefs that continued to persist in parts of rural Germany, Dr H. Malfatti, a professor at the University of Innsbruck, wrote of his conviction that Satan was responsible for paraphysical phenomena, including apparitions, telekinesis and materialisation.[127] In a similar manner, J. Goddfrey Raupert, in a work entitled *Die Geister des Spiritismus, Erfahrungen und Beweise* [*The Ghosts of Spiritualism, Experiences and Proof*], stated his belief that diabolical influences might be at work within the spiritualist milieu. For this reason, he argued, a satisfactory explanation for spiritualism should be a priority for both the church and the scientific community.[128] Such interpretations derived from Catholic doctrine, which forbade conjuring and communication with the spirits of the dead because of the risk of satanic interference.

Catholic concern about spiritualism was not, however, limited to the spiritual pollution attendant upon occultism, but included the moral and physical corruption promoted by darkened spiritualist sittings in which men and women came together to experience the scandalous discourse of ghosts and the immoral behaviour of materialised forms.[129] The close physical proximity of the sexes during spiritualist performances, actively encouraged in the form of hand-holding, and the overtly sexual nature of mediumistic phenomena, often mimicking intercourse or childbirth, were morally and socially dangerous according to the Catholic Church, who forbade their parishioners from attending such gatherings. Furthermore, the Church, mobilising the pathology metaphor, argued that spiritualist experiments were damaging to both physical and mental health, citing as evidence the high incidence of neuroses among both mediums and séance participants.[130] Many mediums, they contended, went mad as a result of their spiritualist activities, their nerves shattering due to the strain, while the over-excitement promoted by séances, they argued, had an adverse effect on the nervous systems of participants. While the Catholic Church continued to prohibit practising Catholics from participating in spiritualist sittings, they argued, as did the Protestant Church, that in spite of such restrictions their parishioners might legitimately take a scientific interest in occult problems.[131]

Although both medical and church groups campaigned vigorously against lay occultism during the Weimar Republic, there remained a certain ambivalence in their attitude towards the occult sciences. There was an implication in their demands, which asked that occult practices be outlawed as long as they were not of scientific worth, that an experimental occultism might be of both philosophical and practical significance. In the medical context, as we have seen in Chapters 2 and 3, doctors expressed considerable interest in both the psychotherapeutic benefits of hypnosis and the insight into both the unconscious and the physical world that experimentation with mediums promised. Indeed, medical professionals argued that they, more than any other group, were best equipped to study such phenomena. Their campaign against occultism, like that of the Protestant and Catholic churches, was based on the threat that occult practitioners posed to their jurisdictional monopoly and to their claims of competence in a field with the potential to be both socially important and financially lucrative.

Those with religious objections to spiritualism and lay occultism did not acknowledge a conflict of interest in the scientific study of the paranormal, claiming that in the spiritual struggle over the 'last questions', parapsychology would act as religion's assistant and ally.[132] Reinhold Michaelis, for example, argued that, while parapsychology could not and should not form the basis of an ethics or religion, its exploration of the soul's hidden depths was of profound *weltanschauliche* significance.[133] Divorcing the study of occultism from the spiritualist hypothesis, religious commentators defined parapsychology as the scientific investigation of abnormal psychical and physical phenomena. The explanation for such occult manifestations, they argued, would be found in the natural rather than spiritual realm. Linking parapsychology to a range of psychological, biological and vitalistic theories they maintained that parapsychology's confinement to observing and describing occult phenomena in naturalistic terms would ensure that it never came into conflict with the teachings of the Church.[134] Josef Dörfler put this most succinctly when he wrote:

> If scientific occultism with its animistic–vitalistic interpretation of mediumistic facts stays within its bounds and sees its tasks as the observation, description and natural explanation of phenomena, without thereby getting into pantheistic ground or above all the field of religion, it will never really be able to come into contradiction with church doctrine. Against occultism as a science the church therefore has no objection.[135]

Clearly in the eyes of Germany's churchmen, parapsychology belonged to a different sphere, but one potentially significant for religion.

The churches' acceptance of parapsychology as different from the occult sciences, proved that the parapsychologists' campaign to demarcate and sanitise their discipline was at least partially successful. Further evidence of this was provided by the belief not only that parapsychology had no religious pretensions, but that it represented an antidote to spiritualism and superstition. Borrowing from contemporary parapsychological theory, Friedrich Walcher, whose book on spiritualism was published by the Evangelische Volksbund [Protestant People's League], argued that so-called spiritualist phenomena were products of the unconscious and deliberate fraud, rather than spirits.[136] Another author, convinced that spiritualism had put itself into competition with Christianity, cited studies by critical occultists including Alfred Lehmann and Max Dessoir as evidence of the fraudulent behaviour of spiritualist mediums.[137] Catholics were no less enthusiastic about parapsychology's potential to eradicate the spiritualist threat than were their Protestant brethren. The Catholic minister G. Bichlmair, for example, in a book entitled *Okkultismus und Seelensorge* [*Occultism and Spiritual Welfare*] (1926) argued, 'the more widespread the pursuit of serious parapsychical research becomes, the more religio-ethical occultism comes into discredit....'[138] In a similar manner, Josef Dörfler, in an article on Catholic attitudes towards occultism, wrote of his conviction that the animistic–vitalistic hypotheses of parapsychologists would prove that occult phenomena hailed not from beyond the border with death, but from beyond the border of the senses, that is, from the unconscious.[139] The churches' embrace of parapsychology and its naturalistic interpretation of occult phenomena enabled their battle against spiritualism to be conducted on a scientific as well as spiritual, moral and social front.

The theories and techniques used to demystify occult phenomena and intended to quash both spiritualists' and lay occultists' claims to religious or scientific expertise were also utilised by those churchmen whose investment in a scientific worldview made them uncomfortable with the miracles upon which Christian faith was founded. Parapsychology's potential to help explain phenomena such as the resurrection or stigmata without recourse to accusations of fraud or allegory made it attractive to members of both the Catholic and Protestant churches, but featured more prominently among Protestant churchmen who had demonstrated a willingness, as early as the Bismarckian and Wilhelmine periods, to adapt the beliefs of the Church to fashions in scientific speculation.[140] While some theologians continued to argue that the saints had performed their miracles independent of the natural or vitalistic forces responsible for occult phenomena, there remained many for whom a naturalistic explanation sat more comfortably than a miraculous one. The resurrection, according to Dr Richard Hoffmann, a professor of Protestant theology at the University of Vienna, could be explained by recourse to the theory of materialisation. Hoffmann found the analogy between Christ's appearance before his disciples and that of mediumistic materialisation a compelling one.[141] Analysing the miracles of the New Testament, Dr Hans Rust, professor of theology at the University of Königsberg, argued for a psychology of religion, believing that many of these events including the resurrection could be explained in terms of hallucination and illusion.[142] While such reinterpretations may have helped quell embarrassment over miracles and their similarity to the spiritualist nonsense the churches were eager to eradicate, they also threatened to dilute religion to the extent that it would become a set of ethical rules, rather than divinely ordained law.[143]

The National Socialist response

Although occultists increasingly faced prosecution for offences such as fraud, assault and bodily harm during the Weimar Republic, parapsychologists tended to remain unscathed by governmental, medical and religious attempts to criminalise or ban occultism, their knowledge and expertise even finding practical applications in fields such as criminology, psychology and geology. In the eyes of Weimar officials, the dangers posed by occultism were of a medical, moral and financial nature, areas in which parapsychology appeared benign. While the spiritual and ideological aspects of occult practices may have been of intense concern to the churches, the state was not motivated to legislate against them for these reasons. The Nazi take-over in 1933, however, altered this situation, the party viewing occultism's dangers in medical, moral, financial and ideological terms, its message of universal brotherhood in direct conflict with the *völkisch* nationalism preached by National Socialism. In this context, parapsychology, which increasingly saw itself not only as an important new science, but as a harbinger of peace, also became subject to state interference.

The 1930s witnessed the introduction of increasingly restrictive legislation against occultists. In 1934, Saxony outlawed the remuneration of fortune telling, its performance in public, and the sale of written material relating to card reading, horoscopes, and dream interpretation.[144] Prussia and Baden followed suit in the second half of the same year.[145] In July 1936, the Regierungspräsident in Hannover [Prime Minister of Hanover] released a police ordinance prohibiting the practice of fortune telling, but allowing for the publication and sale of printed material that took a scientific or cultural–historical approach to the subject.[146] As the decade progressed, however, the National Socialist government took an increasingly hostile stance on occultism in all its forms. A number of talks hosted by the NSD Aerztebund [National Socialist Doctors' Organisation], for example, labelled occultism a 'Volksgefahr' [public hazard] and stressed the need to protect the population, whose susceptibility to such phenomena was heightened by economic crisis, from such morally and politically dangerous forces.[147] Albert Hellwig, who spoke before the NSD Aerztebund in Leipzig during March 1938, expressed similar opinions about the moral, social and economic dangers of occultism, focusing on this occasion on the relationship between quackery and the occult sciences.[148]

While there was some sympathy for occult belief among high-ranking members of the Nazi regime, including Heinrich Himmler (1900–45) and Rudolf Hess (1894–1987), there is little proof that this fascination with the occult affected their decisions or that it provided the motivation for their racist policies.[149] Such sympathies were certainly not widespread, most prominent figures within the regime regarding occultism as an ideological threat. In the course of 1937, this negative stance on occult practice became official when the National Socialist government issued a decree for the protection of the people and the state, which dissolved occult, theosophical and psychical research groups, effectively outlawing occultism.[150] The Nazis' long-held hostility towards occult practice, as a medical, psychological and ideological danger to the German *Volk*, now became manifest not only in official and legal discourse, but also in physical intimidation and arrest. Large numbers of occultists were imprisoned by the Gestapo during the early 1940s, for example, as part of a campaign known as 'Aktion Hess' ['Action Hess'].[151]

Given their approach to occultism, how did the National Socialists respond to parapsychology? While occultists found that laws against fortune telling, card reading and faith healing were swiftly systematised under the Nazis, parapsychologists continued for a long period to remain outside the purview of the law. The National Socialists, like their predecessors, were tolerant of the scientific study of mediumship because it posed no apparent financial or medical threat. They were also loath to dismiss it before they had ascertained whether parapsychology might be of practical or scientific significance to them. This difference between their attitude to occultism and their stance on parapsychology was reflected not only in legal measures, which continued for some time to allow for occult demonstrations and books of a scientific character, but also in the press. Newspapers, which in this period featured articles expounding the dangers of occultism, reported on parapsychological research in a more positive manner. In a letter to Hans Driesch, dated 11 July 1935, for example, Hans Bender wrote that an article with the somewhat exaggerated title of 'The First Clairvoyance Experiments at a German University' had appeared in the *Berliner Zeitung am Morgen* [*Berlin Morning Newspaper*] providing details of his experiments in clairvoyance at the University of Bonn and causing a veritable storm of interest in such research on the part of the press.[152] Newspapers in Bonn, Cologne and Berlin were eager to carry the story, as was the Nazi newspaper, *Völkischer Beobachter* [*National Observer*], that had asked Bender to write them an article.[153]

There is some indication that the National Socialists may have considered sponsoring parapsychological research out of public funds. As Kröner's letters to Driesch indicate, an official within the Propaganda Ministry, one Dr Kittler, head of the Referat Kosmobiologie [Cosmobiology Department], was eager to found a parapsychological study-group, the membership of which would consist of around one hundred of Germany's most prominent parapsychologists, including, it was hoped twenty to thirty university professors.[154] In January 1939, Kröner informed Driesch that preparations had been made to invite the following parapsychologists to join this group: in Berlin, Dr Reismann and Dr Fritsche; in Munich, Dr Tischner, Dr Gerda Walther (1897–1977), Dr Wüst and perhaps Dr Heyer; in Vienna, Professor Schweiger, Gräfin Wassilko (1879–1978) and after certain political difficulties had been cleared up Professor Thirring; as well as Dr Mattiesen and Dr Bender.[155] He concluded his letter by mentioning that he had spoken in Munich to Ernst Schulte-Strathaus, the cultural consultant in the 'Brown House' and an old friend of Schrenck-Notzing, who believed that this parapsychological working group would soon achieve official recognition and become an institute.[156] While there is no proof that this group was ever actually established, perhaps as a consequence of the war, it is not beyond the bounds of possibility that the Propaganda Ministry did seriously consider such a research group. Josef Goebbels (1897–1945), for example, while an opponent of occultism, was interested in the manner in which astrological predictions about the course of the war might be used for propaganda purposes.[157] It seems possible that a group dedicated to parapsychological research might have served a similar purpose.

While the Nazis were more tolerant towards parapsychology than occultism, parapsychologists were not immune from mistreatment or persecution by the regime. Certainly that brand of parapsychology that eschewed experimentation in favour of philosophical speculation was an object of suspicion. A number of researchers of Jewish heritage or suspect political beliefs found themselves ejected from their public service positions in 1933 under the Gesetz zur Wiederherstellung des Berufsbeamtentums [Law for the Restoration of the Professional Civil Service]. Hans Driesch, for example, was forced to retire from the University of Leipzig, ostensibly because he did not possess the requisite educational background (§2 Abs. 1), but in reality for his pacifist beliefs, and T.K. Oesterreich lost his position at the University of Tübingen because his previous political activities made him politically unreliable (§4).[158] Discrimination of this kind was also not unheard of between parapsychologists and within parapsychological societies. In April 1938, for example, Gräfin Zoe Wassilko wrote to Driesch about the unification of the German and Austrian Parapsychological Congress committees. In this letter she stated, 'I myself have been a party member since 1935. Poor Winterstein is unfortunately not an Aryan, even in the best possible case he cannot remain the president of the society.'[159]

Increasingly, during the 1930s, German parapsychologists were prevented from attending international conferences. Some, including Driesch, were denied permission to travel or to give talks in both Germany and other countries because of their political beliefs, but others were prevented from attending conferences because of suggestions that such gatherings were hotbeds of Judaism, Bolshevism and Freemasonry.[160] While this was almost certainly overblown Nazi rhetoric, such congresses did appear to be forums in which pacifist and cosmopolitan ideas were expressed. Richet's and Driesch's exclamations about parapsychology as a foundation for peace and harmony between nations would certainly have been provocative in the German context. It was these aspects of parapsychology, rather than its experimental findings, that posed a threat to or conflicted with Nazi ideology and necessitated restrictions on certain parapsychologists.

Following the outbreak of war in 1939, parapsychologists, who had enjoyed some protection from prosecution and police harassment during the early years of the Nazi regime, also became targets of persecution. Gerda Walther, the former scientific secretary of Schrenck-Notzing, for example, was arrested and held by the Gestapo during the Rudolf Hess special action in June 1941 for her involvement in parapsychological research.[161] Her papers, books and manuscripts relating to occult matters were confiscated and destroyed. While Walther was released quickly, in her opinion because she spoke eight languages and could be usefully employed by the regime, others did not fare so well.[162] Johannes Maria Verweyen (1883–1945), a psychologist and philosopher who had become interested in the philosophical, religious and practical questions surrounding mediumship, died at the Bergen-Belsen concentration camp in 1945 as a result of typhus.[163] His arrest had not been a consequence of his parapsychological research *per se*, but of the ideological implications of his work, which in its emphasis on pacifism and anti-fascism competed with the ideological claims made by the Nazi State.

Conclusion

The death of Schrenck-Notzing in 1929 allowed for a change in focus among German parapsychologists during the 1930s. Abandoning their emphasis on experimentation, these researchers attempted to theorise mediumistic phenomena and to ascertain its meaning. The collapse of materialism under pressure from epistemological changes in the sciences and a resurgence of occult belief in the wake of the war created ideal conditions for this endeavour. In the work of Hans Driesch, in particular, the phenomena of mediumship became linked not only with biology but also once again with the project of establishing a new worldview, in which parapsychology would provide a foundation for pacifism and cosmopolitanism. While under successive Weimar governments parapsychology, in contrast to occultism, did not attract the attention of the police or form the focus of campaigns by the medical community or the churches, under the National Socialists this situation changed. Although there does appear to have been some interest on the part of the Nazis in exploring this nascent science's potential, its philosophical and ideological implications saw it, like occultism, subject to restrictions and bans by the end of the 1930s.

Notes

1. T.K. Oesterreich, 'Parapsychologie in Athen: Der internationale Kongress', *Das Unterhaltungsblatt*, 27 Mai 1930, in: Nachlaß T. K. Oesterreich, 399/10, UAT.
2. *Ibid.*
3. S.H. Mauskopf and M.R. McVaugh, *The Elusive Science* (Baltimore: Johns Hopkins University Press, 1980), 210.
4. Letter from Hans Bender to Hans Driesch, 15 April 1938. Nachlaß 250 Hans Driesch, UBL.
5. Letter from Walther Kröner to Hans Driesch, 4 April 1938. Nachlaß 250 Hans Driesch, UBL.
6. M. Oesterreich, *Traugott Konstantin Oesterreich: Ich-Forscher und Gottsucher: Lebenswerk und Lebensschicksal* (Stuttgart: Fr. Frommanns Verlag, 1954), 1–2.
7. T.K. Oesterreich, *Der Okkultismus im Modernen Weltbild*, 3rd edn (Dresden: Sibyllen-Verlag, 1923), 11–12.
8. *Ibid.,* 12–13.
9. 'Aberglaube – was steckt dahinter?' Hrsg. von der Apologetischen Zentrale, Berlin – Spandau., in: ADW, CA, AC-S 1 Aberglaube.
10. *Ibid.*
11. 'Eine neue, befreiende Weltanschauung', *Revalo-Bund,* in: ADW, CA, AC-S 334 Spiritismus.
12. U.F. Stolzenburg, 'Okkultismus', aus Schweitzer: Das religiöse Deutschland der Gegenwart. 1 Band: Der allgemein religiöse Kreis. Berlin: Hochweg Verlag, in: ADW, CA-S 272 Okkultismus; A. Moll, *Psychologie und Charakterologie der Okkultisten* (Stuttgart: Ferdinand Enke, 1929), 11.
13. Stolzenburg, *op. cit.* (note 12).
14. T.K. Oesterreich, 'Der Okkultismus und die Wissenschaft', *Die Umschau,* 22 (1922), 49–53.
15. Oesterreich, *op. cit.* (note 6).

16. T.K. Oesterreich, 'Entwurf', in: Nachlaß T. K. Oesterreich, 399/14, UAT.

17. T.K. Oesterreich, 'Zur Umgaltung der "Psychishen Studien" in eine "Zeitschrift für Parapsychologie"', in: Nachlaß T. K. Oesterreich, 399/10, UAT.

18. T.K. Oesterreich, 'Die deutsche Philosophie und das Ausland', *Forschungen und Fortschritte: Nachtrichtenblatt der Deutschen Wissenschaft und Technik,* 6, 4 (1930), 52, in: Nachlaß T.K. Oesterreich, 399/10, UAT.

19. *Ibid.*

20. *Ibid.*

21. Oesterreich, *op. cit.* (note 16)

22. *Ibid.*

23. *Ibid.*

24. Oesterreich, *op. cit.* (note 18)

25. Oesterreich, *op. cit.* (note 17)

26. Oesterreich, *op. cit.* (note 7).

27. *Ibid.,* 13–16.

28. T.K. Oesterreich, 'Die Bilanz des wissenschaftlichen Okkultismus', *Neue Presse,* 22 Dezember 1935, in: Nachlaß T. K. Oesterreich, 399/10, UAT.

29. F. Grunewald, *Physikalisch-mediumistische Untersuchungen* (Pfullingen i. Württemberg: Johannes Baum, 1920), 79.

30. *Ibid.,* 79–80.

31. *Ibid.,* 80.

32. *Ibid.*

33. *Ibid.,* 3.

34. A. Gregory, 'Anatomy of a Fraud: Harry Price and the Medium Rudi Schneider', *Annals of Science,* 34 (1977), 451.

35. Letter from A. von Schrenck-Notzing to H. Thirring, 30 November 1925, in: Korrespondenz 1, Nachlaß Albert von Schrenck-Notzing, IGPP.

36. Oesterreich, *op. cit.* (note 7), 16.

37. R. Baerwald, *Okkultismus und Spiritismus und ihre Weltanschauulichen Folgerungen* (Berlin: Deutsche Buchgemeinschaft, 1926), 346–7.

38. 'Die Zukunft, die Frage des Unterganges oder der Aufwärtsentwicklung der europäischen und amerikanischen Kultur hängt davon ab, ob der Mensch die Weltstruktur und seine Stellung in der Welt wieder mit anderen Augen ansehen lernt. Und ich wüsste nicht, was es für Tatsachen geben sollte, die eher dazu angetan sind, ihn dahin zu führen, als die mediumistischen Phänomene. Daher werden sie, wenn sie überhaupt weltanschauliche Ueberzeugungen imstande sind, einen tieferen Einfluss auf das Leben des Menschen und die Gesamtgestaltung und geistige Wiedergeburt der Welt liefern.' T.K. Oesterreich, 'Die Philosophische Bedeutung der mediumistischen Phaenomene', in: Nachlaß T.K. Oesterreich, 399/10, UAT.

39. T.K. Oesterreich, 'Wissenschaft und Mediumismus', in: Nachlaß T.K. Oesterreich, 399/10, UAT.

40. This section has been published in a slightly different form as: H. Wolffram, 'Supernormal Biology: Vitalism, Parapsychology and the German Crisis of Modernity, c. 1890-1933.' *The European Legacy*, 8 (2003), 149–63.

41. H. Driesch, 'Der Okkultismus als neue Wissenschaft', *Psychische Studien*, 50 (1923), 48–50. Driesch was by no means alone in singling out his experimental and theoretical work in biology as a causal factor in epistemological changes within the life sciences. See, for example, V. Mikuška, 'Hans Driesch als Biologe, Philosoph und Okkultist', *Psychische Studien*, 50 (1923), 41–6.

42. Driesch, *ibid.*, 51.

43. *Ibid.*, 52.

44. *Ibid.*, 47. Driesch reiterated this argument in an article that appeared in 1924 in the *Revue Metapsychique*. It was reprinted as H. Driesch, 'Die metapsychischen Phänomene in Rahmen der Biologie', *Psychische Studien*, 52 (1925), 1–14.

45. Driesch contended that at least four other intellectuals had come to the same conclusion about the cause of materialisation. See Driesch, *op. cit.* (note 41), 52; and Driesch, *ibid.*, 14.

46. Driesch notes in his autobiography that his interest in questions of the 'soul-life' dated from 1903. He adds that he first became a corresponding member of the English Society for Psychical Research in 1913. See, H. Driesch, *Lebenserinnerungen: Aufzeichnungen eines Forschers und Denkers in entscheidender Zeit* (Munich: Ernst Reinhardt, 1951), 201.

47. Biology's connection with progressive politics dated from at least the 1830s and 1840s when liberals used biology to prove the naturalness of their political beliefs and the artificiality of institutions such as the state and the Church. See F. Gregory, *Scientific Materialism in Nineteenth Century Germany* (Dordrecht: D. Reidel, 1977); K. Repp, *Reformers, Critics, and the Paths of German Modernity: Anti-Politics and the Search for Alternatives, 1890–1914* (Cambridge: Harvard University Press, 2000); K. Repp, '"More Corporeal, More Concrete": Liberal Humanism, Eugenics, and German Progressives at the Last Fin de Siecle', *The Journal of Modern History*, 72, 3 (2000), 690–3.

48. A. Harrington, *Reenchanted Science: Holism in German Culture from Wilhelm II to Hitler* (Princeton: Princeton University Press, 1996), 25–7.

49. On this change within embryology see M. de Issekutz Wolsky and A.A. Wolsky, 'Bergson's Vitalism in the Light of Modern Biology' in F. Burwick and P. Douglass (eds), *The Crisis in Modernism: Bergson and the Vitalist Controversy* (Cambridge: Cambridge University Press, 1992), 155.

50. Harrington, *op. cit.* (note 48), 48.

51. As Repp points out, however, there existed a stream of biological thought, represented most vividly by August Weismann, which maintained the mechanical nature of organic life. See Repp, 'More Corporeal', *op. cit.* (note 47), 698–700.
52. Wolsky and Wolsky, *op. cit.* (note 49), 155.
53. H. Driesch, *The Science and Philosophy of the Organism,* 2nd edn (London: A. & C. Black, 1929), 34–8.
54. *Ibid.,* 38–40.
55. *Ibid.,* 42–3.
56. Harrington, *op. cit.* (note 48), 50.
57. See H. Driesch, *Analytische Theorie der Organischen Entwicklung* (Leipzig: Wilhelm Engelmann, 1894).
58. F.B. Churchill, 'From Machine-Theory to Entelechy: Two Studies in Developmental Teleology', *History of Biology,* 2, 1 (1969), 171–2.
59. M.G. Ash, *Gestalt Psychology in German Culture, 1890–1967* (Cambridge: Cambridge University Press, 1998), 80.
60. H. Driesch, 'Presidential Address: Psychical Research and Established Science', *Proceedings of the Society for Psychical Research,* 36, 99 (1926), 173.
61. Ash, *op. cit.* (note 59), 81.
62. Elmar Gruber dates Driesch's interest in the publications of the Society for Psychical Research to as early as 1890. See, E. Gruber, 'Hans Driesch and the Concept of Spiritism', *Journal of the Society for Psychical Research,* 49 (1978), 862.
63. H. Driesch, 'Psychical Research and Philosophy' in C. Murchinson (ed.), *The Case For and Against Psychical Belief* (Worcester: Clark University, 1927), 171–2.
64. Driesch, *op. cit.* (note 60), 185–7.
65. Driesch, *op. cit.* (note 46), 152.
66. Gruber, *op. cit.* (note 62), 862.
67. Driesch, *op. cit.* (note 53), 335–6.
68. For an account of Eleanor Sidgwick's involvement with the Society for Psychical Research, see J. Oppenheim, *The Other World: Spiritualism and Psychical Research in England, 1850–1914* (Cambridge: Cambridge University Press, 1985), 120–1.
69. 'Die Bekanntschaft mit Mrs Sidgwick, einer klugen geistvollen Frau, wurde dadurch bedeutungsvoll für mich, daß sie mir jenen Gegenstand näher brachte, der in England Psychical Research, bei uns Parapsychologie… genannt wird, und von dem ich bisher nur wenig wußte, was mich allerdings stark beeindruckt hatte'. Driesch, *op. cit.* (note 46), 152–3.
70. H. Driesch, *Geschichte des Vitalismus* (Leipzig: Johann Ambrosius Barth, 1922), 178–80.

71. H. Bergson, *Mind-Energy: Lectures and Essays,* H. Wildon Carr (trans.), (New York: Henry Holt and Company, 1920), 88–9; 96–7.

72. *Ibid.,* 201.

73. Driesch, *op. cit.* (note 60), 180.

74. 'Zu den physischen Paraphänomenen stand ich skeptischer, obwohl ich 1922 bei Schrenck-Notzing einer Sitzung mit Willi Schneider beigewohnt hatte, die sehr eindrucksvoll gewesen war. Ich hatte keine Betrugsmöglichkeit gefunden… aber völlig genügend im Wissenschaftlichen Sinne waren die Versuchsbedingungen eben doch nicht gewesen'. Driesch, *op. cit.* (note 46), 202.

75. '[D]ie Sitzung mit Rudi hat mich mehr als alles, was ich bisher sah, von der Realität der physichen Phänomene überzeugt. Wiederholt habe ich das Geschehene bei mir überdacht: es ist da wirklich keine Lücke'. Letter from H. Driesch to A. von Schrenck-Notzing, dated 13 May 1928, quoted in A. von Schrenck-Notzing, *Die Phänomene des Mediums Rudi Schneider* (Berlin: Walter de Gruyter & Co., 1933), 119.

76. Driesch, *op. cit.* (note 60), 172. Elmar Gruber links Driesch's election as president of the Society for Psychical Research to his discussion of parapsychology in his *Grundprobleme der Psychologie,* translated into English in 1925 as *The Crisis of Psychology.* See, Gruber, *op. cit.* (note 62), 865.

77. Driesch stated here that 'we may call vitalism a bridge that leads to parapsychology'. Driesch, *op. cit.* (note 60), 175

78. *Ibid.,* 173.

79. H. Driesch, *Psychical Research: The Science of the Supernormal,* T. Bestermann (trans.), (London: G. Bell, 1933), 119.

80. A. von Schrenck-Notzing, 'Die Entwicklung des Okkultismus zur Parapsychologie in Deutschland', *Zeitschrift für Parapsychologie,* 9 (1932), 402–3.

81. A. von Schrenck-Notzing, 'Professor Dr med. et phil. Karl Gruber', in G. Walther (ed.) *Grundfragen der Parapsychologie* (Stuttgart: W. Kohlhammer, 1962), 360. Note that this obituary first appeared in July 1927 in *Zeitschrift für Parapsychologie.*

82. *Ibid.,* 132. This first appeared as an article in *Psychische Studien* in July 1921.

83. Driesch, *op. cit.* (note 46), 218.

84. A. Francé-Harrar, *So war's um Neunzehnhundert: Mein Fin de Siècle* (Munich: Albert Langen & Georg Müller, 1962), 178.

85. *Ibid.,* 182.

86. J. Webb, 'Thomas Mann and the Occult: An Unpublished Letter', *Encounter,* 46, 4 (1976), 24.

87. Driesch, *op. cit.* (note 46), 155.

88. Abschrift VI B 2226. Deutsches Generalkonsulat für China. An das Auswärtige Amt, Berlin. 25 Oktober 1922. Betr.: Empfang von Prof. Driesch

in Schanghai, in: Driesch PA 416 Film 513, UAL; Der Reichsminister des Innern. Abschrift III 4518. Bericht Tokio 21 März 1923, in:, Driesch PA 416 Film 513, UAL.

89. Harrington, *op. cit.* (note 48), 190.

90. Driesch, *op. cit.* (note 60), 181.

91. Driesch, *op. cit.* (note 79), 132–3.

92. Quoted in Harrington, *op. cit.* (note 48), 61.

93. The rhetoric of German holism was appropriated by the National Socialists during the 1930s and many of Driesch's ideas, which had provided a foundation for the broader holistic movement, were used in support of a racist doctrine that he abhorred. See, *Ibid.*, 190.

94. *Ibid.*

95. 'In der er auf die weltanschauliche Bedeutung der psychischen Forschung hinwies und großes Vertrauen in ihre Zukunft bekundete; er ging dann auf allgemeine Fragen über, bekannte sich als überzeugten Pazifisten und wies gerade auch der Parapsychologie eine große Rolle bei der Befriedung der Nationen zu. Beide Male schloß er mit den Worten: '*L'avenir est à nous*' Nach Verabredung mit meinen deutschen Kollegen übernahm ich die Erwiderung; ich bekannte meine volle Übereinstimmung mit allem, was Richet gesagt hatte, und schloß mit den von ihm selbst gebrauchten vertrauensvollen Worten'. Driesch, *op. cit.* (note 46), 239.

96. H. Driesch, 'Der internationale Parapsychologenkongress in Paris', *Unterhaltung und Wissen*, 8 October 1927, in: Nachlaß T.K. Oesterreich 399/10, UAT.

97. Letter from the Ministerium für Volksbildung. A: XVII 509 to Professor Driesch, 12 October 1933, in: Driesch PA 416 Film 513, UAL.

98. Driesch, *op. cit.* (note 46), 275.

99. Letter from W. Kröner to H. Driesch, 4 April 1938, in: Nachlaß 250 Hans Driesch, UBL.

100. *Ibid.*

101. *Ibid.*

102. Letter from the Preussische Minister für Volkswohlfahrt to sämtliche Herren Regierungspräsidenten und den Herren Polizeipräsidenten in Berlin. Betrifft: Verbot der Ausübung und Vorführung der Hypnose durch nicht approbierte Personen. Berlin, den 14 April 1925, in: GStA PK, I. HA Rep. 76 Nr. 1325.

103. 'Alle öffentlichen oder gewerbsmässigen und alle privaten Veranstaltungen über Hypnose, Suggestion, Magnetismus, Okkultismus, Muskellesen und ähnliche Themen sind verboten, sofern sie nicht vom wissenschaftlichen Werte und von der Landespolizeibehörde genehmigt sind.' Letter from der Regierungspräsident. I 13 Nr. 450 to Herrn Minister für Volkswohlfahrt in Berlin. Betrifft: Verbot der Ausübung und Vorführung der Hypnose usw. Berichterstätter: Regierungs und Medizinalrat Dr Mohrmann. Arnsberg, den

27 Mai 1925, in: GStA PK, I. HA Rep. 76 Nr. 1325. Note however that some correspondents objected to the prohibition of private displays of hypnosis, arguing that this would not only be uncontrollable, but would infringe on personal freedoms.

104. Letter from the Reichsminister des Innern. II 9115/24A to Herr Preussicher Minister für Volkswohlfahrt. Berlin, den 14 Januar 1925, in: GStA PK, I. HA Rep. Nr. 1324. On the connection perceived between cinema and hypnotic suggestion and attempts to censor films featuring such subject matter, see S. Andriopoulos, 'Spellbound in Darkness: Hypnosis as an Allegory of Early Cinema', *The Germanic Review*, 77, 2 (2002), 111–12.

105. Founded in Berlin in 1903 this association's stated purpose was to enlighten the public about the dangers posed by quacks to public health. See *Berliner Lokal-Anzeiger*, 1 März 1903; *Berliner Lokal-Anzeiger*, 5 März 1903.

106. Letter from the Deutscher Aerztevereinsbund to the Preussische Ministerium für Volkswohlfahrt, 10 April 1922, in: GStA Pk. I. HA Rep. 76 Nr. 1324.

107. *Ibid.*

108. Letter from the Deutsche Gesellschaft zur Bekämpfung des Kurpfuschertums to the Ministrium des Innern. Berlin, 12 November 1924, in: GStA Pk. I. HA Rep. Nr. 1324.

109. Letter from Regierungs und Medizinalrat Dr Loerch to Herr Minister für Volkswohlfahrt in Berlin, Aachen, 18 Juni 1925, in: GStA PK, I. HA Rep. 76.

110. Letter from Regierungs und Medizinalrat Dr Wegener to the Regierungspräsident, 18 Juni 1925, in: GStA PK, I. HA Rep. 76.

111. Letter from Medizinalrat Dr Dembowski to the Regierungspräsident, Breslau, 6 Juni 1925, in: GStA PK, I. HA Rep. 76.

112. Andriopoulos, *op. cit.* (note 104), 102.

113. Letter from the Ärztliche Verein München to A. von Schrenck-Notzing, Munich 28 August 1920, in: Korrespondenz 3, Nachlaß Albert von Schrenck-Notzing, IGPP.

114. This was particularly the case among the working class in large cities like Berlin where pastoral needs were difficult to meet because of the size of parishes. In working class areas of Berlin, for example, only one per cent of nominal church members attended Sunday services. See D. Blackbourn, *The Long Nineteenth Century: A History of Germany, 1780–1918* (Oxford: Oxford University Press, 1997), 294.

115. M. Pöhlmann, *Kampf der Geister: Die Publizistik der 'Apologetischen Centrale' (1921–1937)* (Stuttgart: Kohlhammer, 1998), 13–15.

116. F. Walcher, *Der Spiritismus* (Stuttgart: Verlag des Evang, Volksbunds, 1922), 7, 20, in ADW, CA, AC-S 1 Aberglaube.

117. 'Aberglaube – was steckt dahinter?', *op. cit.* (note 9).

118. *Ibid.*

119. Walcher, *op. cit.* (note 116).

120. *Ibid.*

121. 'Aberglaube – was steckt dahinter?', *op. cit.* (note 9).

122. E. Zimmermann, 'Der Fluch des Aberglaubens und der Zauberei', ADW, CA, AC-S1 Aberglaube.

123. *Ibid.*

124. Bekämpfung des Wahrsagens im Entwurf StGB. Aus: Die Innere Mission im ev. Deutschland, Heft 4 April 1928), in: ADW, CA, AC-S 1 Aberglaube.

125. J. Dörfler, *Der Spiritismus (Geistererscheinung)*, Apologetische Hefte des katholischen Glaubensapostolates Nr. 3, Graz: Verlag des katholischen Glaubensapostates, 1925, in: ADW, CA, AC-S 334 Spiritismus.

126. *Ibid.*

127. Schrenck-Notzing, *op. cit.* (note 80), 464.

128. *Ibid.*, 466.

129. Dörfler, *op. cit.* (note 125).

130. *Ibid.*

131. X. Pfeiffer, 'Okkultismus und Religion', in: ADW, CA, AC-S 272 Okkultismus.

132. R. Michaelis, 'Parapsychologie und religiöse Erfahrung: Ein Kapitel von den Beziehungen zwischen Okkultismus und Leben', Beilage zur Zeitung, *Der Reichsbote*, 20 September 1931, in: ADW, CA, AC-S 272 Okkultismus.

133. *Ibid.*

134. Dörfler, *op. cit.* (note 125).

135. 'Wenn der wissenschaftliche Okkultismus mit seiner animistisch-vitalistischen Deutung der medialen Tatsachen in seinen Schranken bliebt und seine Aufgaben in der Beobachtung, Beschreibung und natürlichen Erklärung der Erscheinungen sieht, ohne dabei in das pantheistische Fahrwasser oder überhaupt auf das Gebiet der Religion zu geraten, so wird er mit der kirchlichen Lehre niemals wirklich in Widerspruch geräten können. Gegen die Okkultismus als Wissenschaft hat auch die Kirche nichts einzuwenden.' *Ibid.*

136. Walcher, *op. cit.* (note 116).

137. M. Krawielitzki, *Der Spiritismus*, Bad Blankenburg: Buchdruckerei und Verlag Harfe, in: ADW, CA, AC-S 334 Spiritismus.

138. Quoted in Schrenck-Notzing, *op. cit.* (note 80), 463.

139. Dörfler, *op. cit.* (note 125).

140. G.A. Craig, *Germany 1886–1945* (Oxford: Oxford University Press, 1978), 182.

141. Schrenck-Notzing, *op. cit.* (note 80), 504.

142. *Ibid.*, 504–5.

143. Craig, *op. cit.* (note 140), 182–3.

144. Nr. 708 Verbot des Wahrsagens. Ministerium des Innern, 25 October 1934, Nr. I P A: 146 P 3, in: ADW, CA, AC-S1 Aberglaube.

145. *Frankfurter Zeitung*, 11 Dezember 1934.

146. 'Verbot des Wahrsagens in Hannover', *Frankfurter Zeitung*, Nr. 348–9, von 10 Juli 1936. ADW, CA, ACS-S1 Aberglaube.

147. 'Der Volksbetrug der 'Schwarzen Kunst' ', *Der Deutsche*, nr. 107 vom 10 Mai. ADW, CA, AC-S 273 Okkultismus.

148. Letter from A. Hellwig to H. Driesch, 20 March 1938, in: Nachlaß 250 Hans Driesch, UBL.

149. On Nazi interest in the occult, see E. Howe, *Urania's Children: The Strange World of the Astrologers* (London: William Kimber, 1967); N. Goodrick-Clarke, *The Occult Roots of Nazism: Secret Aryan Cults and their Influence on Nazi Ideology – The Ariosophists of Austria and Germany, 1890–1935* (New York: New York University Press, 1985); J. Webb, *The Occult Establishment* (LaSalle: Open Court, 1976).

150. This decree was issued by the head of the SS and German police Heinrich Himmler. Runderlaß des Reichsführers SS und Chef der dt. Polizei im Reichsministerium des Inneren on 20 July 1937; S – PP (II B) Nr.1249/36, *Ministerialblatt des Reichs- und Preußischen Ministeriums des Innern, Ausgabe A* 2 (98), 32 (11 August 1937), 1337–9; C. Treitel, *A Science for the Soul: Occultism and the Genesis of the German Modern* (Baltimore: Johns Hopkins University Press, 2004), 210–42.

151. The Gestapo's involvement was a result of Aktion Hess, a campaign launched against Germany's occultists after Hess's flight to England.

152. Letter from H. Bender to H. Driesch, 11 July 1935, in Nachlaß 250 Hans Driesch, UBL.

153. *Ibid.*

154. Letter from W. Kröner to H. Driesch, 4 April 1938, in Nachlaß 250 Driesch, UBL.

155. Letter from W. Kröner to H. Driesch, 20 January 1939, in Nachlaß 250 Hans Driesch, UBL

156. *Ibid.* On Schulte-Strathaus, who was a member of Hess' staff and an expert on occult subjects, see Howe, *op. cit.* (note 149), 194–5.

157. *Ibid.*, 163–6.

158. Ministerium für Volksbildung. A: XVII 509 to Professor Hans Driesch, 12 Oktober 1933, in: Driesch PA 416 Film 513, UAL; T.K. Oesterreich to Hans Driesch, 30 September 1933, in: Nachlaß 250 Hans Driesch, UBL.

159. 'Selbst bin ich Parteimitglied seit 1935. Der arme Winterstein ist lieder nicht Arier, wenn auch der bestmögliche Fall, trotzdem kann er nicht Vorsitzender der Gesellschaft bleiben.' Letter from Z. Wassilko to H. Driesch 15 April 1938, in: Nachlaß 250 Hans Driesch, UBL.

160. Letter from H. Bender to H. Driesch, 15 April 1938, in Nachlaß 250 Hans Driesch, UBL; Letter from H. Bender to H. Driesch, 16 November 1938, in Nachlaß 250 Hans Driesch, UBL.

161. G. Walther, *Zum anderen Ufer: Vom Marxismus und Atheismus zum Christentum* (Remagen: Otto Reichl, 1960), 474.

162. Grahrath-Wildenroth an Herr Schneider-Schule, 5 December 1945; 'Ergänzungen zum Fragenbogen des American Military Government', in Nachlass Schneider-Schelde, Monacensia Literaturarchiv, München.

163. Walther, *op. cit.* (note 161), 477.

5

Parapsychology in the Courtroom:
Occult Trials, Expertise and Authority
during the Weimar Republic

Introduction

Following the First World War, the courtrooms of the new Republic became both baptisteries and battlegrounds for parapsychologists, transporting questions about the reality of paranormal phenomena, debated up until this time in domestic and scientific spaces, into the public sphere. The prosecution of clairvoyants, such as Claire Reichart – a Munich-based medium who claimed to have foreseen a series of significant political events, including the 1918/19 Revolution, the attack on the socialist leader Erhard Auer and Hitler's failed Putsch – or of hypnotists, like Friedrich Gern – whose somnambulistic spouse divined information about business ventures and unsolved crimes – afforded both a practical application for parapsychology and an audience for its knowledge claims.[1] The judges who tried such cases, often completely ignorant of the scientific literature pertaining to the occult, called upon parapsychologists to advise them in their deliberations. In their capacity as 'Sachverständiger' [expert witnesses], these researchers testified for the existence of the paranormal, proffering evidence of somnambulism and clairvoyance to dramatic effect in courtroom séances. During the 1928 trial of the criminal telepath Elsa Günther-Geffers, for example, such experts helped carry out experiments in the presence of the court in order to establish the veracity of the medium's trance and the accuracy of her prognostications.[2] Conscious of the courtroom's potential as a platform for their professional ambitions, parapsychologists used this forum – ignoring their position as supposedly neutral experts – to publicly campaign for the legitimacy of their nascent discipline.

This 'forensic parapsychology', the occult sibling of the new sub-discipline of forensic psychology, was not, however, without its opponents. Critical occultists such as the jurist Albert Hellwig and the psychiatrist Albert Moll – trained in disciplines on which both occultism and parapsychology encroached – were also routinely asked to provide their expert opinion in occult trials. These men, not only argued against the

233

reality of clairvoyance and other forms of occultism, demonstrating the ease with which such phenomena could be faked, but attacked the epistemological, methodological and theoretical basis of their opponents' claims to expertise in this field. Such testimony transformed the trials of individual occultists like Reichart, Gern and Günther-Geffers into pitched battles between groups of 'experts' over the scientific legitimacy of parapsychology. In several instances, this courtroom debate, which grew increasingly heated and increasingly personal, became the occasion for further legal action. As we shall see, a number of critical occultists found themselves accused of defamation by their courtroom antagonists during the mid- to late 1920s.

This chapter examines the manner in which the mobilisation of parapsychologists and their opponents as expert witnesses allowed the trials of occultists, and the press coverage such trials received, to be utilised by both parties as venues for boundary-work; the intention of which was to claim the cultural authority of science, to establish exclusive rights over the analysis of occult phenomena, and to highlight the absurdity of their opponents' knowledge claims.[3] In so doing, it differs from recent historical studies of occult trials that have analysed the prosecution of occultists in terms of 'liberal despair' over the public's credulity and the threat posed by popular science, as practised in spiritualist séances, to scientists' cultural authority.[4] Concentrating instead on the relationship between diametrically opposed groups of 'experts', each determined to win the right to mould the public's understanding of the occult, this chapter works through the myriad of legal, scientific and professional issues that emerged during the trials of Weimar occultists. The first section provides a brief overview of the relationship between occultism and the law in the German context, highlighting the differing legal responses of the German states and outlining the attempt by certain opponents of occultism to fashion a uniform approach to occult practice within the Reich Criminal Code. The second section looks at the trial of August Drost as an example of the credibility contest that took place between parapsychologists and critical occultists in the courtroom. The third section considers the role of the press in exacerbating this contest, while the final section explores the notion of expertise as it featured in both the Rudloff–Moll trial and the defamation suit against Albert Hellwig.

Occultism and the law

While the Criminal Code of the German Reich did not recognise occultism as a separate or discreet form of criminal activity, it allowed for the prosecution of occult practitioners under legislation dealing with fraud, embezzlement, blackmail, murder, bodily harm, libel and gross misconduct.[5]

In the early twentieth century, charges were brought against occultists for a number of these offences, including defamation, assault and 'fahrlässige Tötung' [negligent homicide].[6] During the Weimar Republic, however, the majority of trials involving occult practitioners resulted from accusations of fraud (§263 Strafgesetzbuch or StGB [Criminal Code]). In most of these cases, the defendant had been involved in Kriminaltelepathie [criminal telepathy] – a practice in which a medium, normally under the guidance of a hypnotist, purported to use their telepathic or clairvoyant powers to help solve crimes either for private citizens or the police.[7] Disgruntled customers or local police authorities, concerned to protect the public from swindlers, launched legal action against these occultists, requesting that the public prosecutor pursue them on charges of fraud.

The 1925 trial of the hypnotist August Drost, one of the earliest and best-known court cases in Germany involving criminal telepathy, centred, as we shall see, on accusations of both fraud and gross misconduct. Drost stood accused of defrauding the citizens of Bernburg in the course of his activities as a self-proclaimed occult detective, a service for which he received money and gifts.[8] Such charges, however, were difficult to prove. Under the Reich Criminal Code, a conviction for fraud depended on establishing that the defendant had acted in bad faith, that is, that he or she had knowingly defrauded their customer.[9] It was insufficient in such cases for the complainant or the prosecution simply to show that information provided by an occultist was incorrect. The court required proof that the accused had offered their services in full knowledge that they, or their medium, did not possess, or did not believe they possessed, the occult powers to which they laid claim. A guilty verdict in such cases did not revolve around the reality of clairvoyance and telepathy, but around the defendant's belief in their reality.

The large number of acquittals in such cases, however, demonstrated the difficulty of establishing either Gutgläubigkeit [good-] or Bösgläubigkeit [bad conscience] on the part of an occultist. Albert Hellwig, a district court director at Potsdam and an expert witness in the case against Drost, acknowledged this problem, writing, 'one can describe this question about good or bad conscience as the central question in all such fraud proceedings. It is also the most difficult question.'[10] In order to ascertain what the accused did or did not believe, Hellwig argued, a thoroughgoing analysis of their personality was necessitated. Only by determining the defendant's credulity in relation to the occult, knowledge of the field, cognisance of common errors, and motives, could this question be answered to the satisfaction of the court.[11] This suggested that the psychiatrist and forensic psychologist, as well as the jurist, had a role to play in occult trials.[12] The release of Drost in the Bernburg case, despite the protestations of Hellwig, was a prime example of the difficulty of establishing the intentions of mediums and their handlers. It also provided ammunition for those critical of the prosecution of occultists under legislation dealing with fraud. These critics, of whom Hellwig was the most prominent, campaigned for a uniform approach to occult practice, demanding that the Reich Criminal Code adopt the more punitive measures towards occultists reflected in the statute books of the southern states.[13]

The criminal codes of a number of the German Länder, including Bavaria, Baden and Hessen,[14] contained provisions for the prosecution of so-called *Gaukelei*, a term perhaps best translated in this context as charlatanry, but which literally connoted travelling showmanship.[15] In Bavaria, for example, transgressions by occultists were pursued under Article 54 of the Bavarian criminal code, a *Gaukelei* paragraph, which stated:

> Whosoever for payment or for the attainment of some other advantage concerns themselves with so-called magic or spirit conjuring, with prophecy, card reading, divination, sign and dream interpretation or other charlatanry of the same kind, will be punished with a fine of up to 150 Marks or with imprisonment.[16]

In Baden and Hessen, these activities were punishable under Articles 68 and 102 of their respective criminal codes, which contained pecuniary measures similar to those found in Bavaria.[17] States, whose statute books included this antiquarian clause, were able to take advantage of it due to an error in Reich legislation that allowed for the ongoing validity of state regulations on crimes, offences, misdemeanours and charlatanry not covered by Reich criminal law.[18] In states that possessed such *Gaukelei* clauses prior to unification, the introduction of a Reich Criminal Code did not necessitate, as it did in other states, the prosecution of occultists under legislation dealing with fraud.

A charge of *Gaukelei* differed significantly from that of fraud in that it presumed *a priori* the non-existence of occult powers and sought to establish guilt or innocence solely on the basis of whether the defendant had accepted remuneration for their services. Clauses such as those found in Bavaria, Baden and Hessen reflected legislators' beliefs that fortune telling and related arts posed a threat to public welfare.[19] Because these practices were understood to be harmful, whether their practitioners believed in them or not, the good or bad conscience of occultists had no bearing on courts' decisions. In Munich during the late 1880s, for example, a woman named Frau Narr was found guilty of *Gaukelei* despite the fact that two expert witnesses gave testimony in which they argued that she had acted in good faith.[20] While the defendant had not asked for payment for her fortune telling, she had accepted small gifts of money, forty or fifty pfennigs at a time; a fact that enabled the court to fine her a hundred Marks.[21] In 1926, the clairvoyant Claire Reichart also appeared before a Munich court charged with fortune telling under Bavaria's *Gaukelei* law. Reichart, whose prognostications about Munich's political life had gained her notoriety, had repeatedly accepted gifts for her prophecies.[22] Despite the impressive list of witnesses and experts who attended her trial, including Erhard Auer, General von Epp and Albert von Schrenck-Notzing, she was fined 100 marks and sentenced to ten days in prison.[23]

In states whose criminal codes included a *Gaukelei* clause, this emphasis on the exchange of money and goods as a measure of guilt provoked outrage on the part of both parapsychologists and occultists, who claimed that the interpretation and application of this law by police was fallacious.[24] *Gaukelei*, they argued, as it was defined in the statute books of the southern states, had never been intended to apply to occultists.[25] On this point there was intense debate during the 1920s between parapsychologists, critical occultists and jurists.[26] *Gaukeleiparagraphen*, parapsychologists maintained, had their basis in the unfounded assumption that paranormal powers did not exist.[27] Carl du Prel, who appeared as an expert witness for Frau Narr, wrote in this regard:

> Whoever may have styled the aforementioned article [54] held the viewpoint of the so-called Enlightenment and of modern materialism. According to this clairvoyance is simply not possible; therefore whoever tells fortunes and accepts payment for it, commits *Gaukelei*.[28]

In a similar manner, the parapsychologist T.K. Oesterreich argued that the concept of *Gaukelei* was the product of an age in which it was widely believed that 'Wahrsagen' [fortune-telling] was a primitive form of superstition. Now, in the twentieth century, he maintained, things were different, many scientists were convinced, on the strength of experiments in the field, that there existed real parapsychical and paraphysical phenomena.[29] In the Gern case, in which Oesterreich appeared as an expert witness, he defined *Gaukelei* as an act in which someone purporting to have occult powers deliberately deceives his or her customer; a reading that interpreted this offence as a special type of fraud.[30] Hellwig disputed Oesterreich's claim on a number of points. Clairvoyance and other so-called occult phenomena were not, he argued, widely recognised by scientists as facts, but were simply espoused as such by a few outsiders.[31] *Gaukelei* was not just a special kind of fraud, because its application was not dependent on the defendant's good faith. It was a law that considered all such acts, whether committed in good or bad conscience, as a danger to public welfare.[32] Until such time as the existence and efficacy of clairvoyance was definitively proven, Hellwig argued, the law must reflect the opinion of the majority, which saw in clairvoyance a threat to public order and health.

On this basis, Hellwig campaigned vigorously throughout the 1920s for harsher penalties against occultists, arguing for the inclusion within the Reich Criminal Code of a *Gaukelei* paragraph.[33] In 1928, for example, he organised a petition, which demanded that the Reichstag implement new legislation to deal with the moral and physical threat posed by fortune telling.[34] This occult art, the signatories claimed, had a damaging effect not only on the public, but also on those who practised it. The petition's sponsors maintained, furthermore, that there existed a tangible link between fortune telling and other forms of criminal behaviour – an attempt to suggest that both professional and non-professional occultists could be counted among the ranks of what Weimar criminalists called 'Berufsvebrecher' [career criminals].[35] The petition argued that the current legislation used to deal with occultists, by which it meant Reich legislation on fraud (§263 StGB), was insufficient to combat this threat.[36] It recommended that the new criminal code – a draft of which became the basis for parliamentary deliberations on penal reform during 1927 – contain a paragraph (§375 StGB) stating 'whoever tells fortunes for financial gain will be punished with up to two years in jail or with a fine. The same penalty will meet those who offer publicly to tell fortunes.'[37] This piece of legislation was intended to put Germany on an equal footing with countries like Switzerland, which had inserted a *Gaukelei* clause into its criminal code in 1918.[38] Hellwig's petition, however, like the process of penal reform in Weimar Germany, ultimately met with little success.[39]

The Drost trial

During the Weimar Republic, a number of high-profile criminal telepaths found themselves in court on charges of fraud; a corollary not only of the rising number of these occult practitioners active in Germany after the First World War, but of the state's increasingly intolerant attitude towards them. As a result of this series of trials, which received extensive coverage in the newspapers of the Republic and later the Reich, a small group of parapsychologists and critical occultists became regulars in the courtroom, providing expert testimony in cases of occult misconduct. The performance of parapsychologists in their capacity as expert witnesses and in their interactions with so-called anti-occultists drew attention to the epistemological fissures within this nascent discipline around the concepts of expertise and authority, concepts that were central also to the series of defamation suits that took place between parapsychologists, critical occultists and mediums during this period. Using the trials of August Drost and Rudloff–Moll as examples, the following sections consider the courtroom as an arena in which expert witnesses and defendants engaged in credibility contests and boundary-work; in some instances fighting to protect their disciplinary borders from those who threatened their cultural authority, and in others attempting to expand these borders in ways that encroached on the cultural authority of others. These proceedings, with their diametrically opposed experts, demonstrate the tensions surrounding parapsychology's claim to scientific legitimacy and the uncertainty during this period surrounding the notion of expertise in nascent fields, including criminology and forensic psychology.

In October 1925, a teacher and itinerant hypnotist by the name of August Drost found himself in the dock of a Bernburg court on charges of fraud and gross misconduct. This rather nondescript man, who supplemented his income as a teacher with the gifts and commissions he received in his capacity as an occult detective and healer, was made famous through his trial and subsequent acquittal and helped popularise the concept of criminal telepathy at all levels of German society.[40] Drost, who for many years had employed a small group of somnambulistic mediums in order to solve crimes, had been arrested in 1924 for accepting payment for what the Bernburg authorities considered deliberate fraud. The case attracted a host of distinguished expert witnesses from Bernburg and Anhalt, as well as from larger cities including Berlin and Munich. These witnesses, who included Albert Hellwig, Rudolf Tischner, and the director of the Bernburg county asylum Professor Heyse, lured, in turn, correspondents from newspapers throughout the country. The trial, which lasted five days, from 12 to 17 October, consisted of the testimony of over one hundred and thirty witnesses and three expert witnesses in relation to forty-five cases of criminal telepathy.[41] On the central issue of Drost's good faith, the court decided, with the support of Tischner and Heyse, that the accused had believed in the clairvoyant powers of his mediums. On this basis he was released without charge.

According to Albert Hellwig, the voice of dissent among the expert witnesses, the Drost case was significant for a number of reasons. Drost's trial, so he argued immediately following the hypnotist's acquittal, provided important material for forensic psychology, a stimulus for occult research, practical and theoretical lessons on points of law, and an opportunity to revive discussion of the volatile relationship between the justice system and the press.[42] Several years after this initial assessment, Hellwig supplemented this list by indicating the historical significance of this case. Drost's trial, while not the first attempt to prosecute a criminal telepath in Germany, was the first such case to receive broad public attention and to inculcate in Germans what Hellwig believed was an unhealthy fascination with criminal telepathy.[43] This trial was important from another perspective also, it demonstrated in its performance in both the courtroom and the press, the many tensions and problems surrounding parapsychology's attempt to gain scientific legitimacy.

Drost's trial was understood, by trial participants and the public alike, less in terms of the defendant's guilt or innocence in relation to charges of fraud and gross misconduct and more in terms of the question of the existence of clairvoyant phenomena.[44] On the day before proceedings were launched in Bernburg, the *Lokalanzeiger Berlin* [*Berlin Local Gazette*] told its readers that the court would consider the very difficult question of whether occult phenomena existed; the defendant's guilt as represented here was of secondary interest.[45] Another newspaper, the *Vossische Zeitung*, argued that this case was not really about Drost, it was occultism, represented by the defence lawyer Dr Winterberg and the homeopathic physician Dr Kröner, over which the true battle would be waged in the course of this trial.[46] The largely successful attempt of the defence to focus the attention of both the court and the public on questions relating to the existence of paranormal powers, rather than on the good or bad faith of the defendant, demonstrated their cognisance of the courtroom's potential as a platform for questions relating to occultism and for the acceptance of parapsychology as a legitimate new science. The testimony of the parapsychologist Rudolf Tischner, for example, related to the defendant's belief in the supernormal detective skills of his mediums as well as to the current state of research on telepathy and clairvoyance. This gap between the court's focus and the polemical aims of expert witnesses allowed parapsychologists to use legal proceedings as a vehicle for their professional and epistemological ambitions.

The court's obligation, as set out by the Strafprozeßordnung [Code of Criminal Procedure], to investigate all evidence deemed relevant to establishing the truth of a case, provided parapsychologists, in their capacity as court-appointed expert witnesses, with an opportunity to present evidence for the reality of paranormal phenomena.[47] In the Tischer case, for example, the court assembled in a room at the Moabit Women's Prison in order to watch Herr Tischer place his wife into a somnambulistic state.[48] The court and expert witnesses then proceeded to ask her questions in order to test her putative powers. An experiment conducted in Zossen during November 1925 with the stage clairvoyant Walther Höpfner was of an even more dramatic nature. In the presence of the judge, the clerk of the court and the public prosecutor, the somnambulistic medium was questioned about a series of thefts. He was asked among other things how many thefts had been carried out and what was stolen. His answers, a series of apparently ungrammatical ramblings, revealed the theft of a number of hens, a gold watch and a carpet by a man of around twenty-eight years with grey-blue eyes, big ears and no moustache.[49] Those questioning him were astounded by

240

his accuracy and by his knowledge of details of which they had been unaware until after further investigation.[50] In Bernburg, Tischner, one of the expert witnesses, conducted an experiment with Drost that he described as an amazing success.[51] Parapsychologists used such experiments and long discourses on the state of parapsychological knowledge to argue both for the reality and efficacy of clairvoyance and the legitimacy of their field. Hellwig grumbled that there was no need for occult experts in such cases, because the pertinent legal questions could be better answered by a forensic psychologist, who would establish the good or bad conscience of the defendant.[52]

The court allowed these experiments and the lengthy explanations of epistemological and methodological matters proffered by expert witnesses in order to ascertain the current state of knowledge about the paranormal and the positions of those for and against the scientific study of the occult.[53] Legally, however, it was concerned solely with ascertaining the defendant's guilt in terms of fraud or *Gaukelei*. This was the case not only in the Drost trial, but in nearly every instance of occult misconduct heard before a German court. In 1889, for example, Carl du Prel wondered why expert witnesses had been called at all in the case of Frau Narr of Munich, given that Article 54 of the Bavarian Legal Code, under which she was prosecuted, regarded any instance of card reading, dream interpretation or clairvoyance as fraud if money had changed hands.[54] The law, in du Prel's opinion, had decided *a priori* that all instances of fortune telling were fraudulent.[55] This dissonance between legal and scientific truth – a feature of many cases in which scientists are asked to testify as expert witnesses – was experienced in Bernburg also, where it was made clear by the judge and the prosecution that it was not the court's place to come to a decision regarding the reality of paranormal phenomena.[56]

> It is not the court's business to decide whether it is scientifically certain that knowledge can be obtained by supernatural means, in particular whether this knowledge can be related to the clearing up of criminal acts. It is also not the court's business to ascertain whether the mediums used by the accused possess the ability to mediate the supernatural in hypnotic states. The court has only to decide whether the accused in the sense of the charge is guilty, first of all of fraud....[57]

Hellwig, who was fully conscious of the manner in which parapsychologists attempted to use such cases as a forum for their beliefs, stressed repeatedly that questions of spiritual or philosophical significance could not be decided in the courtroom. Outside the courtroom, however, the distinction between the court's interest in the good or bad faith of the defendant and their interest in the state of knowledge about the paranormal proved difficult to maintain.

The court's focus on the question of the defendant's guilt or innocence in relation to charges of fraud should have prevented any challenge on the part of parapsychologists or criminal telepaths to the judicial process, but its failure to properly address parapsychologists' attempts to usurp the meaning of such trials led to widespread confusion. Experiments, like those conducted in Moabit, Zossen and Bernburg, clouded the distinction that the court needed to make between its focus on questions of legal truth, and the question of the reality of paranormal phenomena. While the existence of clairvoyance should have remained a non-issue in trials involving criminal telepaths, for many they appeared to confirm it, a problem that was exacerbated by the newspaper coverage these trials received. The concentration of the press on the debate between parapsychologists and critical occultists over the status of occult phenomena tended to obscure for the public the nature of the legal questions involved. When the court declared Drost not guilty on charges of fraud, but warned that the case should stand as an example for those tempted to consult criminal telepaths, for instance, the verdict was widely understood to represent an affirmation of clairvoyance and a triumph for parapsychology.[58] Far from dissuading the public from using criminal telepaths, the court's decision elicited increased interest in occult detection.[59]

The conclusions drawn by the public about the Drost trial were understood by critics such as Hellwig to be the result not only of the machinations of parapsychologists, but also of the inaccurate and exaggerated coverage this case had received in the press.[60] Ignoring the court chairman's pleas for objectivity, the reporters who attended this trial presented a one-sided version of proceedings, choosing to obfuscate the court's focus on the question of fraud, in order to concentrate on the reality of telepathy and clairvoyance. Of the nearly one hundred articles that Hellwig collected on the Drost case, for example, none made explicit the pivotal significance of the defendant's good faith to the court's decision.[61] Coverage of the case also appeared to influence the testimony of witnesses, some of whom had originally reported Drost for fraud but who became increasingly sympathetic and supportive of him in the course of the trial.[62] This was true of the Günther–Gethers case also, where Rudolf Lambert, stated that 'the influence of newspaper reports during this trial on a large number of the witnesses is not to be underestimated.'[63] This less than objective reportage was exclusive neither to small local newspapers nor to the conservative political press but was found in newspapers with both national circulation and leftist agendas. The extent of this coverage, its reception throughout the country and at all levels of society, ensured increased interest in criminal telepathy and minor celebrity for Drost who was bombarded with offers of employment and book and film contracts in the months following his acquittal.

The role of the press

The inaccurate and often misleading nature of newspaper articles on the prosecution of criminal telepaths was due both to a lust for sensation on the part of the press and to deliberate efforts by the prosecution and defence to manipulate the media for polemic purposes. The defence team in Bernburg, for example, installed a representative at the press table and attempted to foster a friendly relationship between the defendant and the media outside the courtroom.[64] This strategy ensured the publication in a large number of newspapers of reports critical of both the court's and prosecution's conduct. These polemical opportunities were exploited not only by parapsychologists, but also by their opponents, who were equally aware of the importance of the press as a platform from which to argue their case. Hellwig, for example, made contributions to a number of high-profile newspapers, including the *Frankfurter Zeitung* [*Frankfurt News*], in order to publicise the prosecution's case and to highlight the nature of the legal questions on which the court's decision was dependent. These articles met with hostility from the parapsychological community, who complained bitterly of Hellwig's prejudicial stance on the case and his attempts to exploit the court's verdict in his ongoing campaign against occultism.[65] This war of words continued long after the defendant's release with talks and articles in a number of specialist forums. In the weeks immediately following Drost's acquittal, for example, Hellwig invited the media to attend a talk at the Psychological Institute established by Albert Moll in Berlin. In the course of this presentation, Hellwig attempted to answer his critics and to strike a deadly blow against occultism in all its forms, reprimanding the press for the role they had played in what he perceived as a miscarriage of justice.[66]

Crime and court reports were some of the most popular and eagerly read columns in the daily press during the Weimar Republic, becoming a site for contemporary juridical debates – a public space in which issues such as the legitimacy of the legal system could be discussed.[67] This use of crime and court reporting was particularly evident in the left-wing press, publications such as the *Weltbühne* [*World Stage*], whose strident critiques of the judiciary sought to combat the political and class prejudice that prevailed within Weimar Germany's judicial system.[68] Such columns, however, were not inevitably political, many catered to the public's appetite for spectacle and excitement, rather than to their sense of moral outrage. The crime scene reports published by daily newspapers tended to be lurid and overdramatised, whipping the public into a frenzy of excitement with a flurry of extra editions that cautioned readers to be on the lookout for burglars and escaped murderers.[69] Newspapers in Berlin, including the *Berliner Zeitung am Mittag* [*Berlin Midday News*], also routinely employed theatrical metaphors in their descriptions of court proceedings, depicting them as dramas or tragedies and casting judges, lawyers and defendants in roles as either heroes or villains.[70] Crime coverage of this nature was, as many contemporaries realised, problematic. The explicit reports of murders that appeared in the press not only exaggerated the statistical significance of violent crime, but often gave the impression of police incompetence.[71] The criminal police, however, while cognisant of these problems, believed it necessary to inform the press as soon as possible after every murder, in the hope of gaining important information from the public.[72] The trials of criminal telepaths, like Drost, which combined the *frisson* elicited by crime with that offered by occultism, provided the drama and spectacle that was the staple of crime and court reporting in Germany's tabloid newspapers.

Hellwig's attempts to redress what he saw as inaccuracies in the coverage of the Drost trial were doubtless a result of his desire to present his perspective to the public, but were equally intended to remind the press of their responsibility both to their readers and their 'Kulturaufgabe' [cultural mission]. Despite his own polemical use of specialist journals and daily newspapers from across the political spectrum, something he freely admitted, Hellwig believed himself entitled to complain of the deficiencies that he saw as hallmarks of the contemporary press in general and of court reports in particular.[73] While court reporters were called upon to provide an unbiased account of events, such impartiality was absent from proceedings in Bernburg, where the parameters of the case had been deliberately obscured by the press in order to focus on questions pertaining to the reality of telepathy and clairvoyance. The irresponsible reportage displayed here, Hellwig contended, was both disruptive of the judicial process and detrimental to public welfare. A lack of objectivity and a fascination with the sensational had, according to Hellwig, long necessitated reform in court reporting.[74] This was a need made more urgent by the trials of criminal telepaths, in which the press's tendency towards sensationalism was exacerbated.

Hellwig's complaints were reflective of a belief that the press was negligent in its attitude towards its role within, and relationship to, the justice system. There was a conviction, widespread during the Weimar Republic, that the press carried a burden of 'public responsibility' equivalent to that of government or parliament.[75] At the root of this theory was the belief that, despite the strain placed on the press' credibility by the war, Germans continued to accept without question ideas expressed in their newspapers.[76] Hellwig wrote in this regard that the press must be aware of the immense suggestive power of the printed word on hundreds of thousands of people who, while incapable of exercising their critical faculties, could easily purchase and read a newspaper.[77] He asked the press to be conscious of their responsibility and to proceed with extreme caution in this extraordinarily delicate and opaque field of inquiry.

Hellwig attempted to demonstrate the press' culpability for the public's 'erroneous' view of criminal telepathy on numerous occasions. The parochial manner in which the Gern case was reported, for example, could not, in his opinion, help but leave the reader with the impression that the medium's clairvoyance had been established beyond all doubt.[78] In this sense, Hellwig argued, the Gern trial was almost identical to that in Bernburg, because in both cases the press had been derelict in their duty to provide objective reportage.[79] In an article, entitled 'The Clairvoyant from Rothenstein' he set about showing just how many inaccuracies the press coverage of such cases contained. The *Thüringer Allgemeine Zeitung* [*Thuringia General News*] reported in January 1925 that the body of a man dressed in a soldier's uniform had been discovered in a shallow grave near the town of Rothenstein.[80] The manner of this discovery was unusual, according to the paper, because the body's location had been provided by a clairvoyant. In consultation with a client, a local farmer, the clairvoyant predicted that the farmer would find a body on his property, a man who had been murdered by communists.[81] Hellwig attempted to verify what this newspaper had printed through an examination of police reports and trance protocols. He found that the clairvoyant had, in fact, told the farmer that he would find something on a forested slope.[82] He made no mention of the fact that it might be a body or that it would be on the farmer's land. Hellwig concluded from this analysis that there existed very little relationship between the reality of such cases and their representation in the media.[83]

Expertise in the courtroom

Newspaper coverage of occult trials introduced the public not only to criminal telepathy, and its possibilities as a form of detection, but also to some of the central epistemological and methodological problems surrounding parapsychology's attempt to become a legitimate science. While those who appeared in the courtroom as expert witnesses on the occult claimed to possess exhaustive knowledge of the paranormal and its study, the issue of expertise remained a constant source of tension between parapsychologists and their antagonists in fields such as psychology, psychiatry and law. This was due in part to a lack of disciplinary consensus on epistemological and methodological matters, including which phenomena should be studied, to which tests they should be subjected, how such phenomena might be explained, and who was best qualified to speak about them authoritatively – a fact most apparent in those arguments that centred on the qualifications and prejudices of court-appointed experts. To some extent, however, the tensions around the issue of expertise and the deconstruction of parapsychological knowledge that took place in such trials were a consequence of the arena and its rules of conduct.

The courtroom is a forum in which scientific credibility is contested and in which assumptions about disciplinary borders and epistemic authority become clouded not only by instances of boundary-work among experts but also by the disjuncture between legal questions and scientific knowledge.[84] First, legal and scientific questions may not coincide. As we have seen in the Drost case, while experts presented evidence for the reality of occultism, the central legal question was the good or bad conscience of the defendant. Second, science and its conjectures are always changing, so the ultimate wrongness or rightness of science in making legal decisions is not as important as other factors, such as clarity, reasonableness and general acceptance by the scientific community.[85] As the occult trials discussed here demonstrate, the appeal to authority and consensus was a more useful tactic for experts and defendants than the use of scientific data. Uncertainty around scientific authority in legal proceedings is not, however, just a result of the disjuncture between legal questions and scientific knowledge or an exclusive feature of trials involving nascent or pseudo-sciences. It is also a consequence of the adversarial nature of expert testimony. While the legal system of Weimar Germany was inquisitorial, the choice of neutral experts by those judges who presided over occult trials became a source of contention between the prosecution and defence. Furthermore, in the civil cases discussed here, which were adversarial, conflicting testimony on the status of parapsychological knowledge and expertise served to make the claims of both sides appear as if they were based on putative facts and a transitory consensus among researchers with specific agendas.[86]

Expert witnesses in German criminal courts during the Weimar Republic were selected at the discretion of a judge, who was also largely responsible for questioning them.[87] As court-appointed officials, these witnesses, who possessed expert knowledge not in the court's possession, were expected to act in an unbiased fashion, supporting neither the prosecution nor the defence.[88] In practice, however, those experts seconded for the purpose of occult trials were almost always aligned with one camp or the other. As a result of such allegiances the neutrality and suitability of expert witnesses in occult cases was frequently contested. During the Drost trial, for example, the defence attempted to have Walther Kröner appointed as an expert witness on the basis that Tischner, Hellwig and Heyse had adopted either a neutral or negative stance towards the defendant. The court chairman responded to this request by reminding counsel for the defence that every expert witness should be neutral and only those who are neutral make suitable expert witnesses.[89] The defence, undeterred, proceeded to protest the inclusion of Hellwig as an expert witness, arguing that his correspondence with Drost while he awaited trial demonstrated the district court director's prejudice against the defendant, not to mention his lack of qualification to pronounce on the occult.[90] Hellwig, for his part, maintained that because the focus of this case was the defendant's good or bad faith, not the reality of his putative powers, experts on occultism were not really needed at all.[91] Indeed, it was his expertise in the law, rather than on the occult, he argued, that made him a suitable expert witness.

The infighting between expert witnesses during the trials of occultists highlighted instabilities and uncertainties within parapsychology around the concepts of expertise and authority that resulted from the lack of epistemological and methodological consensus in this emerging science. It also revealed the desire of other disciplines – including psychology and psychiatry, as represented by Moll, and law, as represented by Hellwig – to claim jurisdiction over the public and forensic analysis of occult phenomena. For this reason, accusations of bias and claims of incompetence peppered the testimony and writings of both parties, their polemics becoming increasingly bitter and increasingly personal throughout the Weimar period. Both parapsychologists and critical occultists attempted to portray their adversaries as intellectually or morally inferior, pointing to the overwhelming evidence for their position and against that of their opponents.[92] Disagreements over what was acceptable behaviour in this field and allegations of insult ultimately led to disputes of a litigious nature between the warring parties. These disputes, which typically took the form of civil proceedings for libel, centred on the question of who was best qualified to pronounce on the occult, indeed who was best suited to shape the scientific and public response to such phenomena.

In July 1925, shortly prior to the Drost trial, the psychiatrist and critical occultist, Albert Moll, appeared before the district court in Berlin-Schönberg charged with having defamed the medium Maria Vollhardt (alias Rudloff).[93] Supported by some of Berlin's most prominent parapsychologists, the plaintiff, the medium's husband, argued that Moll's use of terms such as 'trick', 'manipulation' and 'farce' in reference to Vollhardt's phenomena, was libellous.[94] Moll had published a critical and, in places, satirical account of this medium's phenomena in his book *Der Spiritismus* [*Spiritualism*] (1924) after attending a séance which he believed to have been composed entirely of coarse tricks.[95] In the three-part trial that followed, both parties paraded a series of expert witnesses before the bench, figures including Max Planck (1858–1947), Max Dessoir and Walther Kröner, in order to argue their cases. Moll reproduced for the court a number of the medium's phenomena, pulling a beech-wood tree branch out of the air, for example, while the judge controlled his hands.[96] He also argued that as there existed no consensus within parapsychology over the conditions under which experiments should take place, the appropriate methodological approach or even which phenomena should be studied, he was free to express the opinion he had formed on occultism through four decades of observation and experimentation.[97] Despite the prosecution's best efforts to prove his maliciousness, the charges against Moll were dismissed by the court under §193 of the Reich Criminal Code, a clause intended to safeguard so-called legitimate interests or 'Wahrnehmung berechtigter Interessen' [justifiable differences of opinion].[98]

The significance of these proceedings, as a number of contemporaries were quick to recognise, was not Moll's eventual acquittal, but the use of the courtroom by both the prosecution and the defence as a platform from which to campaign for or against the reality of the paranormal. Albert von Schrenck-Notzing noted in this regard:

> The trial in no way limited itself to the actual facts of the case, rather it turned into a bitter struggle between the opponents and supporters of parapsychology, commanding every means of rhetoric, legalese and specialist knowledge, and considered from this point of view was of universal interest.[99]

This case, which on closer inspection had less to do with Moll's insult of the medium and more to do with his critique of some of Berlin's leading occultists, revolved around parapsychology's claim to scientific status.[100] It also initiated a series of ongoing and increasingly bitter quarrels, in the courtroom and in print, over parapsychological expertise and authority.

The prosecution's argument in the Rudloff–Moll case centred on the question of whether Moll's criticism of Vollhardt, and those occultists who had vouchsafed her phenomena, had gone beyond the acceptable bounds of critique in this field. While the prosecution maintained that this case revolved around libel, the underlying issue appears to have been the status of parapsychology as an emerging science. Admonishing the defence counsel to concentrate on the questions at hand, Rudloff's lawyer outlined the questions on which the court's decision rested:

> The representative of the accused keeps trying to change the focus. This is not about the question of the existence of occult phenomena, rather it is about the accusation of deception; even if the word fraud is not there it is all the same. Is it right that the medium could be accused of such deception or not? Evidence about this must be presented.[101]

Hellwig, who appeared as an expert witness for the defence, agreed with the prosecution that the reality of occult phenomena was not at stake here. However, Moll's guilt or innocence, he argued, was dependent on there being a consensus about the facts within this field:

> We are also in agreement that the case of Rudloff versus Moll can prove nothing for and nothing against the reality of occult phenomena.... But conflict prevails between us over whether occult phenomena, in accordance with the current state of our knowledge, can be viewed as already proven or not.[102]

Moll's comments about Vollhardt's phenomena could not be considered libellous if, as Hellwig contended, the prevailing scientific opinion was that there existed no conclusive proof for the reality of the occult.[103]

The prosecution, in its exposition of the current state of research on occultism, implied that Moll had denied the existence of phenomena that had been accepted and accredited by the scientific community.[104] Rudloff's lawyer, for example, listed the names of sixty persons of scientific, intellectual and cultural repute who had verified the existence of physical phenomena, similar to that exhibited by Vollhardt, in one of Albert von Schrenck-Notzing's publications.[105] He asked Moll whether he disputed the statements of these assorted luminaries, or whether he believed that all of these prominent figures had been deluded.[106] Moll replied that the validity of such results would only be confirmed through extensive repetition of the Baron's experiments. Until such time, he maintained, everyone had the right to express their opinion.[107] In this context, the statements of so-called authorities carried little weight. Quoting one of his correspondents, Hellwig reiterated this point:

> [N]ot the most beautiful protocol, not the authority of the greatest scholars, rather only personal experience is capable of convincing the unprejudiced person. For this reason I maintain that it is pointless when so many parapsychologists hope through books, writings, talks and collections of the statements of authorities etc. to achieve general recognition of the reality of parapsychological phenomena.[108]

What the representatives of parapsychology desperately needed to do, Hellwig maintained, was abandon their fetishism of authority in favour of experimentation that would establish the laws and rules governing occult phenomena.

The reliance within this field on authority was not the only issue over which parapsychologists and critical occultists fought during the course of this trial; the concept of expertise also proved problematic. The prerequisites for, and parameters of, occult expertise became a contentious issue during the Rudloff–Moll trial, where the question of what could legitimately be said about the paranormal and who should be allowed to say it was at stake. While the trials of criminal telepaths had featured questions about the qualifications and prejudices of the expert witnesses, challenges of this nature were more pronounced here. This was because civil proceedings in German courts, unlike criminal cases, were adversarial in nature.[109] As part of his defence Moll, for example, ruthlessly examined Kröner asking questions such as 'Do you know the book by X?', 'Have you read the article in Y?', in an effort to demonstrate what he believed were crucial gaps in this witness' knowledge of the parapsychological cannon.[110] He then proceeded to attack Kröner on the basis that he had long utilised a medium for diagnostic purposes in his homeopathic practice. Lawyers for the prosecution, Herr Tarnowski and Herr Winterberg, similarly attempted to negate the arguments of the philosopher Max Dessoir and the jurist Albert Hellwig, who appeared as expert witnesses for the defence. They sought to undermine the testimony of these experts by relating to the court their disputes and disagreements with prominent occultists.[111] Hellwig's debate with Professor Verweyen in Bonn and his apparent difference of opinion with the criminalist Max Hagemann over the utility of criminal telepathy, were manipulated by the prosecution to imply the dubious nature of his parapsychological expertise.[112] The personal tone of these attacks, which involved accusations not only of lack of experience and competence, but of bad faith and psychological disturbance, saw the Rudloff–Moll trial spark a series of libel suits, the reverberations of which were still being felt during the 1930s.

In November 1925, Hellwig found himself at the centre of two sets of private proceedings. The first was brought against him by the parapsychologist Schröder for comments made in the *Frankfurter Zeitung* in an article entitled 'Geist und Geister' ['Intellect and Ghosts'] and the second was launched by Schröder, Sünner and Winterberg for the use of the term 'objecktive Unverschämtheiten' [objective outrageousness] during the Rudloff–Moll trial.[113] Hellwig's use of this phrase referred to Schröder's selective use of ellipsis in a passage he had quoted from Max Hagemann, deputy head of the Kriminalpolizei, or Kripo [Criminal Police], about the Criminal Investigation Department's use of criminal telepaths. Much had been made by the prosecution during Moll's trial, of Hellwig's negative stance on criminal telepathy and the ostensibly favourable position of the Berlin Criminal Police, as represented by Hagemann, on the use of clairvoyants. Schröder had quoted Hagemann as saying that, 'nevertheless we will not reject the help offered by such persons without further details, because frequently their activities... have led the police on the right track.'[114]

Schröder's use of ellipsis, as Hellwig pointed out, completely altered the meaning of Hagemann's sentence. Between the words 'activities' and 'police' Hagemann had written 'without transcendental powers thereby coming into play'. This was, according to Hellwig, either a conscious distortion of the facts committed in bad faith or an unbelievable misunderstanding.[115] The term 'objective outrageousness', as Moll recalled, was thus used with complete justification to describe the behaviour of Schröder and Sünner, who had attacked Hellwig's honour in full knowledge that their argument was based on a lie.[116]

Both parties attempted through such court proceedings to prove the unsuitability of their opponents as experts on occult matters. Winterberg, Schröder and Sünner, as we have seen, decried Hellwig's lack of knowledge about, and unfounded prejudice against, occultism, while Hellwig countered that these occultists were intellectual children who, like mediums, attempted to distract their opponents with 'Spiegelfechterei' [shadow boxing].[117] This rather uncivilised debate about who should be allowed to shape the scientific and public response to the paranormal was continued through a series of bitter polemics in newspapers and periodicals. Hellwig, for his part, produced a series of pamphlets and newspaper articles that attempted to refute the arguments levelled against him in court and in parapsychological journals including the *Psychische Studien*.[118] He was particularly concerned to answer the accusations made by Schröder in his article 'Pseudoentlarvungen' ['Pseudo-exposures']. In reply to Schröder's accusation that he lacked the experience necessary to pronounce on occult matters, Hellwig pointed to his years of study of the relationship between crime and occultism and to his acceptance by courts, police and journals, in the fields of criminology and medicine, as an expert on the subject.[119] Schröder's implication that jurists lacked the intellectual tools necessary to speak competently on occult questions was also countered by Hellwig. As a result of the lack of epistemological and methodological consensus in this field, he argued, there existed no apprenticeship or course of study that specifically equipped one to deal with parapsychological questions.[120] In the absence of such training, he maintained, the sharp logic and objectivity of jurists made them ideal candidates for expertise in this field.[121]

Bickering of this nature continued well into the 1930s with Kröner's publication of the character study 'Hellwig *ante portas*' (1930) in which he decried the jurist's obstinate disbelief. In this article, Kröner identified two pillars of anti-occultism: the so-called big inquisitor, Moll, and the little inquisitor, Hellwig. He wrote that '[Hellwig] displays an almost rabbit-like fertility in the production of pompous newspaper articles, whose quality stands in inverse proportion to their quantity....'[122] Nearly a decade later, Kröner and Hellwig crossed swords again, this time over Kröner's book *Die*

Wiedergeburt des Magischen [*The Rebirth of Magic*] (1939) in which he described Hellwig as both a 'materialistic enlightener' and a 'medium-eating district court director'.[123] Hans Driesch, whom Kröner had asked to provide a foreword for this book, found himself in the middle of this dispute. In a letter to Driesch, addressing the vitalist's concerns about the personal attacks on Hellwig contained in this book, Kröner wrote:

> As I have already said in 'Hellwig ante portas' and in my correspondence with Hörmann, with Hellwig it is absolutely not a matter of his scientific position on these things, rather it is about his character and his personality.[124]

Hellwig wrote to Driesch asking him whether he agreed with Kröner and whether the attack on 'un-reformable dogmatic nay-sayers' that appeared in his foreword referred to him.[125] Like Kröner, he also argued that he was not opposed to his opponent's scientific position, but that he was concerned with those pathological aspects of his adversary's personality that led him to make personal attacks. Such disputes served only to demonstrate the failure of either group to satisfactorily resolve the questions surrounding the nature of parapsychological authority and expertise during the Weimar Republic.

Civil proceedings between parapsychologists and critical occultists made clear the lack of an epistemological or methodological consensus about the paranormal in Germany. The use and manufacture of authority as well as the nature of expertise in this context were and remained contentious issues in the courtroom throughout the inter-war period. Under these circumstances, where there existed no agreement about which, if any, paranormal phenomena were worthy of study, nor any appropriate methodological approach to the occult nor criteria for parapsychological authority and expertise, it was difficult to maintain that Moll had transgressed the acceptable bounds of critique in this field. Attacks on Hellwig for his unfounded bias and lack of expertise were also difficult to sustain given the lack of consensus about what best qualified one to deal with parapsychological questions, let alone what these questions should be. The increasingly personal nature of these attacks on both sides, intimations of intellectual paucity and mental disturbance, demonstrated the inability of these men to agree upon epistemological and methodological matters. These cases, which appear ultimately to have revolved around the status of parapsychology as a nascent science and who could legitimately pronounce on it, found no adequate resolution in the courtroom during the Weimar Republic.

Conclusion

Parapsychologists' attempts to use the courtroom as a platform for their epistemological and professional ambitions during the Weimar years met with equal measures of success and failure. The trials of occultists accused of fraud or *Gaukelei* afforded parapsychologists an opportunity to present the results of their experimentation to the public and to portray parapsychology as a legitimate new science. Their secondment to the court as expert witnesses also enabled them to meet their opponents head on, pointing to their lack of practical experience and the paucity of their understanding in this field. Judges, however, were ultimately not interested in or capable of deciding the reality of the paranormal, basing their judgements instead on legal criteria such as goodwill and financial gain. While these cases provided the public hearing, in the form of widespread and sensational press coverage, that parapsychologists craved, they ultimately served to expose the epistemic fault lines with which parapsychology in the German context was fraught.

Beyond the publicity they provided for parapsychologists, the trials of criminal telepaths were opportunities for credibility contests and boundary-work between those groups of disciplines which sought jurisdiction over the occult. While for the jurist it was clear that the occultist was a criminal, perhaps an habitual one, the psychiatrist was convinced that he was concerned with a mentally abnormal individual, and the parapsychologist maintained that he dealt with an experimental subject. Just as psychiatrists and jurists were fighting for a monopoly over the criminal in the Republic's courtrooms, so too were psychiatrists, jurists and parapsychologists squabbling over the ambiguous figure of the occultist; linking the trials of Weimar occultists with the disciplinary and professional histories of applied sciences, such as forensic psychology and psychiatry.

Tensions between parapsychologists and critical occultists, apparent in the trials of occultists and criminal telepaths, boiled over in a series of civil proceedings in which authority and expertise formed the crux of their disagreements. The lack of consensus about the epistemological and methodological basis of parapsychology ensured that questions about the nature of parapsychological expertise and the function of authority in this field could not be resolved. It also saw such cases degenerate into personal attacks in which the integrity and mental stability of one's opponent could be questioned. These libel cases revealed, perhaps more starkly than the trials of criminal telepaths like Elsa Günther-Gethers and hypnotists like August Drost, the instabilities within this field around the issues of ontology and epistemology, offering succour to those who wished to analyse the occult in terms of either intellectual error or personal pathology.

Notes

1. On Claire Reichart, see 'Die Hellseherin Claire Reichart', *Stettiner-Abendspost*, Nr. 45, 23 February 1926, in: Nachlaß Albert Hellwig 10/4 Hellsehen allgemein. Korrespondenz, 1914–1929 IGPP; 'Ein neuer Hellseherprozess', *Deutsche Zeitung*, 4 November 1925, in: GStA PK, I. HA Rep. 84a Nr. 10993. On Friedrich Gern and his wife, see T.K. Oesterreich, *Psychologisches Gutachten in einem Hellseherprozess*, (Stuttgart: W. Kohlhammer, 1930), 1.

2. R. Winterberg, 'Der Insterburger Hellseher-Prozeß', *Zeitschrift für Parapsychologie*, 3, 7 (1928), 420–2.

3. Thomas Gieryn has identified the courtroom and the press as arenas 'ripe' for 'juicy' episodes of boundary-work. Both are settings in which tacit assumptions about the contents of science are forced to become explicit and in which credibility is contested. This certainly appears to be the case in the trials of occultists in which parapsychologists and critical occultists appeared as expert witnesses. See T. Gieryn, *Cultural Boundaries of Science: Credibility on the Line* (Chicago: University of Chicago Press, 1999), 24.

4. I am referring here to the work of Corinna Treitel and Benjamin Carter Hett on the early twentieth century trial of the medium Anna Rothe. Treitel has discussed this case as part of her exploration of the relationship between occultism and modernity in Germany, while Hett has considered the Rothe trial in his cultural–historical analysis of criminal trials in Imperial Berlin. See C. Treitel, 'The Culture of Knowledge in the Metropolis of Science: Spiritualism and Liberalism in Fin-de-Siècle Berlin', in C. Goschler (ed.) *Wissenschaft und Oeffentlichkeit in Berlin* (Stuggart: Franz Steiner, 2000), 127–54; B. Carter-Hett, *Death in the Tiergarten: Murder and Criminal Justice in the Kaiser's Berlin* (Cambridge: Harvard University Press, 2004), 153–5.

5. W. Gaudlitz, 'Okkultismus und Strafgesetz', (unpublished PhD dissertation: University of Leipzig, 1932), 6.

6. A. Hellwig, *Okkultismus und Verbrechen: Eine Einführung in die kriminalistischen Probleme des Okkultismus für Polizeibeamte, Richter, Staatsanwälte, Psychiater und Sachverständige* (Berlin: Dr P. Langenscheidt, 1929), 25.

7. For more detailed information on criminal telepathy and its use by the Weimar police, see C. Treitel, *A Science for the Soul: Occultism and the Genesis of the German Modern* (Baltimore: Johns Hopkins University Press, 2004), 143–50; H. Wolffram, 'Crime, Clairvoyance and the Weimar Police', *Journal of Contemporary History*, 44, 4 (2009), 581–601.

8. Drost's case received extensive coverage in the press, in occult and parapsychological journals and in a number of books. See, for example, O. Seeling, *Der Bernburger Hellseher-Prozeß, mit Bild und Schriftprobe des Lehrers*

Drost nebst einem Vorwort von Rechtsanwalt Dr Winterberg (Berlin-Pankow: Linser, 1925).

9. Hellwig, *op. cit.* (note 6), 23.

10. *Ibid.*, 237; Richard Winterberg maintained that the question of good faith, around which the court's decision had revolved in Bernburg, did not appear in the legislation on fraud. He argued that Hellwig had introduced this concept specifically for the prosecution of telepaths, astrologers and clairvoyants. Hellwig countered that every young jurist in the country and many lay people were aware that the law required proof that the defendant did not believe in the reality of the facts in question. See, Winterberg, *op. cit.* (note 2), 417.

11. Hellwig, *ibid.*, 237.

12. *Ibid.*, 237–8.

13. A. Hellwig, 'Hellsehen als strafbare Gaukelei', *Archiv für Strafrecht*, 71 (1927), 125; A. Hellwig, 'Gaukelei nach dem preußischen Allgemeinen Landrecht', *Archiv für Kriminologie*, 31 (1908), 322.

14. According to a 1908 article by Hellwig, Alsace-Lorraine also had a *Gaukelei* clause. Hellwig, 'Gaukelei', *op. cit.* (note 13), 322.

15. These *Gaukeleiparagraphen* by and large existed before Bismarck's 1886 plea to state governments to create new policies for dealing with both foreign and domestic gypsies. While such clauses naturally aimed to prohibit instances of fortune telling by gypsies, they regarded these itinerant travellers as but one species of mountebank among many. For further information on Bismarck's attempt to deal with the gypsy menace see A. Fraser, *The Gypsies*, 2nd edn (Oxford: Blackwell, 1995), 249–50.

16. 'Wer gegen Lohn oder zur Erreichung eines sonstigen Vorteils sich mit angeblichen Zaubereien oder Geisterbeschwörungen, mit Wahrsagen, Kartenschlagen, Schatzgraben, Zeichen- und Traumdeuten oder anderen dergleichen Gaukeleien abgibt, wird an Geld bis zu 150 Mark oder mit Haft bestraft.' Gaudlitz, *op. cit.* (note 5), 28.

17. In Baden a *Gaukeleiparagraph* was included in the statute books as early as 1863, in Hessen in 1855, and in Bavaria in 1871. Prussia during the eighteenth and nineteenth centuries had similar laws, which had ceased to be used by the early twentieth century, see Hellwig, 'Gaukelei', *op. cit.* (note 13), 322–3. Hellwig, *op. cit.* (note 6), 25, fn. 34

18. A. Brieschke, '"Ein so klägliches Bild ist von keinem Kriminaltelepathen bekannt." Ein Hellseher-Prozess in Württemberg in den 1920er Jahren' (unpublished MA thesis: University of Tübingen, 2001), 12.

19. Hellwig, 'Hellsehen', *op. cit.* (note 13), 128.

20. C. du Prel, *Der Somnambulismus vor dem königlichen Landgerichte München I.* (Munich: Knorr & Hirth, n.d), 1–2.

21. *Ibid.*, 1–2.

22. 'Die Hellseherin Claire Reichart', *op. cit.* (note 1).
23. *Ibid.*; 'Kleine Mitteilung' *Zeitschrift für Parapsychologie* 1 (1926), 383.
24. Hellwig, *op. cit.* (note 6), 25.
25. *Ibid.*, 25.
26. Hellwig, 'Hellsehen', *op. cit.* (note 13), 125.
27. Du Prel, *op. cit.* (note 20), 2.
28. 'Wer immer den genannten Artikel stilisirt haben mag, stand auf dem Standpunkt der sogenannten Aufklärung und des modernen Materialismus. Danach ist ein Fernsehen einfach nicht möglich; wer also wahrsagt und sich dafür bezahlen läßt, treibt Gaukelei.' *Ibid.*, 2.
29. Hellwig, 'Hellsehen', op. *cit.* (note 13), 127.
30. *Ibid.*
31. *Ibid.*, 129.
32. *Ibid.*, 128.
33. Hellwig, 'Gaukelei', op. *cit.* (note 13), 322.
34. Winterberg, *op. cit.* (note 2), 425.
35. Bekämpfung des Wahrsagens im Entwurf StGB. Aus: Die Innere Mission im ev. Deutschland, Heft 4 April 1928), in: ADW, CA, AC-S 1 Aberglaube. On the concept of, and concern about, the career criminal in Weimar Germany, see P. Wagner, *Volksgemeinschaft ohne Verbrecher: Konzeption und Praxis der Kriminalpolizei in der Zeit der Weimarer Republik und des Nationalsozialismus* (Hamburg: Christians, 1996), 19–76.
36. *Ibid.*
37. *Ibid.* On attempts to revise the penal code during the Weimar years, see R.F. Wetzell, *Inventing the Criminal: A History of German Criminology, 1880–1945* (Chapel Hill: University of North Carolina Press, 2000), 120–2.
38. Hellwig, 'Hellsehen', *op. cit.* (note 13), 130, n.4.
39. The draft code that became the basis for parliamentary deliberation in 1927 was debated and amended for several years, but was never implemented because of the dissolution of parliamentary government following 1930; Wetzell, *op. cit.* (note 37), 121.
40. Corinna Treitel provides a succinct guide in her book to a number of other criminal telepaths and their trials, see Treitel, *op. cit.* (note 7), 145.
41. Brieschke, *op. cit.* (note 18), 10.
42. A. Hellwig, 'Glossen zum Bernburger Hellseherprozess', *Frankfurter Allgemeine Zeitung,* 31 October 1925, in: GStA Rep. 84a Nr. 10993.
43. Hellwig, *op. cit.* (note 6), 88.
44. 'Hypnotiseur oder Betrüger?', *Vossische Zeitung,* 12 October 1925, in Nachlaß Albert Hellwig 10/4 Korrespondenz 1924–1926, IGPP.
45. 'Ein Medium-Prozeß', *Lokalanzeiger Berlin,* 11 Oktober 1925, in Nachlaß Albert Hellwig 10/4 Korrespondenz 1924–1926, IGPP.
46. 'Hypnotiseur oder Betrüger?' *op. cit.* (note 44).

47. A. Freckmann and T. Wegerich, *The German Legal System* (London: Sweet & Maxwell, 1999), 207. While German judges, who were responsible for the examination of witnesses and experts, decided what evidence was permissible, in practice little, if any, evidence was inadmissible. See E.A. Johnson, *Urbanization and Crime: Germany 1871–1914* (Cambridge: Cambridge University Press, 1995), 44.

48. 'Gericht überprüft Medium', *Germania,* 9 Februar 1937, in ADW, CA, AC-S 273 Okkultismus.

49. Kriminaltelepathischer Versuch durch Amtsgericht Zossen. 17 November 1925, in: Nachlaß Albert Hellwig 10/4 Hellsehen/Fall Höpfner, IGPP.

50. Bemerkungen von Amtsgerichsrat Foerste zu dem kriminaltelepathischen Versuch, 19 November 1925, in Nachlaß Albert Hellwig 10/4 Hellsehen/Fall Höpfner, IGPP.

51. 'Der Freispruch im Drost-Prozeß', *Anhalter Kurier,* 19 October 1925, in GStA Rep. 84a Nr. 10993.

52. Hellwig, *op. cit.* (note 6), 237–8.

53. *Ibid.,* 211.

54. Du Prel, *op. cit.* (note 20), 1.

55. *Ibid.,* 3.

56. 'Der Bernburger Hellseherprozess', *Frankfurter Zeitung,* 17 October 1925; 'Der Bernburger Hellseherprozess', *Frankfurter Zeitung,* 19 October 1925, in GStA Rep. 84a Nr. 10993. On the role of the scientific expert in the courtroom, see the sociological analyses offered in R. Smith and B. Wynne (eds), *Expert Evidence: Interpreting Science in the Law* (London: Routledge, 1989).

57. 'Es ist nicht Sache des Gerichts zu entscheiden, ob wissenschaftlich feststeht, dass auf übernatürlichem Wege Erkentnisse erlangt werden, inbesondere, ob diese Erkentnisse zur Aufklärung von strafbaren Handlungen verwandt werden können. Es ist auch nicht Sache des Gerichts, festzustellen, ob die von den Angeklagten benutzten Medien die Fähigkeit besitzen im hypnotischen Zustande übernatürliche Erkentnisse zu vermitteln. Das Gericht hat nur zu entscheiden, ob sich der Angeklagte im Sinne der Anklage schuldig gemacht hat, zunächst des Betruges…', 'Der Freispruch im Drost-Prozeß', *op. cit.* (note 51).

58. Hellwig, *op. cit.* (note 6), 88. Similarly, Benjamin Hett, in his analysis of the Anna Rothe case, has demonstrated how the court's verdict could be seen to legitimise a belief in the spirit world. See Carter-Hett, *op. cit.* (note 4), 155.

59. Hellwig, *op. cit.* (note 6), 89.

60. In her study of the Gern trial, Angelika Brieschke mentions the unreliable and often ludicrous press coverage the case received. On this basis she decides against the use of newspaper articles as source material. Here it is the very inaccuracy and silliness of the press coverage that interests me because it

was this that helped shape the response of the public to criminal telepathy. Brieschke, *op. cit.* (note 18), 6–7.

61. 'Streiflicher auf den Bernburger Hellseher-Prozess', *Ihr Tag,* 3 November 1925, in GStA Rep. 84a Nr. 10993.

62. Hellwig, *op. cit.* (note 6), 95.

63. '[D]er Einfluß der Zeitungsberichte während dieses Prozesses auf einen großen Teil der Zeugen ist nicht zu unterschätzen.' R. Lambert, 'Der Insterburger Prozeß gegen die hellseherin Frau Günther-Geffers', *Zeitschrift für Parapsychologie,* 4, 4 (1929), 353

64. Hellwig, *op. cit.* (note 6), 94.

65. Der Freispruch im Drost-Prozess', *op. cit.* (note 51).

66. 'Hellwig über den Fall Drost', *Vossische Zeitung,* 30 October 1925, in GStA Rep. 84a Nr. 10993.

67. S.F. Hall, 'The Subject under Investigation: Weimar Culture and the Police', (unpublished PhD dissertation: University of California, Berkeley, 2000), vii.

68. I. Deak, *Weimar Germany's Left-Wing Intellectuals: A Political History of the Weltbühne and Its Circle* (Berkeley: University of California Press, 1968), 122–129; C. Schöningh, *'Kontrolliert die Justiz': Die Vertrauenskrise der Weimarer Justiz im Spiegel der Gerichtsreportagen von Weltbühne, Tagebuch und Vossischer Zeitung* (Munich: Fink, 2000).

69. P. Fritzsche, *Reading Berlin 1900* (Cambridge: Harvard University Press, 1996), 159.

70. *Ibid.,* 158.

71. S.E. Elder, 'Murder Scenes: Criminal Violence in the Public Culture and Private Lives of Weimar Berlin', (unpublished PhD dissertation: University of Illinois, 2002), 4.

72. H.H. Liang, *The Berlin Police Force in the Weimar Republic* (Berkeley: University of California Press, 1970), 115. On the ambiguous relationship between the police and the press, see Elder, *op. cit.* (note 71), 9.

73. Hellwig, *op. cit.* (note 6), 93.

74. *Ibid.,* 94.

75. M. Eksteins, *The Limits of Reason: The German Democratic Press and the Collapse of Weimar Democracy* (London: Oxford University Press, 1975), 71.

76. *Ibid.,* 71.

77. A. Hellwig, 'Der Hellseher von Rothenstein', *Zeitschrift für kritischen Okkultismus und Grenzfragen des Seelenlebens,* 3, 1 (1927), 8.

78. A. Hellwig, 'Ein betrügerischer Kriminaltelepath', *Zeitschrift für kritischen Okkultismus und Grenzfragen des Seelenlebens* 3, 1 (1927), 131.

79. *Ibid.,* 131.

80. Hellwig, *op. cit.* (note 77), 1–2.

81. *Ibid.,* 2.

82. *Ibid.,* 6.

83. *Ibid.*, 1.

84. Gieryn, *op. cit.* (note 3), 24.

85. S.M. Solomon and E.J. Hackett, 'Setting Boundaries between Science and Law: Lessons from *Daubert v. Merrell Dow Pharmaceuticals, Inc.*', *Science, Technology & Human Values*, 21, 2 (1996), 132.

86. *Ibid.*, 149.

87. Freckmann and Wegerich, *op. cit.* (note 47), 196.

88. Johnson, *op. cit.* (note 47), 44.

89. Hellwig, *op. cit.* (note 6), 103.

90. *Ibid.*, 103.

91. Hellwig, 'Hellsehen', *op. cit.* (note 13), 130.

92. W. Kröner, 'Hellwig ante portas!' *Zeitschrift für Parapsychologie*, 5, 10 (1930), 630.

93. For biographical information, see F. Schwab, *Teleplasma und Telekinese: Ergebnisse meiner zweijährigen Experimentalsitzungen mit dem Berliner Medium Maria Vollhardt* (Berlin: Pyramidenverlag, 1923).

94. Niederschrift über meinen gestrigen Zusammenstoss mit den Vertretern des Privatklägers Rudloff in der Beleidigungsklage Rudloff gegen Moll vor dem Amtsgericht Berlin-Schöneberg Abt. 20/21 9. Juli 1925, in: Nachlaß Albert Hellwig 10/4 Korrespondenz 1924–1926, IGPP.

95. A. Moll, *Der Spiritismus* (Stuttgart: Franckh'sche Verlagshandlung, 1924), 37.

96. W. Kröner, 'Epilog zur Moll-Polemik', *Zeitschrift für Parapsychologie*, 1, 3 (1926), 161.

97. Moll disputed the grounds on which he was acquitted in 1926, maintaining it was not possible to commit libel in a context in which the reality of the phenomena in question remained open. See E. Buchner, 'Der Mollprozeß in zweiter Auflage', *Zeitschrift für Parapsychologie*, 3 (1926), 155.

98. A. Hellwig, 'Geist und Geister', *Frankfurter Zeitung*, 26 July 1925, in: Nachlaß Albert Hellwig 10/4 Gerichtssache Moll vs Rudloff, 1925, IGPP.

99. 'Der Prozeß beschränkte sich keineswegs auf den eigentlichen Tatbestand, sondern wuchs sich aus zu einem heftigen, mit allen Mitteln der Rhetorik, der Juristerei und des Fachwissens geführten Kampf zwischen den Gegnern und Anhängern der Parapsychologie und war, unter diesem Gesichtspunkt betrachtet, von allgemeinem Interesse.' A. von Schrenck-Notzing, 'Die Entwicklung des Okkultismus zur Parapsychologie in Deutschland', *Zeitschrift für Parapsychologie*, 7, 7 (1932), 307.

100. Moll's brochure was particularly critical of the séance protocol published by the leading Berlin occultist Dr Friedrich Schwab who had experimented extensively with Vollhardt. See Niederschrift über meinen gestrigen Zusammenstoss mit den Vertretern des Privatklägers Rudloff', *op. cit.* (note 94).

101. 'Der Vertreter des Angeklagten versucht immer den Gesichtpunkt zu verschieben. Es handelt sich nicht um die Frage der Existenz okkulter Phänomene, sondern es handelt sich um den Vorwurf der Täuschung; wenn auch das Wort Betrug nicht darinsteht, ist das gleichgültig. Ist es richtig, dass solche Täuschung dem Medium vorgeworfen werden kann oder nicht? Darüber muss Beweis erhoben werden....' Privatklage Rudloff gegen Moll am 4. Juli 1925, in Nachlaß Albert Hellwig 10/4 Gerichtssache Moll vs Rudloff, 1925, IGPP.

102. 'Einig sind wir auch darin, dass der Prozess Rudloff gegen Moll nichts für und nichts gegen die Echtheit der Okkultisten-Phänomene bewiesen konnte.... Streit aber herrscht zwischen uns darüber, ob die okkulten Phänomene nach dem gegenwärtigen Stande unseres Wissens schon als erwiesen angesehen werden können oder nicht.' A. Hellwig, 'Der Okkultismus im Lichte des Berliner Okkultistenprozesses', in Nachlaß Albert Hellwig 10/4 Gerichtssache Moll vs Rudloff, 1925, IGPP.

103. *Ibid.*

104. Der Mollprozess in der Berufungsinstanz', *Der Okkultismus* 2, 3 (1926), 103–4.

105. This list was derived from A. von Schrenck-Notzing, *Experimente der Fernbewegung*, (Stuttgart: Union Deutsche Verlagsgesellschaft, 1924).

106. Privatklage Rudloff gegen Moll, *op. cit.* (note 101).

107. *Ibid.*, 16–17.

108. '[N]icht die schönsten Protokolle, nicht die Autorität selbst der grössten Gelehrten, sondern nur die eigene Erfahrung den Unvoreingenommen zu überzeugen vermag. Ich halte es deshalb auch für aussichtlos, wenn so manche Parapsychologen zu erreichen hoffen, durch Bücher, Schriften, Vorträge, Zusammenstellungen der Aeusserungen von Autoritäten usw eine allgemeine Anerkennung der Realität der parapsychologischen Erscheinungen zu erzielen.' Hellwig, *op. cit.* (note 102).

109. Freckmann and Wegerich, *op. cit.* (note 47), 146.

110. Buchner, *op. cit.* (note 97), 159.

111. A. Moll to A. Hellwig, 18 July 1925, in: Nachlaß Albert Hellwig 10/4 Korrespondenz 1924–1926, IGPP.

112. Schröder had argued, contrary to Hellwig, in the *Berliner Börsen-Zeitung* that the Berlin police, as represented by Hagemann, were strongly in favour of the use of criminal telepaths. As Hellwig was to point out, however, this impression was only achieved by a dishonest use of ellipsis in a quote from Hagemann. See A. Hellwig, 'Zur Psychologie der Okkultisten', in: Nachlaß Albert Hellwig 10/4 Korrespondenz 1924–1926, IGPP.

113. A. Hellwig to Oberregierungsrat Hagemann, 30 November 1925, in: Nachlaß Albert Hellwig 10/4 Korrespondenz 1924–1926, IGPP.

114. 'Dennoch werde man die angebotene Hilfe solcher Personen nicht ohne weiteres zurückweisen, dann häufig hatte ihre Tätigkeit... die Polizei auf die richtige Fährte gefurht.' Hellwig, *op. cit.* (note 112).
115. *Ibid.*
116. A. Moll to A. Hellwig, 18 July 1925, in: Nachlaß Albert Hellwig 10/4 Korrespondenz 1924–1926, IGPP.
117. Hellwig, *op. cit.* (note 112).
118. A. Hellwig, 'Pseudoentlarvungen', in: Nachlaß Albert Hellwig 10/4 Korrespondenz 1924–1926, IGPP.
119. *Ibid.*
120. *Ibid.*
121. *Ibid.*
122. '[Z]eigte sich um so kregler und entfaltete eine geradezu kaninchenhafte Fruchtbarkeit in der Producktion von hochtrabenden Zeitungsartikeln, deren Qualität in umgekehrter Proportion zur Quantität stand....' Kröner, *op. cit.* (note 92), 631.
123. Kröner, *ibid.*, 630–44; A. Hellwig to H. Driesch, 8 March 1939, in: Nachlaß 250 Hans Driesch, UBL.
124. '[W]ie ich schon in "Hellwig ante portas" und in meinem Briefwechsel mit Hörmann betont habe, handelt es sich bei Hellwig ja garnicht um seine wissenschaftliche Stellungnahme zu den Dingen, sondern um seinen Charkter und seine Persönlichkeit.' W. Kröner to H. Driesch, 8 April 1938, in: Nachlaß 250 Hans Driesch, UBL.
125. A. Hellwig to H. Driesch, 8 March 1939, in: Nachlaß 250 Hans Driesch, UBL.

6

Parapsychology on the Couch:
The Psychology of Occult Belief in Germany

Introduction

In the wake of the 1925 Rudloff–Moll trial, during which the struggle between parapsychologists and their critics to mould the scientific and public responses to occultism had centred on issues of expertise and authority, Albert Hellwig reflected that the proceedings had done little to clarify the question of the reality of occult phenomena, simply casting light on the psychology of certain occult researchers.[1] The insistence of the Berlin occultists, Dr Schröder, Dr Schwab and Dr Sünner, for example, on the veracity of Frau Vollhardt's apports, in spite of compelling evidence to the contrary, served only to convince their adversaries of the pathology of their thought processes as they concerned occult phenomena. Hellwig's observation of the parapsychological psyche, as manifested during this trial, persuaded him of the necessity of a psychological study not only of occult research, as a means of determining the multiple sources of sensory and intellectual error within this field, but also of occult researchers, both individually and in the collective. He wrote:

> All of us who have been critically engaged with occult problems will have experienced that the main difficulty therein lies in that here is a totally different measure than in scientific investigation of other types, everything stands or falls with trust in the personality of the experimenter. Experience shows unfortunately only too often, that even men, from whom one perhaps should not expect it, make bad mistakes without the slightest awareness, as soon as it comes to observation or experiments of an occult kind. The subjective conviction of a researcher stands not seldom in inverse relation to the reliability of their objective principles. It is therefore one of the most important tasks of critical occultism to establish the necessary basis for a psychology of occult research in general and a psychology of the individual occult researchers in particular.[2]

Despite Hellwig's claims that such psychological assessments need not deteriorate into personal attacks, their purpose being to help evaluate parapsychologists' work, the emergence of a psychology of occult belief in Germany served primarily to pathologise and discredit parapsychology and its practitioners.

This chapter attempts to track the emergence of a psychology of occult belief in the German context during the late nineteenth and early twentieth centuries. It argues that the growing emphasis placed on the psychological preconditions for occult belief by academic psychologists represented an attempt to discredit a group that threatened the credibility of their new science.[3] It contends, furthermore, that the failure of psychologists to adequately explain belief in all forms of paranormal phenomena in terms of either fraud or natural causes led to the development of three distinct, but complementary approaches to this problem. The first focused on the intellectual and sensory errors responsible for occult convictions, borrowing heavily from psycho-physics to develop a new sub-discipline known as the psychology of deception and belief. The second utilised the mass psychology of Gustave Le Bon (1841–1931) in order to explain, on the one hand, the positive testimony for the paranormal offered by a number of Germany's most respected cultural and intellectual luminaries and, on the other, the apparently contagious nature of occult belief. The third was a psychoanalytic approach, often used in conjunction with the second, which focused on deep-seated complexes and neurotic predispositions as a means of explaining both parapsychologists' stubborn belief in the occult and their persuasive power over others. Intended to bolster their jurisdictional claims, psychologists' transformation of psychical researchers and parapsychologists from intellectual rivals into objects of psychological inquiry, served ultimately to pathologise occult belief, making literal the pathology metaphor.[4] Not to be outdone, however, parapsychologists performed their own analyses, diagnosing their opponents with a pathological inability to acknowledge the occult. Unable to come to grips with the paranormal on phenomenological terms, this chapter argues, both of these groups chose to combat their opponents' competing knowledge claims with accusations of mental instability.

Psychological societies and experimental psychology

In Germany, the emergence of a psychology of occult belief was intimately connected with the efforts of experimental psychologists to distinguish their nascent science from the study of the paranormal. During the late nineteenth century, as we have seen, there appeared in German cities, including Berlin, Munich and Leipzig, a number of psychological societies dedicated to the experimental study of occult phenomena. These groups, which sought to combat a materialistic view of the mind through an exploration of hypnosis and thought-transference, routinely referred to their study of the unconscious as 'experimental psychology'.[5] The use of this term by those with an interest in somnambulistic and mediumistic phenomena proved problematic, however, for that group of academic psychologists who claimed the same name for the scientific psychology they had founded through the application of an experimental method, derived from physiology, to the study of the mind.[6] These psychologists feared that a connection with occult research would prove damaging to their new science, thwarting both their institutional and professional ambitions. Wilhelm Wundt outlined the problem in his book *Hypnotismus und Suggestion* [*Hypnotism and Suggestion*] (1892) in which he complained that the members of so-called psychological societies, who explored both the secret sciences and the inner life through hypnosis, claimed the term 'experimental psychology' for themselves, almost completely dismissing the contribution of psycho-physics.[7]

During the 1880s and 1890s, the success of experimental psychology as a scientific discipline was by no means assured. As a hybridisation of physiology and philosophy, this new science did not receive the level of sustained support enjoyed by other fields of experimental research, remaining a tenuously supported sub-speciality of philosophy well into the twentieth century.[8] In these circumstances, representatives of experimental psychology were quick to address threats to the scientific credentials of their discipline. The confusion, arising from psychical researchers' use of the term 'experimental psychology' to describe their experiments with paranormal phenomena, for example, posed a threat to the credibility of the new psychology, which forced psychologists such as Wilhelm Wundt and Hugo Münsterberg to publicly address the question of psychology's relationship to psychical research.

The need for experimental psychologists to differentiate their discipline from the scientific study of the paranormal was made more urgent by the German public's growing interest in this area. Shared nomenclature gave the public the impression that academic psychologists had vouchsafed the reality of occult phenomena such as thought-transference – an impression that psychologists feared would undermine their already tenuous position within the German university system. Eager to combat the threat that the taint of occultism posed to their scientific credibility, experimental psychologists sought explanations for the paranormal in terms of either fraud or natural causes. Adopting a phenomenological approach to the paranormal, a number of experimental psychologists, including Münsterberg, began to experiment with hypnosis and thought-transference. Their aim was to condemn 'experimental psychology' as practised by psychical researchers and to demystify the phenomena that they studied. In a paper presented at a meeting of the Akademische Gesellschaft zu Freiburg [Freiburg Academic

Society] in 1889, for example, Münsterberg described experimental psychology as an objective science concerned with examining and measuring mental phenomena, lamenting its confusion with those unmethodical experiments carried out in the darkened cabinets of spiritualists.[9] He went on to list the possible sources of error in those experiments dealing with thought-transference. This ostensibly occult phenomenon, he argued, could be explained in terms of tiny physical cues, emitted by a sender and consciously or unconsciously picked up by a receiver.[10] While Münsterberg did not fundamentally reject the possibility of a transference of thoughts at a distance, he did argue that if it did exist its explanation would lie in the causal laws of science.[11]

Wundt, in contrast, maintained that all occult phenomena were the products of fraud and need not be subjected to scientific analysis. His attendance at an experiment with Henry Slade in 1870, and his participation in the Zöllner debate, had convinced him not only of the entirely fraudulent nature of mediumship and its phenomena but also of the profound difference between mediumistic and psychological experiments.[12] Wundt's uncompromising stance was quite probably the result of his position as one of the founders of experimental psychology; in order to ensure the credibility of his new science he could not afford any accommodation with psychical research.[13] Wundt, who refused to speculate about the causes of such phenomena, rejected the paranormal on ethical, epistemological and methodological grounds. His ethical objection to occult phenomena lay in their relationship with hypnosis, which subsumed one individual's will to that of another. As an early representative of middle-class liberalism in Germany, the freedom of the individual was of fundamental importance to him.[14] Wundt's epistemological concerns about occultism stemmed from a belief in immutable scientific laws. If one were to believe the occultists, he argued, there were two worlds: one the world of Copernicus, Newton and Leibniz, in which there existed universal, unchanging laws; and the other, a world of poltergeists and magnetic mediums, who were capable of altering and manipulating these laws.[15] On the basis that such a world was impossible, he refused even to consider phenomena such as thought-transference. Wundt also identified methodological problems in the 'experimental psychology' of the psychical researchers. Their use of hypnosis as a form of psychological introspection, he argued, flawed their experiments. Hypnosis, Wundt maintained, was an abnormal state like dream or mania and could not, therefore, form the basis of psychological research.[16] Given this conviction, he was openly critical of those psychologists, including Forel, Moll and Münsterberg, who experimented in this field. He believed that such experiments, which often utilised hypnosis, endangered both the mental and physical health of the public and the credibility of experimental psychology.[17] While Wundt refused to acknowledge either the possibility that occult phenomena existed or the need to investigate them experimentally, a number of other experimental psychologists were conscious that an ethical, epistemological or methodological response to these phenomena did not lessen their threat to psychology. These researchers, inspired in part by developments in America, began to develop a new approach to the problem of occultism.

The psychology of deception and belief

Attempts to dismiss psychical research and discourage public interest in the paranormal also occurred in the United States during the late nineteenth and early twentieth centuries, fostered, in part, by Münsterberg, who relocated to Harvard University in 1893.[18] As in the German context, a small group of psychologists, concerned by the threat that psychical research posed to their nascent science and by the public's growing interest in the paranormal, conducted a series of mediumistic experiments in order to prove that occult phenomena were the products of either fraud or natural causes. While this approach helped demonstrate the high incidence of crude trickery in the séance room and the potential for messages and ideas to be transmitted through unconscious muscular movements, it failed, as many of these researchers realised, either to quash interest in the occult or to adequately explain it. This realisation led a number of psychologists, most notably Joseph Jastrow (1863–1944), who received the first doctorate in psychology, to develop a sub-discipline, the psychology of deception and belief.[19] Jastrow's essays in this field claimed that psychology had an authoritative claim to the occult, bringing these apparently irregular phenomena within the realm of normal mental life and demonstrating that misconceptions about them were the result of bad logic and defective observation, both of which tended to stem from inherent mental prepossessions.[20] This change of emphasis – the adoption of a psychological approach to the paranormal rather than a phenomenological one – was also evident in Germany, where those opposed to psychical research demonstrated an eagerness to develop a psychology of occult belief.

Faced with the enigmatic nature of belief in the paranormal, German psychologists, in particular the critical occultists Max Dessoir and Albert Moll, began to concentrate, during the *fin de siècle*, on the question of how seemingly rational people found it possible to believe in the occult. This question marked a movement away from those explanations of the paranormal, favoured by psychologists like Münsterberg and Wundt, that focused either on fraud, to which mediums were believed to be predisposed by an hysterical temperament, or on the naturalistic explanation of these phenomena.[21] Such explanations were replaced by analyses of occult belief in which the psychology of those who provided positive testimony for the existence of occult phenomena played a significant role. In practice, this new approach involved studying the sensory and intellectual errors responsible for such convictions, as well as the mental predisposition and limitations of those who harboured these beliefs. Lapses in concentration, visual illusions and a desire to believe, Dessoir and Moll argued, might all contribute to belief in the paranormal. Extrapolating from both normal and abnormal psychology, in particular from their knowledge of hypnosis and suggestion, these psychologists attempted to explain occult belief in healthy individuals without a history of mental disturbance. This approach firmly established the psychology of deception and belief in Germany within normal psychology.

While it had been typical from the late nineteenth century onwards for psychologists, psychical researchers and critical occultists to assess mediums in pathological or abnormal terms, linking their putative powers to neuroses such as hysteria, an interest in the mental state of those who believed in or studied mediumistic phenomena did not begin to develop until the early twentieth century.[22] The impetus for this development appears, in part, to have been questions that emerged during the trials of mediums accused of fraud about the psychological state of those who provided testimony for the existence of paranormal phenomena.[23] The 1902 trial of the apport medium Anna Rothe (1850–1907), for example, saw psychologists and psychiatrists, formerly interested in the mental state of mediums, focus their attention on the psychology of those spiritualists and occultists who supported and promoted this so-called conduit to the other world.[24] As the author of an article which appeared in *Die Welt am Montag* [*The World on Monday*] in March 1902 jibed:

> The Police rejoice and believe that through the jailing of successful spiritualists they have forcefully put the whole nonsense of spiritualism to rest. An illusionary hope! They should not have jailed Anna Rothe, rather the fourteen fools who believed that her clever conjuring tricks were messages from the fourth dimension.[25]

Indeed, according to Dessoir, who appeared as an expert witness for the prosecution, Frau Rothe's talent lay not in her technical skill as a conjurer, but in her understanding of her audience's psychological weaknesses.[26] These witnesses, who exhibited incapacity neither of the mind nor the senses were, according to the psychologists and critical occultists who studied them, victims not only of their emotional investment in occult questions, but of expectation, both of which tended to diminish and pervert their powers of observation. This heady mixture of anticipation and desire, the critics argued, was not exclusive to those who attended spiritualist séances in the hope of contacting their deceased friends and relatives, but was apparent also in the observational errors made by researchers, who although outstanding in their own fields, remained novices in the study of paranormal phenomena.[27] From these tentative conclusions began to emerge a psychology of sensory error and belief that, by the inter-war period, had begun to mutate, in the hands of certain critics of occultism, into a psychopathology of individual parapsychological researchers.

Conjuring, sensory deception and spiritualism

In an article on the psychology of conjuring, which appeared in the journal *Nord und Süd* [*North and South*] in 1890, Dessoir conducted a psychological analysis of conjuring tricks, extrapolating from this in order to throw some light on the contemporary belief in spiritualism.[28] According to Dessoir, the basis of conjuring was psychological rather than technical, a result not of dexterity, but of the conjurer's understanding of the audience's psychological weaknesses.[29] Conjurers, he maintained, relied on two basic functions of the mental organism as the means of deceiving their audiences: association and imitation. Association worked by establishing for audience members a causal relationship between events. Dessoir argued that when an event B follows directly after another event A, there is a tendency for the observer to expect that when A is repeated B will follow; B thereby becomes associated with A.[30] The simplest form of deception, he maintained, consisted of the use of such expectations to disguise other actions.[31] Dessoir gave the example of a trick in which a collection of beads are placed down the barrel of a pistol and fired at a large wooden box. The conjurer opens the lid of this box to reveal another inside it, which he lifts out and opens to reveal yet another box. As he opens the lid of the third box he pulls a small box containing a set of identical beads from under the table. The audience, however, believe that as with the other two boxes this one has emerged from inside the larger box.[32] Another tool routinely used by conjurers, Dessoir maintained, was distraction. Reliance on the psychological propensity of people to imitate others, he argued, was a particularly effective manner of diverting their attention. In Dessoir's example, the conjurer concentrates his gaze on a person on his right-hand side, causing the audience to turn and look also. With attention diverted from his left side, the conjurer is free to carry out the trick with his left hand.[33]

Many of the psychological insights gained from the study of conjuring, Dessoir maintained, could be applied to spiritualism.[34] Knowledge of paranormal phenomena, he stated, was almost without exception derived from written reports. In other words, most people did not experience these things, rather they read about what certain other people believed they had experienced in séance protocols. By revealing the multiple errors made by observers, the study of conjuring exposed the unreliability of such reports.

> A person sees an orange disappear in the air, without being able to explain the miracle; they are deluded that they have checked eight rings, while they only had two in their hand; they think they have freely pulled a card, that was put into their fingers; they maintain that they held onto an object without letting go, that in reality was situated elsewhere for minutes – and when this person later describes the conjuring tricks to a third party this naturally appears almost inconceivable.[35]

It was the height of naïveté, Dessoir argued, for an observer to maintain that his or her subjective observations mimicked the objective events exactly. In the spiritualist séance, as in the conjuring show, participants made multiple observational errors of which they remained completely unaware. There were, Dessoir maintained, four sources of error associated with the reportage of spiritualist phenomena.[36] The first involved the observer's importation of events that did not happen, but which they are convinced did occur, into the report. He or she claims, for example, to have examined the slate, but did not. The second error revolved around an indiscriminate use of terms. He or she states that they made a thorough examination of the slate, when in fact they looked at it only briefly. Third, the witness confuses the order in which things happened, locating their examination of the slate for instance at an earlier time than it actually happened. The fourth error concerned the tendency of observers not to mention events that they believe are irrelevant.[37] He or she does not mention, for example, that the medium asked them to get up and close the window during the séance.

Elsewhere, Dessoir expanded his psychology of spiritualism beyond the séance protocol, noting the role played by lapses of concentration, interpretative error and mediumistic manipulation in the manufacture of occult belief. He wrote:

> In the majority of cases the observer is deceived neither through actual sleight of hand nor through deception of the senses, rather in a more refined manner he causes himself to be deceived through lapses of attention and errors of interpretation.[38]

Mediums, according to Dessoir, manipulated people's inability to maintain concentration over long periods, distracting observers with conversation and music, and exploiting the portentous atmosphere of the séance room, in order to imbue even the most inconsequential events with significance.[39] Moll also noted the suggestive power of this venue, pointing to the large number of séance participants who espoused belief in the occult both during and immediately after a sitting, but who, with distance from this persuasive milieu, experienced a re-awakening of their critical faculties.[40] Dr Gulat-Wellenburg, for example, who had attended a series of sittings with the medium Eva C. in the home of Albert von Schrenck-Notzing, was initially convinced of the veracity of this medium's phenomena. Shortly after the cessation of these experiments, however, he altered his position, hypothesising that the medium had regurgitated, rather than materialised, the ideoplastic images that issued from her body.[41] Moll contended that a susceptibility to the suggestive atmosphere of the séance room was a result of expectation, the desire to experience something momentous weakening the critical faculties and fostering a credulity on which unscrupulous mediums could prey.[42]

The role of hypnosis and suggestion

While the study of such sensory and intellectual errors remained the basis of the psychology of occult belief, highlighting the specific mechanisms by which individuals came to accept the reality of the paranormal, it was the labile power of hypnosis and suggestion on which critical occultists tended to dwell. These studies looked beyond the observational errors made by those individuals who attended spiritualist séances, to consider the social and cultural milieu in which a belief in the occult was formed. Moll, for example, maintained that the public's belief in occultism could be understood, in part, as a reaction to the spiritual paucity that resulted from the dominance of both scientific and philosophical materialism in Germany during the nineteenth century.[43] Similarly, Dessoir argued that in a scientific age, religion and philosophy were no longer capable of answering the public's ontological questions. In such an age, he maintained, it was unsurprising that occultism, with its promise of proving the immortality of the soul experimentally, would prove attractive for those in search of metaphysical solace.[44] This emphasis on social factors led not only to analyses of the prevailing *Weltanschauung* as a means of explaining belief in the occult, but encouraged the study of occultism from a sociological perspective. Critical occultists now attempted both to explain why a number of Germany's cultural and intellectual luminaries had provided positive testimony for the paranormal, and to account for occultism's penetration of every level of society. They did this primarily by arguing that belief in the paranormal was a form of moral and mental contagion to which all those without the requisite knowledge of conjuring and psychology were susceptible. This social psychological approach to the occult, which developed during the inter-war period in Germany, represented an attempt to explain the spread of occult belief.

The view that belief in the occult was a kind of dangerous malignancy, rather than a benign foible, was nurtured by those concerned to establish a medical monopoly over the use of hypnosis and suggestion and to win the right to mould the scientific interpretation of the occult. This campaign, in which occultism was represented as a distinct threat to public health, was aimed at discrediting those occult practitioners and researchers whose disregard for psychologists' claims obscured the distinct boundaries that this nascent profession wished to establish between psychology and the occult. Occultism, they argued, was easily transmitted not only through direct contact with the contagion, that is, through participation in a séance, but also indirectly, through the written and spoken discourse of occult converts. Critical occultists maintained that the processes of conversion and contagion were a result of a particularly potent and dangerous form of suggestion commonly spread by political or religious fanatics among crowds. This was the line taken by Christian Bruhn, a disciple of Moll or 'Mollschüler', in his 1926 book entitled *Gelehrte in Hypnose [Scholars in Hypnosis]*, in which he identified Albert von Schrenck-Notzing, the primary target of the critical occultists' campaign, as the progenitor of this dangerous mass delusion.[45]

The positive reports of the Schneider mediumship provided by prominent intellectuals including Thomas Mann, Eduard Keyserling (1880–1948), Gustav Meyrink, Hans Driesch and Ludwig Klages, demonstrated for critical occultists, the occult pathogen's infiltration not just of the lower strata, of whom one might expect such irrationalities, but of the upper levels of society.[46] Hellwig bemoaned this fact, writing:

> Experience shows day after day that countless people today are no longer capable of calm and critical thinking as soon as it comes to occult problems. It is truly sad when one sees how even academic men, who have perhaps even made their name in a number of fields of science, completely lose all sense for logic and reason, when it comes to the discussion of such emotional questions.[47]

Over fifty of the nation's most revered intellectuals – doctors, writers and jurists, as well as professors of psychology, physiology, psychiatry, zoology, physics and chemistry – had provided signed statements to the effect that the telekinetic and ectoplasmic phenomena they had witnessed in Schrenck-Notzing's home had taken place under strict experimental conditions. Given the cultural and scientific authority commanded by these important figures, their apparent conviction was difficult to dismiss. If, as the *Magdeburgische Zeitung [Magdeburg News]* insisted, the possibility of error or deception on the part of such luminaries was excluded, how could their testimony be explained?[48] Christian Bruhn's solution to this problem was not to suggest the mental deficiency of these intellectuals, but to hypothesise the sublimation of their intelligence and their reason to a skilful hypnotist, namely the Munich-based parapsychologist Albert von Schrenck-Notzing, whose promotion of physical mediumship among Germany's élite had helped perpetuate the public's interest in occultism. Mann, Keyserling, Meyrink, Driesch and Klages were, according to Bruhn, victims of a 'hypnotische Verzauberung' [hypnotic enchantment] transmitted unconsciously by their charismatic host. This 'enchantment' led not only to the obfuscation of their judgment and the falsification of their memories as they concerned occult phenomena, but as a result of their scientific and cultural authority had a suggestive effect on those with whom they came into contact.[49]

Bruhn used the term hypnosis in a figurative sense to indicate the suggestive influence that Schrenck-Notzing and his laboratory had on séance participants.[50] According to him, the ability of these witnesses to accurately observe their surroundings was actively hindered by the experimental conditions insisted on by Schrenck-Notzing.[51] In the dull red light that dominated such experiments, the black-clad medium, routinely seated in front of the black curtains used to partition the room, became all but invisible. The wild movements of the medium and the loud music that accompanied such séances for up to several hours before the appearance of any occult phenomena, also served to diminish the participants' concentration. Bruhn's analysis, according to an article that appeared in the *Weltbühne* [*World Stage*] during September 1926, made use of a peculiarly modern theory of subjectivity. This theory did not presuppose either the reasonableness of the observing subject or the culpability of external conditions for errors, rather it held that the inner state of the observer was not only capable of, but predisposed to creating false realities.[52] Dreams, fantasies and prejudices, this hypothesis maintained, were deeply embedded in the intellectual process, having a suggestive effect on the way in which the scientific observer perceived reality. Bruhn was irreverent enough to argue that the authority evoked by the *mise en scène* that is Schrenck-Notzing's palatial home and aristocratic title, predisposed the professors who attended his séances to abandon logic in favour of their desire to believe.[53]

According to Bruhn, the belief in the occult that resulted from this suggestive milieu was highly contagious. Schrenck-Notzing's victims, those who had come directly or indirectly into contact with the hypnotic disease manufactured in the Karolinenplatz laboratory, numbered in their thousands.[54] In a manner analogous to the spread of political agitation, Bruhn argued, the occult pathogen was transmitted by the written and spoken discourse of those who attended sittings with the Baron, constituting a serious moral and mental threat to the public.[55] The apparent belief of such figures in the reality of the paranormal and their intellectual and cultural authority had a suggestive effect on those who read their séance protocols or heard them speak. Employing those concepts, including contagion, hypnosis, suggestibility and psychological regression that Gustave Le Bon had identified as the distinguishing characteristics of the psychological crowd, Bruhn provided a dynamic socio-psychological analysis of occult belief among both individuals and groups.

Occult belief and the psychology of the crowd

Le Bon's 1895 book *La psychologie des foules* [known in English as *The Crowd: A Study of the Popular Mind*] expanded upon a number of contemporary studies of mass behaviour to become the most influential early psychology of the crowd.[56] This book, the second of a series of three books on the psychologies of peoples, crowds and socialism, addressed the persistent fear in France of another revolution and instructed the élite on how best to avoid this fatal course.[57] Le Bon characterised the era in which he lived as 'the era of crowds', claiming that the rule of the masses, as epitomised by universal suffrage, would ultimately destroy society.[58] Tantamount to barbarism, he argued, the ascendancy of the crowd as a political force led inevitably to civilisation's reversion to a primitive state.[59] The crowd's task, Le Bon claimed, was not unlike that of a microbe, which speeds the dissolution of a diseased or dead body. The crowd, however, was instrumental in destroying rotten civilisations.[60] In a society like that of nineteenth-century France in which moral, social and political mores were in flux, the destructive potential of the masses created concern. But because crowds were neither essentially mad nor criminal, the solution to this problem had to be political; a psychology of the crowd provided politicians with the tools to govern mass societies.[61] Le Bon, combining several popular hypotheses, provided an analysis of the characteristics of this new and potentially dangerous social and political force.

Le Bon's psychology owed much to a number of contemporary theories and debates. The most significant were Théodule Ribot's (1839–1916) theories of psychological heredity and evolution/dissolution, and the hypnotic suggestion debate that took place between the so-called Salpêtrière and Nancy schools.[62] Ribot believed that mental disturbance was a type of dissolution, a loss of control which saw a reversion to an earlier evolutionary stage. This form of atavism, he maintained, manifested itself in extreme changeability, impulsiveness and lack of willpower. Le Bon used these ideas to argue that while civilised men had more evolved minds than savages and women, under certain circumstances their conscious will and rational thinking might dissolve. This could be the result of a long-term weakening of national character or of a short-term aberration, such as that found in agitated crowds.[63] Of perhaps more significance here, however, were contemporary theories about hypnosis and suggestion. While the Salpêtrière school, headed by Charcot, maintained that hypnosis could only be induced in hysterics, those at Nancy began to argue, during the 1880s, that even people of sound mind were suggestible. Bernheim, for example, stated that hypnotic suggestion, which accentuated ordinary phenomena such as credibility, obedience and excitability, was the act by which an idea was introduced into the brain and accepted by it.[64] Such ideas, he maintained, were also usually translated into action. Bernheim believed furthermore that this effect was best achieved in groups where 'a real suggestive atmosphere' could be created.[65] Le Bon's study of hypnosis and suggestion, which favoured the theories of the Nancy school, led him to conclude that collective states were similar to hypnotic ones.[66]

Critical occultists' mobilisation of crowd psychology helped to elucidate the collective behaviour of occultists and to explain the spread of occult belief. While the social psychology of groups had emerged in response to the increasing importance of the crowd as a political force, its emphasis on suggestion and contagion lent it also to the analysis of occultists. The process of assimilation experienced by the individual within the crowd, for example, bore a striking similarity to the sublimation of the critical faculties that Bruhn had noted among séance participants. Le Bon wrote of this process:

> [A]n individual immersed for some length of time in a crowd in action soon finds himself – either in consequence of the magnetic influence given out by the crowd, or from some other cause of which we are ignorant – in a special state, which much resembles the state of fascination in which the hypnotised individual finds himself in the hands of the hypnotiser. The activity of the brain being paralysed in the case of the hypnotised subject, the latter becomes slave of all unconscious activities of his spinal cord, which the hypnotiser directs at will. The conscious personality has entirely vanished; will and discernment are lost. All feelings and thoughts are bent in the direction determined by the hypnotiser.[67]

This analogy, which Bruhn had used to describe the suggestive state imposed upon séance participants by occultists, was indicative of the link that Le Bon believed existed between the apparently contagious nature of crowd behaviour and suggestion.[68] Critical occultists utilised the concept of contagion, in particular hypnotic or suggestive contagion, to account for the spread of occult belief at every level of society. While crowd psychology provided an elegant model with which to explain the diffusion of belief in the paranormal, it could also be used, as Moll demonstrated, to analyse behaviour within small occult groups.

The psychological crowd, according to Le Bon, need not consist of hundreds or thousands of individuals, in fact, need not involve a physical gathering at all.[69] The distinguishing feature of this entity was a common idea, exacerbated by suggestibility, emotion and the retardation of the observation, and could occur in small groups or among thousands of isolated individuals under the influence of certain violent emotions.[70] One of the examples used by Le Bon to illustrate the suggestibility and credulity of small groups was the spiritualist séance.[71] Even men of learning, he argued, in this situation assumed the characteristics of the crowd with regard to matters outside their field of speciality. He noted here, in particular, an experiment conducted by the English conjurer S.J. Davey, a member of the Society for Psychical Research, in which a number of prominent intellectuals, including Alfred Russel Wallace (1823–1913), observed what they believed were spiritualist phenomena such as slate writing and spirit materialisation.[72] Having examined to their satisfaction the objects and seals used in these experiments, these men became convinced that the phenomena they had experienced were of supernatural origin.[73] After writing and signing reports to this effect, Davey revealed that the phenomena had been the result of a series of very simple tricks. The methods used by Davey were so simple, Le Bon wrote, that it was astonishing that they had succeeded, but the conjurer had such power of mind over those present that he could persuade them that they saw what they did not see.[74] The distinction made by Le Bon between the psychological crowd and the masses, that is, large numbers of people gathered with no common purpose, enabled Moll to apply the principles of crowd psychology to both small groups of occultists and isolated individuals.[75] The unconscious, which Le Bon had argued played a significant role in the behaviour of crowds, was, according to critical occultists, a motivating force among those with a strong interest in the occult, accounting for the often irrational, emotional or fanatical nature of their beliefs. The subconscious juxtaposition of contradictory ideas and the retreat of reason witnessed by Le Bon among crowds were also, according to Moll, distinguishing features of occult groups, whose refusal to accept the necessity of strict control during séances and inability to follow logical argumentation was a concomitant of their abnormal state.[76]

The question of whether the psychological crowd consisted primarily of mentally unstable individuals was answered in the negative by Le Bon, who maintained that the vast majority of those that made up such groups were normal.[77] The idea of a collective mind, dominated by the lowest common denominator, helped explain why ostensibly intelligent people acted violently or irrationally once they became members of a crowd. The temporary madness that subsumed the personalities and the logic of individuals within groups, could also be used to explain the apparent belief of respected intellectuals in something as potentially embarrassing as the occult, without fear of impugning their sanity. While the crowd might not consist primarily of psychotics or neurotics, Le Bon was in no doubt that the figures who led such groups were mentally abnormal. Similarly, critical occultists, such as Moll, argued that belief in the paranormal, as it manifested itself in certain prominent parapsychologists, was inherently pathological.

The figure of the parapsychologist, as characterised by critical occultists – neurotic, combative, superficial, absentminded, credulous and charismatic – was reminiscent of the profile of the mentally unstable individual that Le Bon had identified as the prototypical leader of the crowd. He wrote:

> They are especially recruited from the ranks of those morbidly nervous, excitable, half-deranged persons who are bordering on madness. However absurd may be the idea they uphold or the goal they pursue, their convictions are so strong that all reasoning is lost on them.... The intensity of their faith gives great power of suggestion to their words.[78]

The manner in which prominent parapsychologists' mental derangement lent them persuasive power was noted not only by critical occultists, but also by a number of occult researchers. Walther Kröner, for example, wrote that the majority of the pioneers of occult research were temperamental gentlemen, with an artistic bent and combative nature, whose enthusiasm ran the risk of becoming fanaticism.[79] In order to contain and ultimately eliminate the threat posed by occultism, critical occultists believed it was necessary to understand its aetiology, that is, to gain an insight into the psychology of those individuals who validated and promoted belief in the occult through their research. The attempt of critical occultists, during the inter-war period, to assess the mental health of parapsychologists, most notably their nemesis Schrenck-Notzing, did not, however, represent an abandonment of their interest in the social psychology of occultism, rather a shift of focus to a related area, the study of the unconscious mind and its abnormalities.

Parapsychologists and psychopathology

In his 1929 book *Psychologie und Charakterologie der Okkultisten* [*Psychology and Characterology of Occultists*], Moll rejected the phenomenological approach to the occult in favour of a characterology and psychology of parapsychologists. This analysis was intended, not only to highlight the sensory and intellectual errors responsible for occult belief but also the neuroses and unconscious complexes to which parapsychologists were subject.[80] The failure of parapsychology to gain scientific recognition, Moll argued, had less to do with the nature of its phenomena and more to do with the inadequacies of its researchers, who tended to be lacking in the qualities essential for scientific research.[81] It was for this reason, he contended, that a psychological study focused on the mental state of Germany's leading parapsychologists, rather than a phenomenology of occult events, was the appropriate means of coming to terms with, and eliminating the threat posed by, parapsychology. With chapters entitled 'Oberflächlichkeit, Gedankenlosigkeit, Leichtgläubigkeit der Okkultisten' ['The Superficiality, Absentmindedness, and Credulity of Occultists'] and 'Zur Psychopathologie der Okkultisten' ['Towards a Psychopathology of Occultists'], Moll's book represented the culmination of all the theories that had constituted the psychology of occult belief in Germany. No longer content to assess belief in the paranormal in terms of inattention, misinterpretation, expectation and desire, critical occultists sought the aetiology of such belief in the mental pathology and unconscious conflicts of their adversaries.

While Moll's book attempted the analysis of a number of prominent occultists, it remained focused on one figure in particular, that of Albert von Schrenck-Notzing. The Baron, whose wealth and reputation had enabled him to promote the scientific study of the paranormal among Germany's intellectual and cultural élite, was portrayed by critical occultists as the source of an insidious moral and mental pollutant that posed a significant threat to public health. In his 1929 book *Gelehrte in Hypnose* [*The Scholar in Hypnosis*], Christian Bruhn had contended that the persuasive power through which Schrenck-Notzing spread this contagion was a product not only of his social standing and reputation as a scientist but also of the delusional auto-suggestive state, which fuelled his unshakable belief in the paranormal.[82] Bruhn's portrait of the Baron, reminiscent of the description that Le Bon had provided of those half-deranged persons that form the leadership of crowds, intimated the pathological and perhaps dangerous nature of his personality. As the leader of and metonymic figure for parapsychology in Germany, Schrenck-Notzing remained the focus of critical occultists' psychological analyses and critiques, even after his death in 1929. Moll wrote:

> A man who takes *Fastnacht* jokes for science, who wants to force on others the carnival disguises of hysterical women and other mediums as transfigurations or as teleplasma and as products of the world's unconscious, must also be examined in accordance with the truth after death.[83]

The bitter polemic against the Baron that appeared in Moll's book represented the culmination of psychologists and critical occultists' attempts to combat parapsychologists' knowledge claims, transforming them from intellectual opponents into objects of psychological analysis.

The claim that mental pathology played a significant role in the scientific study of the occult was by no means new in the inter-war period, having first emerged during the 1870s as a response to Zöllner's experiments with the American medium Henry Slade.[84] Moll alerted his readers to the Leipzig astronomer's notoriety in his book on the psychopathology of occult belief, stating, 'As soon as one speaks of the mental state of occultists, most people think of Zöllner, because it is widely maintained that Zöllner was mentally ill'.[85] Moll argued, however, that the psychological peculiarities typical of occultists were of a different order from those exhibited by Zöllner, whose illness was of an hereditary nature and needed to be studied accordingly. The theory adopted by Moll and a number of other critical occultists classified belief in the occult not as a form of madness, consuming victims' personalities and logic in their entirety, but as a type of neurosis, affecting the reason of predisposed individuals in a very specific and limited manner. This approach, which helped explain the behaviour of a number of prominent occult researchers, both complemented critical occultists' writings on the collective behaviour of occultists, and borrowed extensively from psychoanalytic theory.

The psychoanalytic approach

In a letter to the Swiss biologist and parapsychologist Fanny Moser (1872–1953), dated July 1918, Sigmund Freud admitted an interest in occult phenomena that remained unsatisfied because of a lack of personal experience.[86] He mentioned, however, his analysis of two cases of prophecy, from which he had concluded the reality of thought-transference. In spite of this positive analysis, Freud's writings on this topic indicated a deep-seated ambivalence towards the paranormal.[87] In 1921, for example, he gave a paper on psychoanalysis and telepathy in which he stated that it was no longer possible to dismiss the study of occult phenomena. In his 1922 essay on dream and telepathy, however, he claimed that he had no opinion on the reality of telepathy, wishing to remain completely impartial on this topic. In another essay, dated 1933, on dreams and occultism, he retreated somewhat from what he had told Moser, stating that he was not fully convinced of the reality of thought-transference but was ready to be so. Despite this apparent indecision on Freud's part, his psychoanalytic theory was ultimately employed by his followers to argue for the pathology of occult belief.

The Freudian approach to occultism differed from that of experimental psychology, which had tended to concentrate on exposing mediums as deliberate frauds or providing naturalistic explanations for occult phenomena, examining instead the unconscious psychological compulsions and complexes that provoked the behaviour of mediums, occultists and parapsychologists. Psychoanalysts, like most other psychologists, rejected the objective reality of paranormal phenomena, arguing that occult experiences were the result of self-deception and neurosis. The subjective nature of such phenomena was illustrated by Alfred Winterstein who identified the apparitions experienced by certain neurotics as a result of the childhood impressions they had formed of their parents in their nightclothes. The appearance of these ghostly figures to the neurotic adult, according to Winterstein, represented the child's suppressed desire to see the secret, the hidden and the forbidden.[88] Interest in mysticism and occultism, psychoanalysts contended, was linked not only with a fear of death, but also with an unconscious desire to return to the womb, the darkness, comfort and protection of which were recreated in the séance room.[89] The analysis of those individuals who believed themselves possessed of mediumistic powers or who sought to martyr themselves as champions of the paranormal, expanded on these theories.

Mediums, psychoanalysts argued, deluded themselves into believing they possessed paranormal abilities, as a result of a neurotic overestimation of the range of their mental powers.[90] The nature of the mediumistic neurosis, an active rather than passive or inward-turning pathology, compelled mediums to impose their delusional system, that is, the belief that their mental energy was capable of overcoming natural laws, on the outside world. Typically of a combative nature, a result of their narcissistic egocentrism, mediums tended to possess strong suggestive powers, enabling their neurosis to become communicable and their delusions to be taken up by followers with related neuroses.[91] Among those who gathered around these neurotic egoists, according to psychoanalysts, could be found fanatic campaigners for the reality of the occult, whose own neuroses left them highly susceptible to the ideas and dogmas touted by mediums. Possessed of a type of monomania for the occult, these individuals lost the ability to distinguish between their own fantasies and reality. They allowed themselves to be deceived because they wanted to be deceived and deceived themselves, when a medium was not available to do it for them, in order to support their neurotic system, the so-called 'occult complex'.[92] With this diagnosis, psychoanalysts condemned both those who would be labelled spiritualists and those who considered themselves scientists, that is, parapsychologists.

A complex in the psychoanalytic sense was understood to be a group of emotional impulses that, although banished from the conscious mind, continued to influence behaviour. According to psychoanalysts, the successful penetration of the conscious mind by such a complex resulted in a neurosis. The idea of an 'occult complex', first suggested by the critical occultist Graf Carl von Klinckowstroem, utilised this theory, pathologising interest in, and research into, the occult. Moll wrote:

> In recent times one speaks frequently of complexes. Graf Klinckowstroem has spoken of an occult complex, that is, a group of related impulses or over-valued ideas, whereby the impulse manifests itself in the desire to prove the occult under all circumstances. If such complexes exist, then we are dealing with a state that exhibits certain similarities with paranoid delusions.[93]

Moll maintained that the 'occult complex' was analogous to paranoia, a neurosis most often characterised by delusions of grandeur or persecution. People suffering from paranoia, he stated, typically did not lose their ability to reason on every topic, but found themselves unable to employ logic in those areas forming the premises for their specific delusion. This inability to reason on certain subjects, Moll claimed, was apparent among parapsychologists, who even when presented with evidence contrary to their beliefs could not be swayed from the conviction that their occult delusions possessed an objective reality.[94] In defence of this claim, Moll stated that despite the hope that circumstances might exist in which a parapsychologist would admit they were mistaken, such admissions occurred among them as seldom as they did among madmen.[95]

For Klinckowstroem, the obstinate refusal of Schrenck-Notzing to abandon his belief in the reality of his mediums' powers, even in the face of compelling evidence that they had committed fraud, epitomised the occult complex. In a 1928 article on the contemporary status of occult research, he wrote of the Baron's attempts to hinder the discovery of fraud on the part of his mediums, his attempts to reason away the negative observations of others and to discredit those who claimed they had discovered fraud:

> [He] is so strongly prejudiced by the 'occult complex', that he sees in the activities of critics as well as in the publications of those observers who uncover the trick system (like W.J. Vinton in Braunau with the Schneiders), damage done to parapsychological research, instead of recognising that the principal task of every science is to serve the truth.[96]

Schrenck-Notzing's pathological refusal to consider evidence that might undermine his beliefs had been demonstrated not only during his association with the Schneider brothers, but also with the Hungarian medium Ladislaus Lalzlo. Lured to Budapest by reports of Lalzlo's mediumship, Schrenck-Notzing conducted a series of experiments in which he managed to obtain photographs of the ectoplasmic hands and heads that issued from the medium's mouth. Soon after these experiments, Lalzlo was exposed as a fraud after admitting to a colleague that his materialisations were preparations of water and cotton wool that had been hidden in the pockets of his controls. Schrenck-Notzing refused to countenance this exposure, claiming that Lalzlo's phenomena were undoubtedly real and that his admission of guilt was the result of stress.[97]

The belief that the mental state of parapsychologists provided fodder for psychological and psychoanalytic analysis was not limited to critical occultists, but extended to a small number of psychiatrists. The Königsberg psychiatrist Adolf Meyer (1866–1950), for example, argued that given occultists' psychopathic personalities and neurotic temperaments, psychiatrists were the most appropriate group to assess them.[98] Other observers, including the physician Anton Ewald, purported to have noted signs of degeneration and tendencies to hysteria among occultists, arguing that among such neurotics could be found whole companies of psychopaths.[99] These analyses, like those of critical occultists, constituted attempts to discredit and dismiss parapsychologists' knowledge claims by suggesting they were the products of disturbed minds. By transforming parapsychologists from adversaries into objects of psychological analysis, psychologists, psychoanalysts and critical occultists validated and secured their own claims to jurisdiction, expertise and knowledge over the paranormal.[100]

Critique and counter-attack

In the foreword to his 1914 book *Materialisations-Phänomene* [*Phenomena of Materialisation*], Schrenck-Notzing observed that an association with the occult tended to cast doubt on the mental stability of even the most respected intellectuals. He wrote:

> Any dealings with the discredited so-called 'spiritistic' phenomena are attended, even now, by certain disadvantages to the investigator. Not only are his powers of observation, his critical judgment and his credibility brought into question, not only is he exposed to ridicule by the reproach of charlatanism – as, for example, was the famous criminal anthropologist Lombroso – but he even incurs the danger of being regarded as mentally deficient, or even insane, as was the case with the astronomer Zöllner, and the English chemist Crookes.[101]

As the principal target of much of this psychological analysis, Schrenck-Notzing had not only endured accusations of delusion and paranoia, but had shouldered the blame for what many critics saw as the spread of a dangerous moral and mental contagion. The Baron, on his own behalf and as the representative head of parapsychology in Germany, took care to respond to such critiques. To Bruhn's contention that the hypnotic contagion manufactured in his laboratory was responsible for the positive reports received by the Schneider brothers in Vienna, Prague, and London, he reacted with sarcasm and disbelief.[102] How, he asked, could these independent researchers, equipped with a knowledge of conjuring, have fallen victim to his hypnotic powers from so far afield.

The Baron was not alone in his critique of these psychological analyses. The homeopath and occultist Walther Kröner, for example, argued that there were different types of opponents. There were those who were honourable, respecting differences of opinion and capable of differentiating between the person and the subject. There were others, however, concerned solely with portraying their opponents as intellectually or morally inferior.[103] In a letter to Schrenck-Notzing dated 27 July 1925, Kröner outlined his response to such attacks by critical occultists:

> I personally have decided to take up the struggle against Moll and his gang, especially Hellwig, alone and have in fact in the form of a quite severe satirical polemic, psychoanalysed the gentlemen.[104]

Reversing those tactics used against them, parapsychologists attempted to portray their opponents as men plagued by deep-seated and irrational complexes that prevented them from acknowledging evidence for the reality of the occult.

Parapsychologists' responses to the imputation of mental instability tended to take the form of counter accusations. Schrenck-Notzing wrote in 1926, for example:

> [O]ur adversaries have repeatedly expressed the wish to examine the mental state of 'believing' occultists. But they appear in the process to overlook the degree to which their own fanatical refusal to believe blinds them and clouds their judgment.[105]

In a similar manner, Kröner attempted to present the strong aversion to the occult exhibited by Moll and his followers as pathological. He argued, for example, that evidence for the paranormal was such that its existence could only continue to be denied on the basis of either ignorance or neurotic inhibition.[106] Becoming more specific, he wrote:

> It is this, the position of the Moll school, with their confusion of heterogeneous concepts (like the equation of personal questions, specialist questions and questions of principle), that gives the best typical example of an emotional clouding of judgement and through this doggedly held system of errors provides the proof for their own neurotic–dogmatic views.[107]

With such responses, parapsychologists attempted to argue that the critical occultists' fanatical drive to eliminate the scientific study of the occult betrayed the kind of unconscious complexes and neuroses of which they had accused their adversaries.

The link that critical occultists had established between interest in the occult and neurosis was employed by parapsychologists, not only in response to these negativists, but also as a means of divorcing the scientific study of the occult from the taint of spiritualism. Kröner argued, for example, that the neurotic system he had diagnosed among members of the Moll school was replicated almost exactly among extreme adherents to spiritualism and mysticism.[108] While he maintained that both groups were driven by their inner neuroses, he retained some sympathy for the spiritualists. According to Kröner, spiritualism was ultimately constructive, building new ethical and metaphysical systems, while anti-occultism, with its materialistic *Weltanschauung*, was wholly destructive and devoid of moral value. This argument enabled him both to combat those fanatic critics of occultism determined to undermine the scientific study of the occult, and to fight those occultists whose interest in questions of monism and dualism weakened parapsychologists' claims to scientific credibility.

Critical occultists' identification of parapsychologists with spiritualists, as with their equation of occult phenomena and neurotic symptoms, was intended to tar parapsychology as a whole, and representatives of experimental parapsychology in particular, with the same brush as sectarianism and neurosis, relegating the entire field to the realm of self-deception and trickery.[109] According to Kröner, however, the parapsychologist was clearly differentiated from both spiritualists and critical occultists by his even-handed and objective approach to occult phenomena. He wrote:

> What distinguishes the scientist from the emotional occultist is self-criticism, which he remembers in every case and which qualifies him to immediately recognise and eliminate judgment-clouding emotions when they arise.[110]

Viennese parapyschologist Alfred Winterstein (1885–1958) agreed with this assessment, arguing that while the intense interest in or aversion to the occult exhibited by mediums, spiritualists and critical occultists was undoubtedly a result of unconscious processes and rightly the subject of analysis, parapsychologists, whose approach to occultism was scientific, need not undergo such assessment.[111]

Psychoanalysis and parapsychology

While Kröner's embrace of such analyses allowed him to engage in double boundary-work, pathologising the knowledge claims of both critical occultists and spiritualists, he continued to argue that it was ultimately meaningless to consider occult phenomena as the subjective products of neuroses. Like a number of other parapsychologists, including Winterstein, he maintained that psychoanalysis and parapsychology were complementary sciences. While psychoanalysts of the Freudian persuasion would have rejected this claim, a number of others, most notably C.G. Jung, were sympathetic to the view that paranormal phenomena had an objective reality and that psychoanalysis and parapsychology were somehow related.[112] Jung's interest in the connection between psychoanalysis and the paranormal was long standing, his doctoral work, for example, consisting of an analysis of a spiritualist medium.[113] It was his participation in a number of séances with Rudi Schneider, however, that convinced him that parapsychology provided access to the unconscious.[114]

Psychoanalysis, which had revealed mental phenomena to which experimental psychologists had remained oblivious, was applicable to neuroses and related unconscious processes, including ecstasy, somnambulism and mediumship. Only the conscious mind, Kröner argued, was slave to the five senses. Space, time and self did not harness the unconscious like they did the upper levels of consciousness, the normal phenomena of these lower levels being of a parapsychological nature. The absence of time and space in this realm enabled telepathic messages, for example, to be sent and received simultaneously.[115] The physical phenomena of mediumship, he argued, were also a product of the unconscious, issuing from the vegetative zone. Kröner maintained that a psychoanalytic understanding of parapsychology would lead to its acceptance by science. He wrote:

> In truth the occult is nothing other than a psychological split, the intrusion of a natural process into a higher plane of consciousness. And this recognition removes the last intellectual resistance, which could hinder the scientific acceptance of parapsychology, after one is forced to come to terms with the phenomena.[116]

The tools with which critical occultists hoped to dismantle the scientific pretensions of parapsychologists were used by men like Kröner to prove the objective reality of occult phenomena. To his mind, psychoanalysis and occultism, united in parapsychology, would form the most important scientific discipline of the future, a triumph that could not be prevented even by 'Dunkelmänner' [obscurantists] like Albert Moll.[117]

Conclusion

The volatile relationship and fierce credibility contests that took place between psychology and parapsychology in Imperial and inter-war Germany were a result of both shared nomenclature and shared territory. Psychologists and parapsychologists both claimed to possess definitive knowledge of, and epistemic authority over, the mind that was achieved through empirical investigation, making it difficult for the German public to differentiate between them. By maintaining that parapsychologists' knowledge claims were a result of an underlying mental pathology, psychologists were able to dismiss their competitors' pretensions to expertise and authority, and to affect their transformation into objects of psychological inquiry. Psychologists, psychoanalysts and critical occultists legitimated their claims to jurisdiction over the mind by pathologising and analysing their adversaries.

The evolution of the psychology of occult belief from a phenomenology to a psychopathology, during the first decades of the twentieth century was a result of psychologists' and critical occultists' desire to eliminate the threat posed by parapsychology and of their growing interest in both social psychology and psychoanalysis. Reflective of contemporaries' concerns about the crowd and the individual as agents within the modern world, these approaches to the problem of occultism had a resonance which critical occultists hoped would guide public interest away from the paranormal and towards psychology. The unconscious complexes and suggestive powers that formed the basis of these psychological approaches to occultism had their precursors in medical hypnotists' campaigns against lay hypnotists and itinerant occultists during the late nineteenth century. These same men, now labelled critical occultists, continued their battle, subtly altering their rhetoric to accommodate contemporary theories and concerns.

The theories with which critical occultists attempted to combat occultism, psychoanalysis in particular, were also used by parapsychologists to counter their opponents' accusations of neurosis and to establish the objectivity of occult phenomena. The counter-accusations levelled by parapsychologists sought not only to pathologise the disbelief of critical occultists but to discredit in a similar manner the inconvenient and embarrassing beliefs of spiritualists. Parapsychologists they claimed, were representatives of scientific impartiality and reason and possessed the only true and objective knowledge pertaining to the occult. As bastions of this knowledge, they re-emphasised the objective reality of occult phenomena and argued that psychoanalysis, the weapon with which both groups sought to annihilate each other, held the key to validating and explaining the paranormal. Critical occultists and parapsychologists, in their eagerness to discredit their opponents' knowledge claims, transformed the psychology of occult belief from an analysis of the sensory and intellectual errors contributing to belief in the paranormal to an assessment of individual researchers' mental pathologies.

The movement towards a psychopathology of occult belief (or disbelief) during the first decades of the twentieth century demonstrated the inability of either party to come to terms with the paranormal on phenomenological grounds. By ignoring the nature of the phenomena and concentrating on the mental state of those that claimed their reality or unreality, it was possible to avoid the intractable epistemological questions that arose from the empirical study of the paranormal. It was clear from this process of psycho-pathologisation, that characterised the evolution of the psychology of occult belief in Germany, that the question of who should have the right to mould the public and scientific responses to paranormal phenomena, and to assign their meaning, remained as fraught as it had been during the late nineteenth century.

Notes

1. 'Psychologische Glossen zu dem Berliner Okkultistenprozess. Landgerichtsdirektor Dr Albert Hellwig in Potsdam', in: Nachlaß Albert Hellwig 10/4, Gerichtssache Moll vs Rudloff, 1925, IGPP.

2. 'Jeder von uns, der sich kritisch mit okkultistischen Problemen befasst hat, wird die Erfahrung gemacht haben, dass die Hauptschwierigkeit darin liegt, dass hier in ganz anderem Masse als bei wissenschaftlichen Untersuchungen anderer Art alles mit dem Vertrauen auf die Persönlichkeit des Experimentators steht und fällt. Die Erfahrung zeigt leider nur allzu oft, dass auch Männer, von denen man es an und für sich vielleicht nicht erwarten sollte, sobald es sich um Beobachtungen oder Experimente okkulter Art handelt, schwere Fehler machen, ohne dass sie es im geringsten gewahr werden. Die subjektive Ueberzeugungen eines Forschers steht nicht selten im umgekehrten Verhältnis zur Verlässlichkeit ihrer objektiven Grundlagen. Es ist deshalb eine der wichtigsten Aufgaben des kritischen Okkultismus, die erforderlichen Unterlagen zur Psychologie der okkultischen Forschung im allgemeinen und zur Psychologie der einzelnen okkultischen Forscher im Besonderen zu schaffen.' *Ibid.*

3. Sofie Lachapelle has argued that physical manifestations of religiosity, including possession, stigmata and mediumship, were potentially detrimental to nascent disciplines such as psychiatry and psychology during the mid to late nineteenth century. This was because these disciplines were constructed on the assumption that the human mind and its phenomena could be explained physiologically. See S. Lachapelle, 'A World Outside Science: French Attitudes Towards Mediumistic Phenomena, 1853–1931', (unpublished PhD dissertation: University of Notre Dame, 2002), 154.

4. D. Hess, *Science in the New Age: The Paranormal, Its Defenders and Debunkers, and American Culture* (Madison: University of Wisconsin Press, 1993), 62.

5. See for example, A. von Schrenck-Notzing, *Über Hypnotismus und Suggestion* (Augsburg: Wirthschen, 1889), 38.

6. B. Wolf-Braun, 'Zur Rezeptionsgeschichte der Parapsychologie im Rahmen der akademischen Psychologie: die Stellungnahmen von Wilhelm Wundt (1832–1920) und Hugo Münsterberg (1863–1916)' in J. Jahnke, *et al.* (eds), *Psychologiegeschichte - Beziehungen zu Philosophie und Grenzgebieten*, (Munich: Profil Verlag, 1998), 413.

7. W. Wundt, *Hypnotismus und Suggestion* [1892], 2nd edn (Leipzig: Wilhelm Engelmann, 1911), 5.

8. M.G. Ash, *Gestalt Psychology in German Culture, 1890–1967* (Cambridge: Cambridge University Press, 1998), 18.

9. Wolf-Braun, *op. cit.* (note 6), 408.

10. Münsterberg's theory was derived from that of Wilhelm Preyer who had conducted an extensive number of experiments in this area. See W. Preyer, 'Telepathie und Geistersherei in England', *Deutsche Rundschau* 26 (1886), 30–51; W. Preyer, *Die Erklärung des Gedankenlesens nebst Beschreibung eines neuen Verfahrens zum Nachweise unwillkürlicher Bewegungen* (Leipzig: T. Grieben, 1886).

11. Wolf-Braun, *op. cit.* (note 6), 409.

12. K.B. Staubermann, 'Tying the Knot: Skill, Judgment and Authority in the 1870s Leipzig Spiritistic Experiments', *British Journal for the History of Science*, 34 (2001), 78.

13. This is a similar argument to that made by Marshall and Wendt in M.E. Marshall and R.A. Wendt, 'Wilhelm Wundt, Spiritism, and the Assumptions of Science', in W.G. Bringmann and R.D. Tweney (eds), *Wundt Studies: A Centennial Collection* (Toronto: C.J. Hogrefe, 1980), 165.

14. Wolf-Braun, *op. cit.* (note 6), 410.

15. Wundt, *op. cit.* (note 7), 8–9.

16. *Ibid.*, 9–10.

17. *Ibid.*, 7.

18. D.J. Coon, 'Testing the Limits of Sense and Science: American Experimental Psychologists Combat Spiritualism, 1880–1920', *American Psychologist*, 47, 2 (1992), 143–51.

19. *Ibid.*, 149.

20. J. Jastrow, *Fact and Fable in Psychology* (London: Macmillan and Co., 1901), viii–ix.

21. Coon, *op. cit.* (note 18), 149.

22. For an example of a psychiatric assessment of a medium, see Dr Neumann's analysis of the clairvoyant Ludwig Kahn in 1908, in U. Schellinger, 'Faszinosum, Filou und Forschungsobjekt: Das erstaunliche Leben des Hellsehers Ludwig Kahn (1873–c.1966)', *Die Ortenau*, 82 (2002), 434–7. Lachapelle, in the French context, has argued that psychiatry and psychology

legitimised mediumistic phenomena by rejecting mystical interpretations of them and presenting them as pathological. She provides an interesting discussion of the association between spiritism and mental illness and the attempts of some French psychologists to use the study of mediumship in the construction of their theories of personality. See Lachapelle, *op. cit.* (note 3), 154–218.

23. B. Wolf-Braun, 'Zur Geschichte der Parapsychologie in der Weimarer Republik: Deutungen des Mediumismus', (Report for the Institut für Grenzgebiete der Psychologie und Psychohygiene, University of Bonn, 2002), 8.

24. For a contemporary account of the Rothe case, see Erich Bohn, *Der Fall Rothe: Eine criminal-psychologische Untersuchung* (Breslau: S. Schottlaender, 1901).

25. 'Die Polizei triumphirt und glaubt durch die Verhaftung der efolgreichen Spiritistin dem ganzen Unwesen des Spiritismus energetisch zu Leibe gegangen zu sein. Trügerische Hoffnung! Nicht Anna Rothe hätte sie verhaften sollen, sondern die vierzehn Thoren, die an ihre geschickten Taschenspielerstücke als Kundgebungen aus Dimension 'vier' glaubten', 'Zur Verhaftung Anna Rothes', *Die Welt am Montag*, 1902, in: GStA PK, I. HA Rep. 89 Nr. 15340.

26. M. Dessoir, *Vom Jenseits der Seele: Die Geheimwissenschaften in kritischer Betrachtung*, 3rd edn (Stuttgart: Ferdinand Enke, 1919), 174.

27. Wolf-Braun, *op. cit.* (note 23), 9.

28. M. Dessoir, 'Zur Psychologie der Taschenspielerkunst', *Nord und Süd*, 52 (1890), 194–221.

29. *Ibid.*, 212.

30. *Ibid.*, 207.

31. *Ibid.*, 207–8.

32. *Ibid.*, 208.

33. *Ibid.*, 211.

34. *Ibid.*, 218.

35. 'Eine Person sieht eine Apfelsine in der Luft verschwinden, ohne sich das Wunder erklären zu können, sie wähnt acht Ringe geprüft zu haben, während sie nur zwei in der Hand gehabt hat, sie meint eine Karte frei zu ziehen, die ihr in die Finger gesteckt wurde, sie behauptet einen Gegenstand unablässig festgehalten zu haben, der in Wirklichkeit sich auf Minuten anderswo befand – und wenn sie dann nachher einem Dritten die Taschenspielerkunststücke schildert, erscheinen diese natürlich schier unbegreiflich.' *Ibid.*, 218.

36. *Ibid.*, 219.

37. Moll, in particular, linked the problem of conversion to suggestion. See A. Moll, *Psychologie und Charakterologie der Okkultisten* (Stuttgart: Ferdinand Enke, 1929), 97.

38. 'In der Mehrzahl der Fälle wird der Beobachter weder durch eigentliche Taschenspielerei noch durch Trugwahrnehmungen getäuscht, sondern er wird in feinerer Weise veranlaßt, sich selbst durch Lücken der Aufmerksamkeit und Irrtümer der Deutung zu täuschen.' Dessoir, *op. cit.* (note 26), 189–90.

39. *Ibid.,* 192–3.

40. Moll, *op. cit.* (note 37), 96.

41. M. von Kemnitz, *Moderne Mediumforschung: Kritische Betrachtungen zu Dr von Schrenck-Notzing's 'Materialisationsphaenomene'* (Munich: J. F. Lehmann, 1914), 63–96; A. von Schrenck-Notzing, *Der Kampf um die Materialisationsphänomene* (Munich: Ernst Reinhardt, 1914), 18–47.

42. Moll, *op. cit.* (note 37), 87.

43. *Ibid.,* 11.

44. Dessoir, *op. cit.* (note 28), 217.

45. See C. Bruhn, *Gelehrte in Hypnose: Zur Psychologie der Überzeugung und des Traumdenkens,* (Hamburg: Parus, 1926).

46. These reports appeared primarily in Schrenck-Notzing's book *Experimente der Fernbewegung,* which dealt with the physical mediumship of Willy Schneider.

47. 'Die Erfahrung zeigt Tag für Tag, dass unzählige Menschen heute nicht mehr imstande sind ruhig und kritisch zu denken, sobald es sich um okkultistische Probleme handelt. Es stimmt traurig, wenn man sieht, wie selbst akademisch gebildete Männer, die sich vielleicht sogar auf manchen Gebieten der Wissenschaft einen Namen gemacht haben, vollkommen allen Sinn für Logik und Vernunft verlieren, wenn es sich um die Erörterung derartig gefühlsbetoner Fragen handelt.' 'Zur Psychologie der Okkultisten', in: Nachlaß Albert Hellwig 10/4, Gerichtssache Moll vs Rudloff, 1925, IGPP

48. 'Gelehrte in Hypnose: Das Uebersinnliche und seine Kritiker', *Magdeburgische Zeitung,* 11 Juni 1926, in: GStA Rep. 84a Nr. 10993.

49. A. von Schrenck-Notzing, 'Die Gelehrtenhypnose des Dr Christian Bruhn', in *Die Physikalischen Phänomene der grossen Medien* (Stuttgart: Union Deutsche Verlagsgesellschaft, 1926), 275.

50. Moll, *op. cit.* (note 37), 96.

51. R. Arnheim, 'So ist es! Ist es so?' *Die Weltbühne,* XXII. 37 (14 September 1926), 416.

52. *Ibid.,* 416.

53. *Ibid.,* 417.

54. Schrenck-Notzing, *op. cit.* (note 49), 275.

55. Moll, *op. cit.* (note 37), 98.

56. G. Le Bon, *The Crowd: A Study of the Popular Mind* [1895], 2nd edn (Atlanta: Cherokee, 1982), xv–xvi; S. Muscovici, *The Age of the Crowd: A Historical Treatise of Mass Psychology*, J.C. Whitehouse (trans.) (Cambridge: Cambridge University Press, 1985), 55.

57. J. Ginneken, *Crowds, Psychology, and Politics 1871–1899* (Cambridge: Cambridge University Press, 1992), 172, 174.

58. Le Bon, *op. cit.* (note 56), xv–xvi.

59. *Ibid*, xviii.

60. *Ibid.*, xviii– xix.

61. Muscovici, *op. cit.* (note 56), 80.

62. Ginneken, *op. cit.* (note 57), 138.

63. *Ibid.*, 141.

64. *Ibid.*, 144.

65. Moscovici, *op. cit.* (note 56), 82–3.

66. *Ibid.*, 81.

67. Le Bon, *op. cit.* (note 56), 11.

68. *Ibid.*, 11

69. *Ibid.*, 2–3.

70. *Ibid.*

71. In his later work on the psychology of belief (1911), Le Bon again derived his examples from psychical research, looking at how seemingly sceptical scientists, in particular Charles Richet, had had their rationality overturned by belief when they experimented with mediums. See M.B. Brower, 'The Fantasms of Science: Psychical Research in the French Third Republic, 1880–1935' (unpublished PhD dissertation: Rutgers University, 2005), 257–9.

72. Le Bon, *op. cit.* (note 56), 25.

73. *Ibid.*, 26.

74. *Ibid.*

75. Moll, *op. cit.* (note 37), 98.

76. *Ibid.*, 101.

77. Le Bon, *op. cit.* (note 56), xix.

78. *Ibid.*, 113–14.

79. Kröner quoted in Moll, *op. cit.* (note 37), 114.

80. *Ibid.*, 4.

81. *Ibid.*, 3.

82. Schrenck-Notzing, *op. cit.* (note 49), 275–6.

83. 'Ein Mann, der Fastnachtsscherze als Wissenschaft hinnahm, der die Faschingsvermummungen hysterischer Weiber und anderer Medien als Transfiguration oder Teleplasma und als Produkt des Unbewußten der Welt aufoktroyieren wollte, muß auch nach dem Tode wahrheitsgemäß beleuchtet werden.' Moll, *op. cit.* (note 37), 4.

84. See J.K.F. Zöllner, *Wissenschaftliche Abhandlungen*, Vol. III (Leipzig: L. Staackmann, 1879).

85. Moll, *op. cit.* (note 37), 95.

86. E. Bauer, 'Ein noch nicht publizierter Brief Sigmund Freuds an Fanny Moser über Okkultismus und Mesmerismus', *Freiburger Universitätsblätter*, 25, 93 (1986), 97.

87. *Ibid.*, 106–9.

88. A. Winterstein, 'Die Bedeutung der Psychoanalyse für die Parapsychologie', *Zeitschrift für Parapsychologie*, 7 (1930), 426.

89. *Ibid.*, 427.

90. W. Kröner, 'Parapsychologie und Psychoanalyse', *Zeitschrift für Parapsychologie*, 2 (1926), 99–100.

91. *Ibid.*, 100.

92. *Ibid.*, 100–1.

93. 'In neuer Zeit spricht man häufig von Komplexen. Graf Klinckowstroem hat vom okkultistischen Komplex gesprochen, d.h. einer Gruppe zusammengehöriger affektbetoner oder überwertiger Vorstellungselemente, wobei der Affekt sich in dem Wunsche zeigt, unter allen Umständen Okkultes zu beweisen. Wenn solche Komplexe bestehen, handelt es sich um einen Zustand, der gewisse Ähnlichkeiten mit paranoischen Wahngebilden zeigt.' Moll, *op. cit.* (note 37), 112–13.

94. *Ibid.*, 101.

95. *Ibid.*, 109.

96. '[I]st so stark im "okkultistischen Komplex" befangen, dass er in der Tätigkeit der Kritiker sowie Veröffentlichungen solcher Beobachter, die Tricksystem aufdecken (wie W.J. Vinton in Braunau bei Schneiders), eine Schädigung der parapsychologischen Forschung erblickt, anstatt einzusehen, dass die vornehmste Aufgabe einer jeden Wissenschaft die ist, der Wahrheit zu dienen Graf Carl v. Klinckowstroem, 'Der gegenwärtiger Stand der okkulter Forschung,' *Unsere Welt: Illustrierte Zeitschrift für Naturwissenschaft und Weltanschauung*, 20. Jahrg. Dezember 1928 Heft 12, 370, in: ADW, CA, AC-S 272 Okkultismus.

97. 'Schrenck-Notzings 2x entlarvtes Medium', *Welt am Sonntag*, 8 July 1932, in: ZA Personen Schrenck-Notzing, SdArMü.

98. Moll, *op. cit.* (note 37), 114–15.

99. *Ibid.*, 115.

100. The 'psychologisation' and 'pathologisation' of the paranormal also helped diminish the threat posed to notions of subjectivity and identity. Hayward has written about this in the British context, see R. Hayward, *Resisting History: Religious Transcendence and the Invention of the Unconscious* (Manchester: Manchester University Press, 2007).

101. A. von Schrenck-Notzing, *Phenomena of Materialisation: A Contribution to the Investigation of Mediumistic Teleplastics*, E. E. Fournier d'Albe (trans.), (London: Kegan Paul, Trench, Trubner & Co., 1920), v.

102. Schrenck-Notzing, *op. cit.* (note 49), 278–9.

103. W. Kröner, 'Hellwig ante portas!', *Zeitschrift für Parapsychologie*, 5 (1930), 630.

104. 'Ich persönlich habe mich entschlossen, den Kampf gegen Moll und Konsorten, speziell Hellwig, von mir allein aus aufzunehmen und zwar in der Form einer ganz scharfen satyrischen Streitschrift, die Herrn einmal psychoanalysiert.' Letter from W. Kröner to A. von Schrenck-Notzing, 27 July 1925, in: Korrepondenz Berlin Folder, Nachlaß Schrenck-Notzing, IGPP.

105. 'Unsere Herrn Gegner haben wiederholt den Wunsch geäußert, den Geisteszustand 'gläubiger' Okkultisten untersuchen zu lassen. Sie scheinen dabei aber den Grad ihrer eigenen fanatischen Negativgläubigkeit zu übersehen, der sie verblendet und ihr Urteil trübt.' A. von Schrenck-Notzing, 'Einleitung', *Die Physikalischen Phänomene der grossen Medien*, (Stuttgart: Union Deutsche Verlagsgesellschaft, 1926), 6.

106. Kröner, *op. cit.* (note 90), 102

107. 'Es ist dies der Standpunkt der Schule Molls, die mit ihrer Vermischung heterogener Begriffe (wie der Gleichsetzung von Personal-, Sach-, und Prinzipienfragen) das typische Beispiel einer affektiven Urteilstrübung zum besten gibt und durch dieses zäh festgehaltene Fehlleistungssystem den Beweis für ihre neurotisch-dogmatische Einstellung liefert.' *Ibid.*, 103.

108. *Ibid.*, 103.

109. *Ibid.*, 102

110. 'Was jedoch den Wissenschaftler von Gefühlsokkultisten unterscheidet, ist die Selbstkritik, die er in jedem Falle behält, und die ihn befähigt, affektive Urteilstrübungen beim Auftauchen sofort zu erkennen und zu beseitigen.' *Ibid.*

111. Winterstein, *op. cit.* (note 88), 422, 436.

112. See C.G. Jung, *Memories, Dreams, and Reflections*, Aniela Jaffé (ed.), R. and C. Winston (trans.), (London: Flamingo, 1961).

113. C.G. Jung, *Zur Psychologie und Pathologie sogenannter occulter Phänomene* (Leipzig: Oswald Mutze, 1902).

114. D. Bair, *Jung: A Biography* (Boston: Little, Brown and Company, 2003), 167, 329; F.X. Charet, *Spiritualism and the Foundations of C.G. Jung's Psychology* (Albany: State University of New York Press, 1993).

115. Kröner, *op. cit.* (note 90), 111.

116. 'In Wahrheit ist das Okkulte nichts anderes als ein seelischer Spaltungsvorgang, das Eindringen eines naturgemäßen Prozesses in eine höhere Bewußtseinszone. Und diese Erkenntnis beseitigt den letzten

Denkwiderstand, der die wissenschaftliche Anerkennung der Parapsychologie hindern könnte, nachdem man gezwungen ist, sich mit der Phänomenik abzufinden.' *Ibid.*, 110.

117. *Ibid.*, 113.

Conclusion

On the borders of science

In the preface to his 1908 book *Verbrechen und Aberglaube* [*Crime and Superstition*], the district court director and outspoken critic of parapsychology Albert Hellwig wrote, 'It sounds like a paradox, but is nevertheless true, that the border areas of science are almost more interesting than the individual branches of science themselves'.[1] While Hellwig was concerned here with the intersection of criminology and anthropology in the field of 'kriminelle Aberglauben' [criminal superstition], his observation might have referred just as well to those nascent sciences, psychical research and parapsychology, to which he dedicated so much of his life. The peculiar fascination that these disciplines exercised on Hellwig, who became relentless in his critique of their proponents, was equally apparent among a number of his contemporaries, whose attraction to, or repulsion from, the scientific study of the paranormal also seemed to result from their border status. As we have seen, it was the desire to create a discipline that expanded the frontiers of science, in particular those of psychology, which led to the emergence of psychical research in Germany during the late nineteenth century. Similarly, it was the trespass on the borders and epistemic authority of other disciplines throughout the Imperial and inter-war periods that led opponents of psychical research and parapsychology to launch a counter-attack. This took the form of a psychology of occult belief that naturalised paranormal phenomena and pathologised parapsychologists, thus repelling the epistemic and ontological threat that they posed to the borders of science.

As *The Stepchildren of Science* has tried to show, critics and proponents alike during the late nineteenth and early twentieth centuries, maintained the conviction that psychical research and parapsychology were 'Grenzgebiete der wissenschaftlichen Forschung' [border areas of scientific research].[2] For critics, who placed the emphasis on the words 'border area' rather than on 'scientific research', the border status of psychical research and parapsychology derived from their inability to meet the basic requirements for scientific status. Lack of consensus on the phenomenological, epistemological and methodological basis of these disciplines, they argued, excluded them from the scientific sphere. For proponents of these nascent sciences, however, the term 'border area' connoted the pioneering project on which they had embarked. Concerned with those phenomena, including materialisation, telekinesis and clairvoyance, which fell outside the scope of psychology, biology and physics, these researchers sought to expand science's frontiers. In so doing, their aim was to overturn the one-sided materialistic *Weltanschauung* that, they contended, dominated German philosophy and science to the detriment of society and culture. Research with somnambulists and mediums, those individuals with the ability to produce paranormal phenomena, would, they maintained, provide the foundation for a more 'vollständige Weltanschauung' [complete worldview] on which scientific reform and philosophical renewal could be based.[3]

The emergence of these self-confessed border sciences precipitated, as we have seen, a range of bitter and largely irresolvable boundary disputes. These confrontations took place not only with the sciences on which psychical research and parapsychology encroached, but also with the occult philosophies from which they wished to distinguish themselves. The foundation of the Psychologische Gesellschaft in Munich and the Gesellschaft für Experimental-Psychologie in Berlin, for instance, led to a series of debates with physiological psychologists over the use of the term 'experimental psychology' and the validity of hypnosis as a means of accessing the unconscious. These same societies also became the site for an argument between occultists and psychical researchers over the spiritist or animist interpretation of paranormal phenomena, which culminated in the split of the Psychologische Gesellschaft; a separation that physically demarcated and epistemologically sanitised the psychical researchers' nascent discipline. In the decades that followed, such credibility contests occurred in a wide variety of venues, including the stage, the laboratory and the courtroom, but nonetheless continued to centre on similar problems, in particular, the nature of scientific authority and expertise.

The performance of these debates in public arenas such as the courtroom and the stage ensured that psychical research and parapsychology, like their occult siblings, became matters of interest not only to the scientific and medical communities, but also to the churches and the state. For the scientific and medical communities, whose increasing specialisation and professionalisation during the late nineteenth century were intended to ensure their monopolies of scientific knowledge and healthcare, the apparent threat posed by psychical research and parapsychology was equivalent to that of the scientific dilettantism and lay medicine with which these disciplines overlapped. Pressure from these communities to dismiss or prohibit these practices was such that scientists and doctors with an interest in the paranormal felt it necessary to engage in rigorous self-policing. The emergence of 'critical occultism' at the *fin de siècle*, for example, was a result of such self-regulation on the part of those physicians whose interest in the paranormal threatened to undermine their advocacy of medical hypnosis. For the churches and the state, however, psychical research and parapsychology were less problematic. While occultism represented a threat to the body and the soul, which was combated with a range of legal measures and religious admonitions, the scientific study of the paranormal appeared, at least until the late 1930s, largely benign. Such tolerance on the part of the churches and the state was evidence that the boundary-work undertaken by these nascent disciplines had been at least partially successful in distinguishing them from the occult sciences.

Using the tools of intellectual and cultural history, as well as the theoretical perspectives provided by the sociology of science, this book has sought to make explicit what many of those contemporaries who wrote about psychical research and parapsychology implied – that, depending on one's perspective, the true significance of, or dilemma posed by, these disciplines was to be located in their border status. This approach has allowed an analysis of psychical research and parapsychology in the German context that goes beyond that of recent studies in which occultism and the scientific study of the paranormal are seen largely as manifestations of underlying social, cultural and political anxieties. Using such analyses as a foundation, this book has concentrated instead on the complex negotiations and bitter disputes that typify discipline formation in most fields, but which are particularly messy when a nascent science encroaches on its neighbours' territory and threatens the assumptions on which they are based. Concentrating on the multiple boundary disputes that surrounded the emergence of psychical research and parapsychology in Germany, *The Stepchildren of Science* has tried to demonstrate how scientific authority and expertise were constructed in the Imperial and inter-war periods and the manner in which these so-called pseudo-sciences helped both their practitioners and their opponents highlight, negotiate and remedy methodological and epistemological problems within the contemporary sciences. In so doing, this book has sought to confirm what Hellwig contended, that the border areas of science are almost as interesting, some might argue more interesting, than the individual branches of science themselves.[4]

Notes

1. 'Es klingt paradox, trifft aber doch zu, daß die Grenzgebiete der Wissenschaften fast noch interessanter sind als die einzelnen Wissenszweige

selber.' A. Hellwig, *Verbrechen und Aberglaube: Skizzen aus der volkskundlichen Kriminalistik* (Leipzig: B.G. Teubner, 1908), v.
2. A. Hellwig, 'Pseudoentlarvungen', in: Nachlaß Albert Hellwig 10/4 Korrespondenz 1924–1926, IGPP.
3. W. Hübbe-Schleiden, 'Aufruf und Vorwort', *Sphinx*, 1 (1886), 4.
4. Hellwig, *op. cit.* (note 1), v.

Bibliography

Archival material

Archiv, Diakonisches Werk der Evangelischen Kirche in Deutschland, Berlin.
Apologetische Centrale des Central-Ausschusses für die Innere Mission
ADW, CA AC-S   1–3 [Aberglaube, 1928–1936]
272–273 [Okkultismus, 1925–1937]
334 [Spiritismus, 1922–1933]

Evangelisches Zentralarchiv, Berlin.
Bestand 7. Generalia (Evangelischer Oberkirchenrat)
3946 [Die spiritistiche und scientistische Bewegung, 1901–1934]
Bestand 14. Königliches Consistorium der Provinz Brandenburg
823 [Spiritismus, Scientismus, Gebetsheilung usw, 1897–1939]
Geheimes Staatsarchiv Preussischer Kulturbesitz, Berlin.
Rep. 76 Kultusministerium, Vc Wissenschaftssachen
Sekt. 1 Tit. XI Teil V C
Nr. 48 [Die Wünschelrute, 1911–1934]
Rep. 76 Kultusministerium, VIIIB Jüngere Medizinalregistratur
Nr. 1324 [Anwendung des Hypnotismus und des Magnetismus zu Heilzwecken, 1881–1927]
Nr. 1325 [Anwendung der Hypnose durch nicht approbierte Vertreter der Heilkunde, 1902–1925]
Nrn. 1327–1332 [Ausübung der Heilkunde durch Laien (Kurpfuscher), Bde. 1–6 1894–1927]
Rep. 84a Justizministerium
Nr. 10992 [Hypnose und Suggestion, 1897–1931]
Nr. 10993 [Hypnose und Suggestion. Äußerungen der Presse, 1925–1929]
Rep. 89 Geheimes Zivilkabinett, Jüngere Periode
Nr. 15340 [Scientismus und Spiritismus, 1902]

Archiv, Institut für Grenzgebiete der Psychologie und Psychohygiene, Freiburg
Nachlaß 10/4 Albert Hellwig, not indexed.
Nachlaß Albert von Schrenck-Notzing

Bibliography

Universitätsarchiv, Leipzig

   PA 0416 0513 Hans Driesch

Universitätsbibliothek Sondersammlungen, Leipzig

   Nachlaß 250 Hans Driesch

Bayerisches Hauptstaatsarchiv, Munich.

   Sammlung Rehese P1853 [Dr. Karl Gruber]
   Sig Personen 4086 [Dr. Karl Kemmerich]
   Sig Personen 4466 [Albert Freiherr v. Dr. med.
   Schrenck-Notzing]

Staatsarchiv, Munich

Polizeidirektion München

   5610 [Okkultische Gesellschaft e.V., 1925–1930]
   7104 [Hypnose, 1929–1940]
   7107 [Hellseherei, 1924–1947]

Stadtarchiv, Munich

   ZA Okkultismus

ZA Personen Gruber, Karl

   ZA Personen Schrenck-Notzing, Albert

Stadtbibliothek, Munich

Monacensia Literaturarchiv

   Autographensammlungen Rudolf Tischner
   Nachlaß Schneider-Schelde
   Sammlung Karl du Prel
   Sammlung Max Kemmerich [L 4400–4401]
   Sammlung Albert von Schrenck-Notzing

Universitätsarchiv, Tübingen

   Nachlaß 399 T. K. Oesterreich

Bibliography

Periodicals: psychical research and parapsychology

Der Okkultismus: Erste illustrierte Monatsschrift zur Aussprache und Aufklärung über
*   alle Zweiggebiete und Auffassungen des Okkultismus und verwandter Richtungen*
Proceedings of the Society for Psychical Research
Psychische Studien
Sphinx: Monatsschrift für die geschichtliche und experimentale Begründung der
*   übersinnlichen Weltanschauung auf monistischer Grundlage.*
Wissenschaftliche Zeitschrift für Okkultismus
Zeitschrift für kritischen Okkultismus und Grenzfragen des Seelenlebens
Zeitschrift für Parapsychologie
Zentralblatt für Okkultismus: Monatsschrift zur Erforschung der gesamten
*   Geheimwissenschaften.*

Other newspapers and periodicals

Archiv für Kriminalanthropologie
Archiv für Kriminologie
Archiv für Strafrecht
Berliner medizinische Wochenschrift
Kriminalistische Monatshefte
Nord und Süd
Philosophische Studien
Vierteljahrsschrift für gerichtliche Medizin und offentliches Sanitätswesen
Die Weltbühne

Published primary sources

Aksakov, A., 'Prospectus', *Psychische Studien*, 1 (1874), 1–6.

_____ 'Mein in einen Glückauf- und Vorwärts- Ruf zum Neuen Jahre 1878
   verwandeltes Abscheidswort an meine Leser', *Psychische Studien*, 4 (1878),
   1–4.

_____ 'Kritische Bemerkung über Dr Eduard von Hartmann's Werk: 'Der
   Spiritismus'', *Psychische Studien*, 13 (1886), 17–22; 62–76; 109–25;
   161–79; 210–20; 259–71; 305–16; 356–68; 406–14; 453–64; 501–16;
   548–65.

_____ 'Meine photograpischen Experimente in London', *Psychische Studien*, 14
   (1887), 1–13.

Bibliography

Amereller, K., 'Das Krall'sche Institut für Tierpsychologie und parapsychologische Forschung, München', *Zeitschrift für Parapsychologie*, 3 (1929), 165.

Arnheim, R., 'So ist es! Ist es so?', *Die Weltbühne*, 22, 37 (1926), 415–18.

Bärwald, R., *Okkultismus und Spiritismus und ihre weltanschaulichen Folgerungen* (Berlin: Deutsche Buch-Gemeinschaft, 1926).

Bernheim, H., *Suggestive Therapeutics: A Treatise on the Nature and Uses of Hypnotism*, Christian Herter (trans.), 2nd edn (Edinburgh: Young J. Pentland, 1890).

Bohn, E., *Der Fall Rothe: Eine criminal-psychologische Untersuchung* (Breslau: S. Schottlaender, 1901).

Bruhn, C., *Gelehrte in Hypnose: Zur Psychologie der Überzeugung und des Traumdenkens* (Hamburg: Parus, 1926).

Buchner, E., 'Der Mollprozeß in zweiter Auflage', *Zeitschrift für Parapsychologie*, 1, 3 (1926), 154–69.

Büchner, L., *Kraft und Stoff oder Grundzüge der natürlichen Weltordnung*, 21st edn (Leipzig: Theod. Thomas, 1904).

Dessoir, M., 'Mr Henry Slade in Berlin', *Psychische Studien*, 13 (1886), 97–100.

———— 'Eine Sitzung mit Herrn Slade in Berlin', *Sphinx*, 1, 1 (1886), 191–4.

———— 'Experiments in Muscle-Reading and Thought-Transference', *Proceedings of the Society for Psychical Research*, 4 (1886–87), 111–26.

———— *Bibliographie des modernen Hypnotismus* (Berlin: C. Duncker, 1888).

———— 'Experiments in Thought-Transference', *Proceedings of the Society for Psychical Research*, 5 (1888–89), 355–7.

———— 'Die Parapsychologie', *Sphinx*, 7 (1889), 341–4.

———— 'Zur Psychologie der Taschenspielerkunst', *Nord und Süd*, 52 (1890), 194–221.

———— *Das Doppel-Ich*, 2nd edn (Leipzig: Ernst Günther, 1896).

———— *Vom Jenseits der Seele: Die Geheimwissenschaften in kritischer Betrachtung*, 3rd edn (Stuttgart: Ferdinand Enke, 1919).

———— *Buch der Erinnerung*, 2nd edn (Stuttgart: Ferdinand Enke, 1947).

Driesch, H., *Analytische Theorie der Organischen Entwicklung* (Leipzig: Wilhelm Engelmann, 1894).

_____ 'Der Okkultismus als neue Wissenschaft', *Psychische Studien,* 50 (1923), 47–58.

_____ 'Die metapsychischen Phänomene in Rahmen der Biologie', *Psychische Studien,* 52 (1925), 1–14.

_____ 'Presidential Address: Psychical Research and Established Science', *Proceedings of the Society for Psychical Research,* 36, 99 (1926), 171–86.

_____ *The Science and Philosophy of the Organism,* 2nd edn (London: A. & C Black, 1929).

_____ *Psychical Research: The Science of the Supernormal,* T. Bestermann (trans.), (London: G. Bell, 1933).

_____ *Lebenserinnerungen: Aufzeichnungen eines Forschers und Denkers in entscheidender Zeit* (Munich: Ernst Reinhardt, 1951).

du Prel, C., *Der Kampf um's Dasein am Himmel: Versuch einer Philosophie der Astronomie,* 2nd edn (Berlin: Denicke, 1876).

_____ 'Problem: Medium oder Taschenspieler?' Der Stand der Streitfrage' *Sphinx,* 1 (1886), 362–70.

_____ 'Wohin führt der Hypnotismus?', *Psychische Studien,* 15 (1888), 10–15.

_____ 'Über die Bedeutung der transcendentalen Psychologie', *Sphinx,* 5 (1888), 366–76.

_____ 'Übersinnliche Gedankenübertragung', *Sphinx,* 5(1888), 24–31.

_____ *Die vorgeburtliche Erziehung als Mittel zur Menschenzüchtung: Ein Beitrag zur Lösung der socialen Frage* (Jena: Costenoble, 1889).

_____ *The Philosophy of Mysticism,* 2 vols, C.C. Massey (trans) (London: George Redway, 1889).

_____ 'Unser Zweck', *Sphinx,* 11, 61 (1891), 2–4.

_____ 'Über den Einfluß psychischer Faktoren im Okkultismus', *Sphinx,* 15 (1893),1–29.

_____ *Die Entdeckung der Seele durch die Geheimwissenschaften* (Leipzig: Ernst Günthers, 1894).

_____ 'Programm für experimentellen Okkultismus', *Sphinx,* 18, 95 (1894), 23–33.

_____ *Experimentalpsychologie und Experimentalmetaphysik* (Leipzig: Max Altmann, 1905).

du Prel, C. (*cont...*), *Nachgelassene Schriften* (Leipzig: Max Altman, 1911).

_____ *Das Rätsel des Menschen: Eine Einführung in das Studium der Geheimwissenschaften,* H. Fritzsche (ed.) (Wiesbaden: Hermann Glock, 1950).

_____ *Der Somnambulismus vor dem königlichen Landgerichte München I* (Munich: Knorr & Hirth, n.d).

Fechner, G., *Erinnerungen an die letzten Tage der Odlehre und ihres Urhebers* (Leipzig: Breitkopf & Härtel, 1876).

Francé-Harrar, A., *So war's um Neunzehnhundert: Mein Fin de Siècle* (Munich: Albert Langen & Georg Müller, 1962).

Gruber, K., *Okkultismus und Biologie: Gesammelte Aufsätze aus dem Nachlaß* (Munich: Drei Masken Verlag, 1930).

Grunewald, F., *Physikalisch-mediumistische Untersuchungen* (Pfullingen i. Württ.: Johannes Baum Verlag, 1920).

Gulat-Wellenburg, W. von, Graf C. von Klinckostroem, and H. Rosenbusch, *Der Physikalische Mediumismus* (Berlin: Ullstein, 1925).

Hansen F.C.C. and A. Lehmann, 'Über unwillkürliches Flüstern: Eine kritische und experimentelle Untersuchung der sogenannten Gedanken-Übertragung', *Philosophische Studien,* 11 (1895), 471–530.

Hartmann, E. von, *Der Spiritismus* (Leipzig: Wilhelm Friedrich, 1885).

_____ 'Geister oder Halluzinationen?' *Sphinx,* 4 (1887), 8–17.

Heidenhain, R., *Hypnotism or Animal Magnetism: Physiological Observations,* 4th edn, L.C. Woolridge (trans.) (London: Kegan Paul, Trench & Co, 1888).

Hellwig, A., 'Gaukelei nach dem preußischen Allgemeinen Landrecht', *Archiv für Kriminologie,* 31 (1908), 322–3.

_____ *Verbrechen und Aberglaube: Skizzen aus der volkskundlichen Kriminalistik* (Leipzig: B. G. Teubner, 1908).

_____ *Okkultismus und Wissenschaft unter besonderer Berücksichtigung der Telekinese und der Materialisationen* (Stuttgart: Ferdinand Enke, 1926).

_____ 'Ein betrügerischer Kriminaltelepath', *Zeitschrift für kritischen Okkultismus und Grenzfragen des Seelenlebens,* 3, 1 (1927), 130–7.

_____ 'Hellsehen als strafbare Gaukelei', *Archiv für Strafrecht,* 71 (1927), 124–30.

_____ 'Der Hellseher von Rothenstein', *Zeitschrift für kritischen Okkultismus und Grenzfragen des Seelenlebens,* 3, 1 (1927), 1–8.

Bibliography

_____ *Okkultismus und Verbrechen: Eine Einführung in die kriminalistischen Probleme des Okkultismus für Polizeibeamte, Richter, Staatsanwälte, Psychiater und Sachverständige* (Berlin: Dr P. Langenscheidt, 1929).

_____ 'Erik Jan Hanussen als psychographologischer Sachverständiger', *Archiv für Kriminologie,* 90 (1932), 119–28.

Hornung, H., 'Die forensische Bedeutung des Hellsehens und der Gedankenübertragung', *Archiv für Kriminologie,* 76 (1924), 247–88.

Hübbe-Schleiden, W., 'Aufruf und Vorwort', *Sphinx,* 1 (1886), 1–4.

_____ 'Objektivität sogenannter Materialisationen, Alexander Aksakof wider Eduard von Hartmann', *Sphinx,* 4 (1887), 107–26

Hulisch, A., 'Nochmals Slade in Berlin', *Psychische Studien,* 13 (1886), 145–9.

Jahresbericht der Psychologischen Gesellschaft in München 1888/1889 (Munich: Knorr & Hirth, 1889).

Jastrow, J., *Fact and Fable in Psychology* (London: Macmillan and Co., 1901).

Jung, C.G., *Zur Psychologie und Pathologie sogenannter occulter Phänomene* (Leipzig: Oswald Mutze, 1902).

_____ *Memories, Dreams, and Reflections,* A. Jaffé (ed.) R. and C. Winston (trans.), (London: Flamingo, 1961).

Kemnitz, M., *Moderne Mediumforschung: Kritische Betrachtungen zu Dr. von Schrenck-Notzings 'Materialisationsphaenomene'* (Munich: J.F. Lehmann, 1914).

Kiesewetter, C., *Geschichte des neueren Okkultismus: Geheimwissenschaftliche Systeme von Agrippa von Nettesheim bis zu Karl du Prel* (Leipzig: Wilhelm Friedrich, 1891).

Kröner, W., 'Epilog zur Moll-Polemik', *Zeitschrift für Parapsychologie,* 1, 3 (1926), 160–9.

_____ 'Parapsychologie und Psychoanalyse', *Zeitschrift für Parapsychologie,* 2 (1926), 99–114.

_____ 'Hellwig ante portas!' *Zeitschrift für Parapsychologie,* 5, 10 (1930), 630–44.

Lambert, R., 'Der Insterburger Prozeß gegen die Hellseherin Frau Günther-Geffers', *Zeitschrift für Parapsychologie,* 4 (1929), 229–39; 269–86; 339–59.

Le Bon, G., *The Crowd: A Study of the Popular Mind,* 2nd edn (Atlanta: Cherokee, 1982).

Bibliography

Lodge, O., 'Address by the President', *Proceedings of the Society for Psychical Research*, 17 (1902), 37–57.

Maier, F., 'Neues von der Schlaftänzerin', *Psychische Studien*, 31, 5 (1904), 235–318.

Mann, T., *Three Essays*, H.T. Lowe-Porter (trans) (London: Adelphi, 1932).

Mikuška, V., 'Hans Driesch als Biologe, Philosoph und Okkultist', *Psychische Studien*, 50 (1923), 41–6.

Moll, A., *Der Rapport in der Hypnose: Untersuchungen über thierischen Magnetismus* (Leipzig: Otto Dürr, 1892).

_____ *Gesundbeten: Medizin und Okkultismus* (Berlin: Hermann Walther, 1902).

_____ 'Ueber Heilmagnetismus und Heilmagnetiseure in forensischer Beziehung', *Vierteljahrsschrift für gerichtliche Medizin und offentlichesSanitätswesen*, 35 (1907), 1–21.

_____ *Hypnotism: Including a Study of the Chief Points of Psycho-Therapeutics and Occultism*, 4th edn A.F. Hopkirk (trans.) (London: Walter Scott, 1909).

_____ *Der Spiritismus* (Stuttgart: Franckh'sche Verlagshandlung, 1924).

_____ *Psychologie und Charakterologie der Okkultisten* (Stuttgart: Ferdinand Enke, 1929).

_____ *Perversions of the Sex Instinct: A Study of Sexual Inversion*, M. Popkin (trans.), (Newark: Julian Press, 1931).

_____ *Ein Leben als Arzt der Seele: Erinnerungen* (Dresden: Carl Reissner, 1936).

Oesterreich, T.K., *Der Okkultismus im modernen Weltbild*, 3rd edn (Dresden: Sibyllen-Verlag, 1923).

_____ *Psychologisches Gutachten in einem Hellseherprozess* (Stuttgart: W. Kohlhammer, 1930).

Offner, M., 'Die deutsche Gesellschaft für psychologische Forschung', *Sphinx*, 11, 66 (1891), 333–6.

Preyer, W., *Die Erklärung des Gedankenlesens nebst Beschreibung eines neuen Verfahrens zum Nachweise unwillkürlicher Bewegungen* (Leipzig: Grieben, 1886).

_____ 'Telepathie und Geisterseherei in England', *Deutsche Rundschau*, 26 (1886), 30–51.

'Programm der Gesellschaft für Experimental-Psychologie zu Berlin', *Sphinx*, 5 (1888), 296–300.

Bibliography

'Programm der psychologischen Gesellschaft in München', *Sphinx*, 2, 1 (1887), 32–6.

'Rechtsprechung', *Kriminalistische Monatshefte*, 3 (1929), 45–6.

Schrenck-Notzing, A. von, *Telepathische Experimente des Sonderausschusses der Psychologischen Gesellschaft zu München* (Leipzig: T. Griebens, 1887).

—— 'Übersinnliche Eingebung in der Hypnose', *Sphinx*, 3, 18 (1887).

—— *Hypnotische Experimente: Comité-Bericht der Psychologischen Gesellschaft in München* (Leipzig: Oswald Mutze, 1888).

—— *Über die praktische Bedeutung des Hypnotismus* (Augsburg: Wirthschen, 1889).

—— *Über Hypnotismus und Suggestion* (Augsburg: Wirthschen, 1889).

—— 'Experimental Studies in Thought-Transference', *Proceedings of the Society for Psychical Research*, 7 (1891–2), 3–22.

—— *Die Bedeutung der hypnotischen Suggestion als Heilmittel* (Berlin: Deutsches Verlagshaus,1895).

—— 'Beiträge zur forensischen Beurtheilung von Sittlichkeitsvergehen mit besonderer Berücksichtigung der Pathogenese psychosexualler Anomalien', *Archiv für Kriminalanthropologie*, 1 (1898), 5–25, 137–60.

—— *Die gerichtlich medicinische Bedeutung der Suggestion: Vortrag gehalten gelegentlich des zweiten internationalen Congresses für experimentellen und therapeutischen Hypnotismus in Paris (August 1900)* (Leipzig: F.C.W. Vogel, 1900).

—— *Die Traumtänzerin Magdeleine G.: Eine psychologische Studie über Hypnose und dramatische Kunst* (Stuttgart: Ferdinand Enke, 1904).

—— *Der Kampf um die Materialisationsphänomene* (Munich: Ernst Reinhardt, 1914).

—— *Phenomena of Materialisation: A Contribution to the Investigation of Mediumistic Teleplastics*, E.E. Fournier d' Albe (trans.), (London: Kegan Paul, Trench, Trubner & Co., 1920).

—— 'Albert von Keller als Malerpsychologe und Metapsychiker', *Psychische Studien*, 48 (1921), 193–215.

—— *Experimente der Fernbewegung* (Stuttgart: Union Deutsche Verlagsgesellschaft, 1924).

Schrenck-Notzing, A. von (*cont...*), 'Ein elektrischer Apparat für Medienkontrolle', *Zeitschrift für Parapsychologie,* 9 (1926), 513–16.

_____ *Die Physikalischen Phänomene der grossen Medien* (Stuttgart: Union Deutsche Verlagsgesellschaft, 1926).

_____ 'Die Entwicklung des Okkultismus zur Parapsychologie in Deutschland', *Zeitschrift für Parapsychologie,* 1 (1932), 37.

_____ *Die Phänomene des Mediums Rudi Schneider* (Berlin: Walter de Gruyter & Co., 1933).

_____ *Grundfragen der Parapsychologie,* G. Walther (ed.), (Stuttgart: W. Kohlhammer, 1962).

Schwab, F., *Teleplasma und Telekinese: Ergebnisse meiner zweijährigen Experimentalsitzungen mit dem Berliner Medium Maria Vollhart* (Berlin: Pyramidenverlag, 1923).

Sebottendorff, R. von. *Bevor Hitler Kam* (Munich: Grassinger, 1933).

Seeling, O., *Der Bernburger Hellseher-Prozeß, mit Bild und Schriftprobe des Lehrers Drost nebst einem Vorwort von Rechtsanwalt Dr Winterberg* (Berlin-Pankow: Linser, 1925).

_____ 'Verbot der Beschäftigung von sogen: Kriminaltelepathen', *Zeitschrift für Parapsychologie,* 4, 7 (1929), 401–4.

Sellin, C., 'Eduard von Hartmann und die Materialisationen', *Sphinx,* 1 (1886), 289–304.

Statuten der Psychologischen Gesellschaft in München (Munich: n.p. 1887).

Statuten der Psychologischen Gesellschaft in München (Munich: n.p. 1889).

Sünner, P., 'Ein Beitrag zur Frage des Zusammenhanges zwischen Hysterie und Mediumismus', *Zeitschrift für Parapsychologie,* 5 (1931), 265–77.

Tischner, R., *Geschichte der Parapsychologie: Von Mitte des 19. Jahrhundrets bis zum ersten Drittel des 20. Jahrhunderts* (Tittmanig: Walter Pustet, 1960).

Tucholsky, K., *Gesammelte Werke,* M. Gerold-Tucholsky and F.J. Raddatz (eds), Vol. V, (Reinbek bei Hamburg: Rowohlt, 1975).

Walther, G., *Zum anderen Ufer: Vom Marxismus und Atheismus zum Christentum* (Remagen: Otto Reichl, 1960).

Winterberg, R., 'Der Insterburger Hellseher-Prozeß', *Zeitschrift für Parapsychologie,* 3, 7 (1928), 415–26.

Bibliography

Winterstein, A., 'Die Bedeutung der Psychoanalyse für die Parapsychologie', *Zeitschrift für Parapsychologie*, 7 (1930), 421–36.

Wittig, C., 'Eduard v. Hartmann über den Spiritismus' *Psychische Studien*, 10 (1884), 244–5.

Wundt, W., *Der Spirtismus eine sogenannte wissenschaftliche Frage* (Leipzig: Wilhelm Engelmann, 1885).

_____ *Lectures on Human and Animal Psychology*, J.E. Creighton and E.B. Titchener (eds), 2nd edn (London: Swan Sonnenschein & Co., 1894).

_____ *Essays*, 2nd edn (Leipzig: Wilhelm Engelmann, 1906).

_____ *Outlines of Psychology*, C. Hubbard Judd (ed.), 3rd edn (London: Williams & Norgate, 1907).

_____ *Principles of Physiological Psychology*, E. Titchener (trans.), 5th edn (London: Swan Sonnenschein & Co., 1910).

_____ *Hypnotismus und Suggestion*, 2nd edn (Leipzig: Wilhelm Engelmann, 1911).

Zöllner, J.K.F., *Wissenschaftliche Abhandlungen*, Vol. III (Leipzig: L. Staackman, 1879).

Zweig, S., *The World of Yesterday* (London: Cassell and Company, 1945).

Secondary sources

Unpublished secondary reports/conference papers

Bluma, L., 'Techniken der Kommunikation zwischen Wissen und Spekulation', Paper presented at Grenzgänge-Wissenschaftliches und okkultes Wissen im 19. und 20. Jahrhundert, Ruhr-Universität Bochum, 11.12.1999 Wolf-Braun, B. 'Mesmerismus, Hypnotismus und die Parapsychologische Forschung: 'Rapport' und 'Mentalsuggestion' als Gegenstand der Wissenschaft im ausgehenden 19. und frühen 20. Jahrhundert', Final report for the Institut für Grenzgebiete der Psychologie und Psychohygiene, University of Bonn, 1999.

_____ 'Zur Geschichte der Parapsychologie in der Weimarer Republik: Deutungen des Mediumismus', Report for the Institut für Grenzgebiete der Psychologie und Psychohygiene, University of Bonn, 2002.

Bibliography

Dissertations

Besser, I. 'Presse des neueren Okkultismus in Deutschland von 1875 bis 1933' (unpublished PhD dissertation: University of Leipzig, 1945).

Brower, M.B. 'The Fantasms of Science: Psychical Research in the French Third Republic, 1880–1935' (unpublished PhD dissertation: Rutgers University, 2005).

Brieschke, A. '"Ein so klägliches Bild ist von keinem Kriminaltelepathen Bekannt": Ein Hellseher-Prozess in Württemberg in den 1920er Jahren' (unpublished MPhil dissertation: University of Tübingen, 2001).

Eberhardt, M. 'Die Kriminalpolizei, 1933–1939' (unpublished MPhil dissertation: University of Konstanz, 1999).

Elder, S.E. 'Murder Scenes: Criminal Violence in the Public Culture and Private Lives of Weimar Berlin' (unpublished PhD dissertation: University of Illinois, 2002).

Gaudlitz, W. 'Okkultismus und Strafgesetz' (unpublished PhD dissertation: University of Leipzig, 1932).

Hall, S.F. 'The Subject under Investigation: Weimar Culture and the Police' (unpublished PhD dissertation: University of California, Berkeley, 2000).

Kaiser, T., 'Zwischen Philosophie und Spiritismus: Bildwissenschaftliche Quellen zur Leben und Werk des Carl du Prel' (unpublished MPhil dissertation: Universität Lüneburg, 2005).

Kurzweg, A. 'Die Geschichte der Berliner "Gesellschaft für Experimental-Psychologie" mit besonderer Berücsictigung ihrer Ausgangssituation und des Wirkens von Max Dessoir' (unpublished PhD dissertation: Free University of Berlin, 1976).

Lachapelle, S. 'A World Outside Science: French Attitudes Towards Mediumistic Phenomena, 1853–1931' (unpublished PhD dissertation: University of Notre Dame, 2002).

Monroe, J. 'Evidence of Things Not Seen: Spiritism, Occultism and the Search for a Modern Faith in France, 1853–1925' (unpublished PhD dissertation: Yale University, 2002).

Teichler, J.U. '"Der Charlatan strebt nicht nach Wahrheit, er verlangt nur nachGeld": Zur Auseinandersetzung zwischen naturwissenschaftlicher Medizin und Laienmedizin im deutschen Kaiserreich am Beispiel von Hypnotismusund Heilmagnetismus' (unpublished PhD dissertation: University of Leipzig, 1999).

Bibliography

Treitel, C. 'Avatars of the Soul: Cultures of Science, Medicine, and the Occult in Modern Germany' (unpublished PhD dissertation: Harvard University, 1999).

Sharp, L.L., 'Rational Religion, Irrational Science: Men, Women, and Belief in French Spiritism, 1853–1914' (unpublished PhD dissertation: University of California at Irvine, 1996).

Verter, B., 'Dark Star Rising: The Emergence of Modern Occultism, 1800–1950' (unpublished PhD dissertation: Princeton University, 1997).

Williams, J.P. 'The Making of Victorian Psychical Research: An Intellectual Elite's Approach to the Spiritual World' (unpublished PhD dissertation: University of Cambridge, 1984).

Published secondary sources

Anderson, M.L. 'The Limits of Secularization: On the Problem of the Catholic Revival in Nineteenth-Century Germany', *The Historical Journal*, 38, 3 (1995), 647–70.

Andriopoulos, S. 'Spellbound in Darkness: Hypnosis as an Allegory of Early Cinema', *The Germanic Review*, 77, 2 (2002), 102–16.

Ash, M.G. 'Academic Politics in the History of Science: Experimental Psychology in Germany, 1879–1941', *Central European History*, 13, 3 (1980), 255–86.

_____ *Gestalt Psychology in German Culture, 1890–1967: Holism and the Quest for Objectivity* (Cambridge: Cambridge University Press, 1998).

Baer, U., 'Photography and Hysteria: Towards a Poetics of the Flash', *Yale Journal of Criticism*, 7, 1 (1994), 41–78.

Bair, D., *Jung. A Biography* (Boston: Little, Brown and Company, 2003).

Barnes, B. and S. Shapin (eds), *Natural Order: Historical Studies of Scientific Culture* (Beverly Hills: Sage Publications, 1979).

Barrow, L., 'Socialism in Eternity: The Ideology of Plebeian Spiritualists, 1853–1913', *History Workshop*, 9 (1980), 37–69.

_____ *Independent Spirits: Spiritualism and English Plebeians, 1850–1910* (London: Routledge & Kegan Paul, 1986).

Bauer, E., 'Ein noch nicht publizierter Brief Sigmund Freuds an Fanny Moser über Okkultismus und Mesmerismus', *Freiburger Universitätsblätter*, 25, 93 (1986), 93–110.

Bauer, E. (*cont...*), 'Periods of Historical Development of Parapsychology in Germany: An Overview', *Proceedings of the Parapsychological Association 34th Convention* (Petaluma: Parapsychological Association, 1991).

Berg, M. and G. Cocks (eds.), *Medicine and Modernity: Public Health and Medical Care in Nineteenth- and Twentieth-Century Germany* (Cambridge: Cambridge University Press, 1997).

Bessel, R., *Germany after the First World War* (Oxford: Clarendon Press, 1993).

Besser, J., 'Die Vorgeschichte des Nationalsozialismus in neuem Licht', *Die Pforte: Monatsschrift für Kultur*, 2, 21/22 (1950), 763–84.

Blackbourn, D. and G. Eley, *The Peculiarities of German History: Bourgeois Society and Politics in Nineteenth-Century Germany* (Oxford: Oxford University Press, 1984).

_____ *The Long Nineteenth Century: A History of Germany, 1780–1918* (New York and Oxford: Oxford University Press, 1998).

Bossenbrook, W., *The German Mind* (Detroit: Wayne University Press, 1961).

Braude, A., *Radical Spirits: Spiritualism and Women's Rights in Nineteenth-Century America* (Boston: Beacon Press, 1989).

Bringmann, W.G. and R.D. Tweney (eds), *Wundt Studies: A Centennial Collection* (Toronto: C.J. Hogrefe, 1980).

Bunge, M., 'A Skeptic's Beliefs and Disbeliefs', *New Ideas in Psychology*, 9, 2 (1991), 131–50.

_____ 'What is Science? Does it Matter to Distinguish it from Pseudoscience? A Reply to my Commentators', *New Ideas in Psychology*, 9, 2 (1991), 245–83.

Burrow, J.W., *The Crisis of Reason: European Thought, 1848–1914* (New Haven: Yale University Press, 2000).

Burwick, F. and P. Douglass (eds), *The Crisis in Modernism: Bergson and the Vitalist Controversy* (Cambridge: Cambridge University Press, 1992).

Bynum, W.F., R. Porter and M. Shepherd (eds), *The Anatomy of Madness: Essays in the History of Psychiatry*, Vol III (London: Routledge, 1988).

Cahan, D., 'The Industrial Revolution in German Physics, 1865–1914', *Historical Studies in the Physical Sciences*, 15, 2 (1985), 1–65.

Chadwick, O., *The Secularization of the European Mind in the 19th Century* (Cambridge: Cambridge University Press, 1975).

Bibliography

Charet, F.X., *Spiritualism and the Foundations of C.G. Jung's Psychology* (Albany: State University of New York Press, 1993).

Churchill, F.B., 'From Machine-Theory to Entelechy: Two Studies in Developmental Teleology', *History of Biology*, 2, 1 (1969), 165–85.

Collins, H.M., and T.J. Pinch, *Frames of Meaning: The Social Construction of Extraordinary Science* (London: Routledge & Kegan Paul, 1982).

Coon, D.J., 'Testing the Limits of Sense and Science: American Experimental Psychologists Combat Spiritualism, 1880–1920', *American Psychologist*, 47, 2 (1992), 143–51.

Crabtree, A., *From Mesmer to Freud: Magnetic Sleep and the Roots of Psychological Healing* (New Haven and London: Yale University Press, 1993).

Craig, G.A., *Germany 1886–1945* (Oxford: Oxford University Press, 1978).

Daim, W., *Der Mann, der Hitler die Ideen gab. Jörg Lanz von Liebenfels*, 3rd edn (Vienna: Ueberreuter, 1994).

Deak, I., *Weimar Germany's Left-Wing Intellectuals. A Political History of the Weltbühne and Its Circle* (Berkeley: University of California Press, 1968).

De Certeau, M., *The Possession at Loudun*, M.B. Smith (trans.), (Chicago: University of Chicago Press, 1990).

Dixon, J., 'Sexology and the Occult: Sexuality and Subjectivity in Theosophy's New Age', *Journal of the History of Sexuality*, 7, 3 (1997), 409–33.

———— *Divine Feminine: Theosophy and Feminism in England* (Baltimore: Johns Hopkins University Press, 2001).

Eksteins, M., *The Limits of Reason: The German Democratic Press and the Collapse of Weimar Democracy* (Oxford: Oxford University Press, 1975).

Ellenberger, H., *The Discovery of the Unconscious: The History and Evolution of Dynamic Psychiatry* (New York: Basic Books, 1970).

Emsley, C. and B. Weinberger (eds), *Policing Western Europe: Politics, Professionalism, and Public Order, 1850–1940* (New York: Greenwood Press, 1991).

Fischer, A. (ed.), *Im Reich der Phantome: Fotografie des Unsichtbaren* (Ostfildern-Ruit: Cantz, 1997).

Franekel, E., *Deutschland und die westlichen Demokratien* (Stuttgart: Kohlhammer, 1964).

Fraser, A., *The Gypsies*, 2nd edn (Oxford: Blackwell, 1995).

313

Bibliography

Freckmann, A. and T. Wegerich, *The German Legal System* (London: Sweet & Maxwell, 1999).

Freytag, N., *Aberglauben im 19: Jahrhundret: Preußen und seine Rheinprovinz zwischen Tradition und Moderne (1815–1918)* (Berlin: Duncker & Humblot, 2003).

Fritzsche, P., *Reading Berlin 1900* (Cambridge: Harvard University Press, 1996).

Fullerton, R., 'Towards a Commercial Popular Culture in Germany: The Development of Pamphlet Fiction, 1871–1914', *Journal of Social History*, 12, 4 (1979), 489–511.

Gauld, A., *The Founders of Psychical Research* (New York: Schocken Books, 1968).

—— *A History of Hypnotism* (Cambridge: Cambridge University Press, 1992).

Gerth, H.H. and C. Wright Mills (eds), *Max Weber: Essays in Sociology* (Oxford: Oxford University Press, 1958).

Gieryn, T.F., *Cultural Boundaries of Science: Credibility on the Line* (Chicago: University of Chicago Press, 1999).

Ginneken, J. van., *Crowds, Psychology, and Politics 1871–1899* (Cambridge: Cambridge University Press, 1992).

Goldstein, J., *Console and Classify: The French Psychiatric Profession in the Nineteenth Century* (Cambridge: Cambridge University Press, 1987).

Goodrick-Clarke, N., *The Occult Roots of Nazism: Secret Aryan Cults and their Influence on Nazi Ideology: The Ariosophists of Austria and Germany, 1890–1935* (New York: New York University Press, 1985).

Gordon, M., *Erik Jan Hanussen: Hitler's Jewish Clairvoyant* (Los Angeles: Feral House, 2001).

Goschler, C. (ed.), *Wissenschaft und Oeffentlichkeit in Berlin* (Stuttgart: Steiner, 2000).

Gregory, A., 'Anatomy of a Fraud: Harry Price and the Medium Rudi Schneider', *Annals of Science*, 34 (1977), 449–549.

Gregory, F., *Scientific Materialism in Nineteenth Century Germany* (Dordrecht: D. Reidel, 1977).

Gruber, E., 'Hans Driesch and the Concept of Spiritism', *Journal of the Society for Psychical Research*, 49 (1978), 861–74.

Hacking, I., 'Telepathy: Origins of Randomization in Experimental Design', *Isis*, 79 (1988), 427–51.

Bibliography

'Hans Bender im Gespräch mit Johannes Mischo (1983)', *Zeitschrift für Parapsychologie und Grenzgebiete der Psychologie*, 33 (1991), 6–16.

Hatfield, G., 'Wundt and Psychology as Science: Disciplinary Transformations', *Perspectives on Science*, 5, 3 (1997), 349–82.

Harrington, A., *Reenchanted Science: Holism in German Culture from Wilhelm II to Hitler* (Princeton: Princeton University Press, 1996).

Harris, R., *Murders and Madness: Medicine, Law, and Society in the Fin de Siècle* (Oxford: Clarendon Press, 1989).

Hau, M., *The Cult of Health and Beauty in Germany: A Social History, 1890–1930* (Chicago: University of Chicago Press, 2003).

Hayward, R., *Resisting History: Religious Transcendence and the Invention of the Unconscious* (Manchester: Manchester University Press).

Hazelgrove, J., *Spiritualism and British Society between the Wars* (Manchester: Manchester University Press, 2000).

Hett, B.C., *Death in the Tiergarten: Murder and Criminal Justice in the Kaiser's Berlin* (Cambridge: Harvard University Press, 2004).

Hess, D., *Science in the New Age: The Paranormal, Its Defenders and Debunkers, and American Culture* (Madison: University of Wisconsin Press, 1993).

Hillman, R., 'A Scientific Study of Mystery: The Role of the Medical and Popular Press in the Nancy-Salpêtrière Controversy on Hypnotism', *Bulletin of the History of Medicine*, 39, 2 (1965), 163–82.

Herrmann, D.B., *Karl Friedrich Zöllner* (Leipzig: B.G. Teubner, 1982).

Hertz, F., *The German Public Mind in the Nineteenth Century: A Social History of German Political Sentiments, Aspirations and Ideas*, E. Northcott (trans.), (London: George Allen & Unwin, 1975).

Holden, P. (ed.), *Women's Religious Experience* (London: Croom Helm, 1983).

Howe, E., *Urania's Children: The Strange World of the Astrologers* (London: William Kimber, 1967).

Jahnke, J. *et al.*, *Psychologiegeschichte: Beziehungen zu Philosophie und Grenzgebieten: Passauer Schriften zur Psychologiegeschichte*, Vol. XII (Munich: Profil, 1998).

Jefferies, M., *Imperial Culture in Germany, 1871–1918* (New York: Palgrave Macmillan, 2003).

315

Jelavich, P., *Munich and Theatrical Modernism: Politics, Playwriting, and Performance, 1890–1914* (Cambridge: Harvard University Press, 1985).

_____ *Berlin Cabaret* (Cambridge: Harvard University Press, 1993).

Johnson, E.A., *Urbanization and Crime: Germany 1871–1914* (Cambridge: Cambridge University Press, 1995).

Kaes, A., *M* (London: BFI Publishing, 2000).

Kelly, A., *The Descent of Darwin: The Popularization of Darwinism in Germany, 1860–1914* (Chapel Hill: University of North Carolina Press, 1981).

Kocka, J., 'Asymmetrical Historical Comparison: The Case of the German *Sonderweg*', *History and Theory*, 38, 1 (1999), 40–50.

Kraus, R.H., *Beyond Light and Shadow: The Role of Photography in Certain Paranormal Phenomena: An Historical Survey* (Munich: Nazraeli Press, 1995).

Krieger, L., *The German Idea of Freedom* (Boston: Beacon Press, 1957).

Kselman, T., *Death and Afterlife in Modern France* (Princeton: Princeton University Press, 1993).

Kuhns, D.F., *German Expressionist Theatre: The Actor and the Stage* (Cambridge: Cambridge University Press, 1997).

Lange, F.A., *History of Materialism and Criticism of its Present Importance*, Vol. II, E.C. Thomas (trans.), 2nd edn,(London: Kegan Paul, Trench, Trubner, & Co., 1892).

Langwiesche, D., *Liberalism in Germany*, C. Banerji (trans.), (London: Macmillan Press, 2000).

Laurence, J.R. and C. Perry, *Hypnosis, Will and Memory: A Psycho-legal History* (New York: Guilford Press, 1988).

Leahey, T.H. and G.E. Leahey, *Psychology's Occult Doubles: Psychology and the Problem of Pseudoscience* (Chicago: Nelson-Hall, 1983).

Lepenies, W., *Between Literature and Science: The Rise of Sociology*, R.J. Hollingdale (trans.), (Cambridge: Cambridge University Press, 1988).

Liang, H.H., 'The Berlin Police in the Weimar Republic', *Journal of Contemporary History*, 4, 4 (1969), 157–72.

_____ *The Berlin Police Force in the Weimar Republic* (Berkeley: University of California Press, 1970).

Bibliography

Linse, U., *Geisterseher und Wunderwirker: Heilsuche im Industriezeitalter* (Frankfurt am Main: Fischer, 1996).

_____ 'Der Spiritismus in Deutschland um 1900', in M. Bassler and H. Châtellier (eds), *Mystik, Mystizismus und Moderne in Deutschland um 1900* (Strasbourg: Presses Universitaires de Strasbourg, 1998), 95–113.

_____ 'Das Buch der Wunder und Geheimwissenschaften: Der spiritistische Verlag Oswald Mutze in Leipzig im Rahmen der spiritistischen Bewegung Sachsens', in M. Lehmstedt and A. Herzog (eds), *Das Bewegte Buch: Buchwesen und soziale, nationale und kulturelle Bewegungen um 1900* (Wiesbaden: Harrassowitz, 1999), 219–44.

Loers, V. (ed.), *Okkultismus und Avantgarde: Von Munch bis Mondrian, 1900–1915* (Frankfurt: Schirn Kunsthalle, 1995).

Luttenberger, F., 'Friedrich Zöllner, der Spiritismus und der vierdimensionale Raum', *Zeitschrift für Parapsychologie und Grenzgebiete der Psychologie,* 19 (1977), 195–214.

Mauskopf, S.H. and M.R. McVaugh, *The Elusive Science: Origins of Experimental Psychical Research* (Baltimore: Johns Hopkins University Press, 1980).

McVaugh, M. and S.H. Mauskopf, 'J.B. Rhine's *Extra-Sensory Perception* and its Background in Psychical Research', *Isis,* 67 (1976), 161–89.

Meyer-Renschhausen, E. and A. Wirz, 'Dietetics, Health Reform and Social Order: Vegetarianism as a Moral Physiology: The Example of Maximilian Bircher-Benner (1867–1939)', *Medical History,* 43 (1999), 323–41.

Mitchell, I., 'Marxism and German Scientific Materialism', *Annals of Science,* 35 (1978), 382–3.

Moore, R.L., *In Search of White Crows: Spiritualism, Parapsychology and American Culture* (Oxford: Oxford University Press, 1977).

Moscovici, S., *The Age of the Crowd: A Historical Treatise of Mass Psychology,* J.C. Whitehouse (trans.), (Cambridge: Cambridge University Press, 1985).

Mosse, G.L., 'The Mystical Origins of National Socialism', *Journal of the History of Ideas,* 22 (1961), 81–96

_____ *The Crisis of German Ideology: Intellectual Origins of the Third Reich* (London: Weidenfeld and Nicolson, 1964).

Murchinson, C. (ed.), *The Case For and Against Psychical Belief* (Worcester: Clark University, 1927).

Bibliography

Nicolas, S. and L. Ferrand, 'Wundt's laboratory at Leipzig in 1891', *History of Psychology*, 2, 3 (1999), 194–203.

Noakes, R. J., 'Telegraphy is an Occult Art: Cromwell Fleetwood Varley and the Diffusion of Electricity to the Other World', *British Journal for the History of Science*, 32 (1999), 421–59.

_____ 'The "Bridge Which is Between Physical and Psychical Research": William Fletcher Barrett, Sensitive Flames, and Spiritualism', *History of Science*, xlii (2004), 419–64.

_____ 'Ethers, Religion and Politics in Late-Victorian Physics: Beyond the Wynne Thesis', *History of Science*, xliii (2005), 1–41.

_____ 'Cromwell Varley Frs, Electrical Discharge and Victorian Spiritualism', *Notes & Records of the Royal Society*, 61 (2007), 5–21.

Oesterreich, M., *Traugott Konstantin Oesterreich: Ich-Forscher und Gottsucher Lebenswerk und Lebensschicksal* (Stuttgart: Fr. Frommanns Verlag, 1954).

Oppenheim, J., *The Other World: Spiritualism and Psychical Researchi n England, 1850–1914* (Cambridge: Cambridge University Press, 1985).

Owen, A., *The Darkened Room: Women, Power and Spiritualism in Late Victorian England* (London: Virago Press, 1989).

_____ *The Place of Enchantment: British Occultism and the Culture of the Modern* (Chicago: University of Chicago Press, 2004).

Parot, F., 'Psychology Experiments: Spiritism at the Sorbonne', *Journal of the History of the Behavioral Sciences*, 29 (1993), 22–8.

Pick, D., *Faces of Degeneration: A European Disorder, c.1848– c.1918* (Cambridge: Cambridge University Press, 1989).

Pilkington, R. (ed.), *Men and Women of Parapsychology: Personal Reflections* (Jefferson: McFarland & Company, 1987).

Pinch, T.J., 'Normal Explanations of the Paranormal: The Demarcation Problem and Fraud in Parapsychology', *Social Studies of Science*, 9, 3 (1979): 329–48.

Pöhlmann, M., *Kampf der Geister: Die Publizistik der 'Apologetischen Centrale' (1921–1937)* (Stuttgart: Kohlhammer, 1998).

Puschner, U., W. Schmitz and J.H. Ulbricht (eds), *Handbuch zur 'Völkischen Bewegungen' 1871–1918* (Munich: K.G. Saur, 1996).

Pytlik, P., *Okkultismus und moderne: Ein kulturhistorisches Phänomen und seine Bedeutung für die Literatur um 1900* (Munich: Schöningh Verlag, 2005).

Bibliography

Raia, C.G., 'From Ether Theory to Ether Theology: Oliver Lodge and the Physics of Immortality', *Journal of the History of the Behavioral Sciences*, 43, 1 (2007), 19–43.

Rausch, A., *'Okkultes' in Thomas Manns Roman Der Zauberberg* (Frankfurt am Main: Peter Lang, 2000).

Repp, K., '"More Corporeal, More Concrete": Liberal Humanism, Eugenics, and German Progressives at the Last Fin de Siecle', *Journal of Modern History*, 72, 3 (2000), 683–730.

_____ *Reformers, Critics, and the Paths of German Modernity: Anti-Politics and the Search for Alternatives, 1890–1914* (Cambridge: Harvard University Press, 2000).

Reuveni, G., 'Reading Sites as Sights of Reading: The Sale of Newspapers in Germany before 1933 - Bookshops in Railway Stations, Kiosks and Street Vendors', *Social History*, 27, 3 (2002), 273–87.

Robinson, D.N., *An Intellectual History of Psychology*, 3rd edn (London: Arnold, 1995).

Roth, M., 'Hysterical Remembering', *Modernism/Modernity*, 3, 2 (1996), 1–30.

Sawicki, D., *Leben mit den Toten: Geisterglauben und die Entstehung des Spiritismus in Deutschland, 1770–1900* (Munich: Schöningh, 2002).

Schellinger, U., 'Faszinosum, Filou und Forschungsobjekt: Das erstaunliche Leben des Hellsehers Ludwig Kahn (1873–*ca.*1966)', *Die Ortenau*, 82 (2002), 434–7.

Schnädelbach, H., *Philosophy in Germany, 1831–1933*, E. Matthews (trans.), (Cambridge: Cambridge University Press, 1984).

Schöningh, C., *'Kontrolliert die Justiz': Die Vertrauenskrise der Weimarer Justiz im Spiegel der Gerichtsreportagen von Weltbühne, Tagebuch und Vossischer Zeitung* (Munich: Fink, 2000).

Schoonover, K., 'Ectoplasms, Evanescence, and Photography' *Art Journal*, 62, 3 (2003), 31–43.

Scull, A. (ed.), *Madhouses, Mad-Doctors and Madmen: The Social History of Psychiatry in the Victorian Era* (London: Athlone Press, 1981).

Smith, H.W. (ed.), *Protestants, Catholics and Jews in Germany, 1800–1914* (Oxford: Berg, 2001).

Smith, R. and B. Wynne (eds), *Expert Evidence: Interpreting Science in the Law* (London: Routledge, 1989).

Bibliography

Solomon, S.M. and E.J. Hackett, 'Setting Boundaries between Science and Law: Lessons from *Daubert v. Merrell Dow Pharmaceuticals, Inc.*', *Science, Technology & Human Values*, 21, 2 (1996), 131–56.

Staubermann, K.B., 'Tying the Knot: Skill, Judgement and Authority in the 1870s Leipzig Spiritistic Experiments', *British Journal for the History of Science*, 34 (2001), 67–79.

Stern, F., *The Politics of Cultural Despair: A Study in the Rise of the German Ideology* (Berkeley: University of California Press, 1961).

Stromberg, W.H., 'Helmholtz and Zoellner: Nineteenth-Century Empiricism, Spiritism and the Theory of Space Perception', *Journal of the History of the Behavioral Sciences*, 25 (1989), 372–80.

Treitel, C., *A Science for the Soul: Occultism and the Genesis of the German Modern* (Baltimore: Johns Hopkins University Press, 2004).

Tucker, J., 'Photography as Witness, Detective, and Impostor: Visual Representation in Victorian Science' in B. Lightman (ed.), *Victorian Science in Context* (Chicago: University of Chicago Press, 1997), 378–408.

Turner, F.M., *Between Science and Religion: The Reaction to Scientific Naturalism in Late Victorian England* (New Haven: Yale University Press, 1974).

_____ 'The Victorian Conflict between Science and Religion: A Professional Dimension', *Isis*, 69, 3 (1978), 356–76.

Vondung, K. (ed.), *Das wilhelminische Bildungsbürgertum: Zur Sozialgeschichte seiner Ideen* (Göttingen: Vandenhoeck & Ruprecht, 1976).

Wagner, P., *Volksgemeinschaft ohne Verbrecher: Konzeptionen und Praxis der Kriminalpolizei in der Zeit der Weimarer Republik und des Nationalsozialismus* (Hamburg: Christians, 1996).

Waldrich, H.P., *Grenzgänger der Wissenschaft* (Munich: Kösel, 1993).

Walkowitz, J., 'Science and Séance: Transgressions of Gender and Genre in Late Victorian London', *Representations*, 22, 2 (1988), 3–29.

Wallis, R., 'Science and Pseudo-Science', *Social Science Information*, 24, 3 (1985), 585–601.

Wallis, R. (ed.), *On the Margins of Science: The Social Construction of Rejected Knowledge*, Sociological Review Monograph No. 27 (Keele: University of Keele Press, 1979).

Webb, J., *The Occult Underground* (La Salle: Open Court Publishing, 1974).

Bibliography

_____ *The Occult Establishment* (La Salle: Open Court Publishing, 1976).

_____ 'Thomas Mann and the Occult: An Unpublished Letter', *Encounter*, 46, 4 (1976), 21–4.

Wegner, G., 'Das Leben des Georg von Langsdorff: Turner, Revolutionär und Wissenschaftler', *Zeitschrift des Breisgau-Geschichtsvereins: 'Schau-ins-Land'*, 111 (1992), 79–94.

Weindling, P., 'Medical Practice in Imperial Berlin: The Casebook of Alfred Grotjahn', *Bulletin of the History of Medicine*, 61 (1987), 391–410.

_____ *Health, Race and German Politics between National Unification and Nazism, 1870–1945* (Cambridge: Cambridge University Press, 1989).

Wetzell, R.F., *Inventing the Criminal: A History of German Criminology, 1880-1945* (Chapel Hill: University of North Carolina Press, 2000).

Winkelmann, O., 'Albert Moll (1862–1939) als Wegbereiter der Schule von Nancy in Deutschland', *Praxis Psychotherapie*, 10, 1 (1965), 1–7.

Winter, A., *Mesmerized: Powers of Mind in Victorian Britain* (Chicago: University of Chicago Press, 1998).

Winter, J., *Sites of Memory, Sites of Mourning: The Great War in European Cultural History* (Cambridge: Cambridge University Press, 1995).

Wolf-Braun, B., '"Was jeder Schäferknecht macht, ist eines Ärztes unwürdig": Zur Geschichte der Hypnose im wilhelminischen Kaiserreich und in der Weimarer Republik (1888–1932)', *Hypnose und Kognition*, 17 (2000), 135–52.

Wolffram, H., 'Supernormal Biology: Vitalism, Parapsychology and the German Crisis of Modernity, *c*.1890–1933', *The European Legacy*, 8 (2003), 149–63.

Wynne, B., 'Physics and Psychics: Science, Symbolic Action, and Social Control in Late Victorian England' in B. Barnes and S. Shapin (eds), *Natural Order: Historical Studies of Scientific Culture* (Beverly Hills: Sage Publications, 1979), 167–86.

Reference Works

Killy, W. and R. Vierhaus, (eds), *Deutsche Biographische Enzyklopädie* (Munich: K. G. Saur, 1998).

Shepard, L. (ed.), *Encyclopedia of Occultism and Parapsychology*, 2 vols, 3rd edn (Detroit: Gale Research, 1991).

Index

A

Abel, Ambrosius 70
academia
    medical practitioners 96, 101
    parapsychology 176
    psychical research constitution
        57–8
    psychological societies 265
acquittals, occult trials 235, 239
adolescent mediums 147, 150, 160,
    162
adversarial legal system 246, 250
aetiology, occult belief 277–8
afterlife
    religious beliefs 215
    spirit photography 153
    spiritualism 156, 214
    see also death
Aksakov, Aleksandr 41–3, 52, 61–2,
    135
anaesthetic drugs 86, 107, 110
Anglo-Saxon nations 194–5
animal magnetism 21, 46
    see also mesmerism
animism 42
    hypnosis and 84, 108–9
    Karolinenplatz experiments 13
    Psychologische Gesellschaft split
        69, 71
    religious views 217–18
    spiritism *vs* 22, 37, 156–7
Apologetische Centrale (Centre for
    Apologetics) 214
applied psychology 137
apports 263, 268
Ariosophy 20, 63
aristocracy involvement 57

artistic creativity
    occultism and 22
    spiritualism and 51
    Traumtänzerin 112–19
Ärztliche Gesellschaft für
    Parapsychologische Forschung
    (Medical Society for
    Parapsychological Research)
    213
association theory 269
Aster, Ernst 145
atavism 274
Athens congress 191
atomic energy 195–6
Auer, Erhard 237
Austria
    Ariosophy 63
    medium contracts 164
    mesmerism 85–6
    Nazism 222
authority 296–7
    courtroom contexts 238–9, 246–7,
        249, 252–3
    experimental parapsychology
        169–74
    intellectual error theory 272–4
    psychology and 267, 272–4
    see also expertise/expert witnesses;
        power relations
auto-suggestive states 278
automatic writing 110–11, 157–8,
    175–6

B

bacteriology 153
'bad faith' in fraud cases 235, 237,
    240–2, 246

Index

Printed in the United States
by Baker & Taylor Publisher Services